A PRIMER OF
clinical psychiatry

A PRIMER OF
clinical psychiatry

2nd edition

Dr David J Castle
MBChB MSc MD DLSHTM GCUT FRCPsych FRANZCP

Dr Darryl Bassett
MB BS BSc FRANZCP Dip Psychother European
Certificate in Anxiety and Depression

Dr Joel King
MBBS MPsych FRANZCP Cert Child Adol Psych

Dr Andrew Gleason
MBBS (Hons) BSc FRANZCP

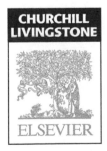

CHURCHILL
LIVINGSTONE

ELSEVIER

Sydney Edinburgh London New York Philadelphia St Louis Toronto

Churchill Livingstone

is an imprint of Elsevier

Elsevier Australia. ACN 001 002 357
(a division of Reed International Books Australia Pty Ltd)
Tower 1, 475 Victoria Avenue, Chatswood, NSW 2067

ELSEVIER

National Library of Australia Cataloguing-in-Publication Data

Title:	A primer of clinical psychiatry / David J Castle … [et al.]
Edition:	2nd ed.
ISBN:	9780729541572 (pbk.)
Notes:	Includes index.
Subjects:	Psychiatry.
Other Authors/Contributors:	Castle, David J.
Dewey Number:	616.89

Publishing Director: Luisa Cecotti
Developmental Editor: Neli Bryant
Project Managers: Liz Malcolm, Nayagi Athmanathan
Edited by Margaret Trudegeon
Proofread by Gabrielle Challis
Cover design by Tania Gomes
Internal design by Stan Lamond
Index by Robert Swanson
Typeset by Toppan Best-set Premedia Limited
Moved to digital printing 2016

CONTENTS

Foreword   ix

Preface   x

Acknowledgements   xi

Contributors and Reviewers   xii

About the authors   xiv

How to use this book   xvii

Part 1   1

Chapter 1   A HISTORY OF PSYCHOLOGICAL MEDICINE   2

Chapter 2   ETHICS AND PSYCHIATRY   26

Part 2   THE TOOLS OF PSYCHIATRY   35

Chapter 3   THE PSYCHIATRIC INTERVIEW AND MENTAL STATE EXAMINATION   36

Chapter 3   *CASE-BASED LEARNING:* A MAN NAMED JAKE   46

Chapter 4   PHYSICAL EXAMINATION AND SPECIAL TESTS   50

Chapter 4   *CASE-BASED LEARNING:* JAKE RETURNS   57

Part 3   THE SYNDROMES OF PSYCHIATRY   61

Chapter 5   CLASSIFICATION   62

Chapter 6 ORGANIC PSYCHIATRY 71
Chapter 6 *CASE-BASED LEARNING:* A NURSE NAMED SAM 88

Chapter 7 SCHIZOPHRENIA AND RELATED DISORDERS 93
Chapter 7 *CASE-BASED LEARNING:* A MOTHER AND DAUGHTER, KAREN AND MELISSA 107

Chapter 8 DEPRESSIVE DISORDERS 112
Chapter 8 *CASE-BASED LEARNING:* AN ELDERLY MAN NAMED FRED 127

Chapter 9 BIPOLAR AND RELATED DISORDERS 131
Chapter 9 *CASE-BASED LEARNING:* A HUSBAND NAMED LAWRENCE 143

Chapter 10 ANXIETY AND POST-TRAUMATIC DISORDERS 147
Chapter 10 *CASE-BASED LEARNING:* AN ELECTRICIAN NAMED SCOTT 157

Chapter 11 THE OBSESSIVE-COMPULSIVE DISORDERS 162
Chapter 11 *CASE-BASED LEARNING:* A STUDENT NAMED STEPHEN 168

Chapter 12 EATING DISORDERS 172
Chapter 12 *CASE-BASED LEARNING:* A MEDICAL STUDENT NAMED PAT 181

Chapter 13 SOMATISATION AND THE SOMATOFORM DISORDERS 184
Chapter 13 *CASE-BASED LEARNING:* A WIFE NAMED MARGARET 194

Chapter 14 PERSONALITY DISORDERS 198
Chapter 14 *CASE-BASED LEARNING:* A WOMAN NAMED STEPHANIE 209

Chapter 15 BIOLOGICAL TREATMENTS 214
Chapter 15 *CASE-BASED LEARNING:* A STORE MANAGER NAMED NEAL 258

Chapter 16 THE PSYCHOTHERAPIES 264
Chapter 16 *CASE-BASED LEARNING:* STEPHEN RETURNS 280

Chapter 17 DEALING WITH PSYCHIATRIC EMERGENCIES 283
Chapter 17 *CASE-BASED LEARNING:* A DIALYSIS PATIENT NAMED
        KEN 293

Part 4   SPECIAL GROUPS 297

Chapter 18 CHILD AND ADOLESCENT PSYCHIATRY 298
Chapter 18 *CASE-BASED LEARNING:* A MOTHER NAMED KATE 313

Chapter 19 OLD AGE PSYCHIATRY 317
Chapter 19 *CASE-BASED LEARNING:* A DAUGHTER NAMED SOPHIA 327

Chapter 20 FORENSIC PSYCHIATRY AND RISK ASSESSMENT 332
Chapter 20 *CASE-BASED LEARNING:* AN ACADEMIC NAMED ALI 339

Chapter 21 DUAL DISABILITY 344
Chapter 21 *CASE-BASED LEARNING:* A MAN NAMED MICHAEL 357

Chapter 22 SUBSTANCE USE DISORDERS 362
Chapter 22 *CASE-BASED LEARNING:* A PATIENT NAMED PETER 379

Index 385

Foreword

Students of medical disciplines are under increasing pressure to understand and process core information regarding a range of topics from basic science through to clinical treatments. The world of psychiatry is no exception, especially with the rapid expansion of knowledge about the causation and treatment of psychiatric and psychological problems. In this fast-moving world, textbooks that can act as a 'one-stop shop' and provide a comprehensive overview of the discipline, with up-to-date information as well as clinical grounding, are extremely useful.

The second edition of *A Primer of Clinical Psychiatry* by David J Castle, Darryl Bassett, Joel King and Andrew Gleason is a perfect example of this. Comprising 22 chapters, the book provides the core knowledge required for mastering skills such as performing a psychiatric interview and structuring a history, together with how to carry out a mental state examination and decide on relevant physical examinations and investigations. Individual chapters cover the history of psychiatry, ethics and the current classification structure of psychiatric diagnostic systems. There are discrete chapters dedicated to explaining the major psychiatric disorders such as schizophrenia, affective disorders, anxiety disorders and substance abuse. There are comprehensive chapters on biological and non-biological treatments, with useful clinical tips and worked case examples. Specialist topics written by experts cover old age psychiatry, child psychiatry, dual disability and forensic psychiatry.

Each clinical chapter is enhanced by a customised 'case-based learning' module, which allows readers to undertake an experiential learning process relevant to their particular needs, with cross-references to the core text. This comprehensive and clearly written book is perfectly aimed at the knowledge requirements of medical students, but will also be of use to GPs (the very comprehensive medication information will be of particular use to this group) and any other student of psychiatry (psychologists, social workers, nurses and occupation therapists).

Professor Ian Everall
Cato Professor and Head
Department of Psychiatry
The University of Melbourne

Preface

This is the second edition of a textbook of clinical psychiatry that is concise yet comprehensive and readily accessible. It aims to provide an easy entry to the pertinent facts of clinical psychiatry for medical students and students of mental health disciplines; a resource for established clinicians, including GPs, and also a brief yet thorough overview for the more advanced psychiatric trainee or mental health professional. New chapters in this edition include a synopsis of the history of psychiatry and ethical aspects of psychiatry.

Throughout the text there is a particular focus on providing readers with a clinically applicable skill and knowledge set. Liberal use of fact boxes and summary lists ensure that readers will have at their fingertips the facts required for an understanding of the core elements of clinical psychiatry, including basic clinical skills and an overview of the syndromes of psychiatry. Each clinical chapter has a customised case-based learning module that allows learnings to be cemented and placed in a clinical context.

To effect coherence of approach and minimal overlap between chapters, the bulk of the core text has been written by Drs Castle and Bassett, who are experienced psychiatrists with expertise in a broad range of clinical and research areas. The psychiatric interview and mental state examination and clinical investigations relevant to psychiatry are covered in some detail. All of the major syndromes of psychiatry are addressed, covering epidemiology, aetiology and clinical aspects, and including discussion of specific treatment approaches. A separate section reviews, more generally, biological and psychosocial aspects of treatment in psychiatry, with worked case examples. A chapter on psychiatric emergencies is included in this section.

This second edition includes role-play scenarios aligned with each of the main subject areas. Drs King and Gleason have done the lion's share of the work in this regard and have provided students with an opportunity to gain a unique understanding of psychiatry, as well as rehearse for their clinical exams.

To ensure that special topics are up-to-date and relevant, experts in particular fields have authored specialist chapters, including 'Old age psychiatry', 'Child and adolescent psychiatry', 'Substance use disorders', 'Dual disability' and 'Forensic psychiatry'. All chapters have numerous brief clinical vignettes to bring the text to life and demonstrate the diversity of expression of mental illnesses.

We hope this book will be a useful guide to the discipline of clinical psychiatry.

David Castle, Darryl Bassett, Joel King and Andrew Gleason

Acknowledgements

The preparation of the second edition of this book has again been founded upon the wisdom, knowledge and experience of my co-editor, Professor David Castle. *A Primer of Clinical Psychiatry* arose from his concept and we are pleased to see that it has been well received. Drs Joel King and Andrew Gleason have joined us with their substantial contribution of training-focused case material, raising the quality of the book even further. Dr Sherylee Bassett has again provided a tower of strength for me and also generously provided a chapter on the history of psychiatry. Finally I thank Dr Joe Cardaci for his generous provision of the SPECT scans included in the book.

Darryl Bassett
29 June 2012

I am delighted to have the opportunity to work with Darryl Bassett in producing a second edition of this book. The first edition was well reviewed and has proven very popular with medical students in particular. This new edition is greatly enhanced by the addition of case-based learning material attached to each clinical chapter: for these we are most grateful to Drs Andrew Gleason and Joel King, who have shown initiative and innovative thinking and with whom we have greatly enjoyed working. We also expressly thank colleagues who contributed to the specialist chapters.

David J Castle
29 June 2012

We are honoured that Professors David Castle and Darryl Bassett invited us to contribute to this text. We must thank the medical students whom we have taught over the last three years. Their participation and insights into early versions of this book's role-play scenarios have proven invaluable. Our surgical and medical colleagues, namely Mr Daniel Spernat, Dr Eric Cheah and Dr Sarah Garner, provided advice when the scenarios stepped outside of pure psychiatry.

Joel King and Andrew Gleason
29 June 2012

Contributors and Reviewers

Robert Adler MB BS, PhD, MCrim (Forensic Psychology), FRACP, FRANZCP

Consultant Forensic Psychiatrist, Adolescent Forensic Health Service, Royal Children's Hospital, Melbourne

David Ames BA, MD, FRCPsych, FRANZCP

Professor of Ageing and Health, University of Melbourne; Director National Ageing Research Institute

Michael Baigent MBBS, FRANZCP, FAChAM

Associate Professor, Department of Psychiatry, Flinders University, and Drug and Alcohol Services, South Australia

Sherylee Bassett BA(Hons), PhD

Former Lecturer and Tutor in Classics and Ancient History, University of Western Australia and University of Adelaide

Chad Bennett BSc(Hons), MBBS, MRCPsych, FRANZCP

Clinical Director, Victorian Dual Disability Service, St Vincent's Hospital, Melbourne

Peter Bosanac MBBS(Melb), MMed(Psychiatry), MD, Grad Dip Mental Health Science (Clinical Hypnosis), FRANZCP

Director of Clinical Services, St Vincent's Mental Health, Melbourne; Senior Lecturer in Psychiatry, University of Melbourne

Nicola Lautenschlager MD, FRANZCP

Professor of Psychiatry of Old Age, Academic Unit for Psychiatry of Old Age, St. Vincent's Health, Department of Psychiatry, University of Melbourne

Samantha Loi MBBS, MPsych, FRANZCP, Cert Old Age Psych

Consultant Psychiatrist, St Vincent's Aged Mental Health; Lecturer, University of Melbourne

Dan Lubman BSc(Hons), MB ChB, PhD, FRANZCP, FAChAM

Director, Turning Point Alcohol and Drug Centre; Professor of Addiction Studies and Services, Monash University

Katinka Morton MBBS, MBioethics, FRANZCP, Cert Child Adol Psych

Consultant Psychiatrist, Forensicare; RANZCP Director of Training, Victoria's Western Region; Honorary Clinical Associate Professor, University of Melbourne

Daniel O'Connor MD, FRANZCP

Professor of Old Age Psychiatry, Monash University

Alessandra Radovini MBBS, DPM, FRANZCP, Cert Child Adol Psych

Director Mindful, Centre for Training and Research in Developmental Health, Department of Psychiatry, the University of Melbourne; Senior Lecturer, Department of Psychiatry, the University of Melbourne; Clinical Director, headspace, National Youth Mental Health Foundation

Michael Salzberg MBBS, MD, FRANZCP

Director of Consultation-Liaison Psychiatry, St Vincent's Hospital, Melbourne; Associate Professor, Department of Psychiatry, University of Melbourne

Danny Sullivan MBBS, MBioeth, MHlthMedLaw, MRCPsych, FRANZCP

Consultant Forensic Psychiatrist, Assistant Clinical Director, Victorian Institute of Forensic Mental Health; Adjunct Senior Lecturer, School of Psychology and Psychiatry, Monash University

Reviewers

Timothy Francis BSc, MBBS, FRACGP

General Practitioner, Nambucca Heads, New South Wales

Catherine Franklin MBBS, MPhil, Cert Cons Liaison Psych, FRANZCP

Consultant Psychiatrist, Queensland Centre for Intellectual and Developmental Disability; School of Medicine, University of Queensland, Queensland

Laura Gray BSc, PhD

Lecturer, School of Medicine, Deakin University

Philippa Hay MBChB, MD, DPhil, FRANZCP

Foundation Chair of Mental Health, University of Western Sydney

Hugh Kildea MBBS, Dip(Obst)RCOG, JP, FRACGP

Medical School Clinical Skills Coordinator, Medicine, Learning and Teaching Unit, Faculty of Health Sciences, University of Adelaide

About the authors

Professor David Jonathan Castle MBChB MSc MD DLSHTM GCUT FRCPsych FRANZCP is currently Chair of Psychiatry at St Vincent's Health and the University of Melbourne. He is a former MRC Research Scholar at the South African Institute for Medical Research, MRC Research Fellow at the London School of Hygiene and Tropical Medicine (where he gained an MSc in epidemiology), and has trained both in clinical research and psychiatry at London's prestigious Maudsley Hospital and Institute of Psychiatry. His strong commitment to teaching is reflected in his completion of the Graduate Certificate in University Teaching from the University of Melbourne in 2011.

Professor Castle's clinical and research interests include schizophrenia and related disorders, cannabis abuse and bipolar disorder. A specific area of interest is the medical care of people with a mental illness. He is also pursuing his work on OCD spectrum disorders, notably body dysmorphic disorder. He has been successful in attracting substantial grant funding from a variety of different sources, and has strong local, national, and international research links. He has received a number of awards for his work, most recently (2011) the Senior Research Award from the Royal Australian and New Zealand College of Psychiatrists.

Professor Castle has published around 400 articles and book chapters, and has produced 17 books aimed at clinical, academic and lay audiences. His book, *Marijuana and Madness* (co-edited with Prof Sir Robin Murray, UK), was the British Medical Association's Mental Health Book of the Year in 2005. He is on a number of advisory boards and editorial boards, and is a regular reviewer for over 30 national and international scientific journals. He also shows a strong commitment to feeding back information to the populations he studies, and is regularly invited to present at scientific, local and lay meetings.

Dr Darryl Bassett MB BS BSc FRANZCP Dip Psychother is currently a Consultant Psychiatrist in full-time private practice. In 2010 Dr Bassett was appointed Adjunct Professor of Psychiatry in the School of Medicine at the University of Notre Dame, WA, and Clinical Associate Professor of Psychiatry in the School of Psychiatry and Clinical Neurosciences at the University of Western Australia. His current research interests are in the pathophysiology of bipolar disorders. He has particular interest in bipolar disorders, schizophrenia and the psychiatry of physical illness. His current intellectual interests are in psychopharmacology and the neurobiology of mental illness.

Dr Bassett graduated in science and medicine in Queensland. After several years of general medicine he trained in psychiatry in South Australia and received the RANZCP College Medallion after completing his fellowship examinations. He became a Research Fellow in psychiatry before moving into a mixed private and general hospital psychiatric practice, and also gained a Graduate Diploma in Psychotherapy. His clinical interests at that time were in the psychiatric aspects of chronic pain, the management of major mood disorders, the psychiatry of physical illness and individual psychotherapy. Later, he took responsibility for a bipolar disorders clinic in a large mental hospital. Throughout this time he was also heavily involved in the teaching of psychiatric trainees and in the examinations conducted by the RANZCP.

Dr Bassett also continued to research, working jointly with academic psychiatrists and clinical psychologists. His research interests have included chemical carcinogenesis, responses to facially expressed emotion in schizophrenia, the interface between depressive disorders and chronic pain, process in psychotherapy, the management of chronic pain, beliefs in the paranormal among sufferers of bipolar disorders, and illness validation. During his time in Adelaide he founded a psychiatric intensive care unit in a private hospital and spent three years heavily involved in the management of acutely psychotic patients. He moved to Western Australia in 2000 to slow down! He was awarded the European Certificate in Anxiety and Depressive Disorders in July 2012 by the University of Maastricht.

Dr Joel King MBBS MPsych FRANZCP Cert Child Adol Psych is currently a Consultant Child and Adolescent Psychiatrist at Eastern Health and the Melbourne Clinic. He obtained his medical degree from the University of Adelaide and trained in psychiatry at St. Vincent's Hospital and the Austin Hospital. He is an Honorary Senior Fellow with the University of Melbourne and Past President of the Victorian Branch of the Australian and New Zealand Association of Psychiatrists in Training. He is involved in the teaching of psychiatry at both undergraduate and postgraduate levels and created a role-play based teaching series, which he began teaching to medical students in 2010.

Dr Andrew Gleason MBBS (Hons) BSc FRANZCP is currently a Consultant Psychiatrist at the Melbourne Health Aged Persons' Mental Health Program. He studied medicine and science at the University of Sydney and completed advanced training in neuropsychiatry at the Royal Melbourne Hospital. He has taught medical students from the University of Melbourne and the University of Sydney, as well as interns, residents and registrars.

How to use this book

Nearly every chapter is followed by a role-play scenario. The exceptions are Chapters 1, 2 and 5. These role-play scenarios are similar to the Observed Structured Clinical Examination (OSCE) stations used by many medical schools and in postgraduate clinical examinations. The names and characters are fictional, but represent realistic scenarios.

Students can practise the scenarios in their own time with a colleague to familiarise themselves with the chapter's material and relevant clinical skills that are pertinent to both real clinical interactions and exams. Students may find that this is best achieved by working in pairs, because every role-play scenario requires two participants: one to play the doctor ('candidate') and the other to play the patient, relative, or health professional ('actor'). Chapter 7 is the only exception, requiring two students as actors.

The scenarios can also be practised as part of a clinical tutorial, with a psychiatrist or psychiatry registrar facilitating. This will provide students with access to expert feedback and discussion of relevant material.

Each scenario contains instructions, which include a description of the setting and the task. This is followed by a description of the actor's role and a model answer. The actor should read the entire scenario and memorise the role as much as possible in order to portray the character accurately. Dressing the part may assist in this.

The actor should set up the room, place a copy of the instructions where the candidate can read them, and act as the timekeeper. Once the actor is ready, the candidate has 2 minutes to read the instructions before the station begins, and 10 minutes to complete the task. Some chapters include examiner's questions. The actor should play the examiner and ask these questions to the candidate. To avoid confusing the candidate, the actor may move their chair to a different position and clearly state that they are now playing the examiner. After the role-play is finished, both the candidate and the actor should read the model answer and refer back to the chapter if necessary. The candidate and actor may wish to come back at a later stage and switch the roles to obtain another perspective of the scenario.

The scenarios are not merely a test of content of the chapter they accompany. The model answers are guides to facilitate further learning. They are not intended to represent the only correct answer. In most cases, the model answers are set at a level above what would be expected of a medical student, although at times we have indicated the minimum that would be expected. Furthermore, the model answers generally represent more than would be possible in a ten minute interaction. Some of this material is preceded with the heading 'For the more advanced learner'. This is again intended to assist the student in thinking broadly rather than just aiming to 'tick the answer boxes'. Where possible, it will be helpful for students to discuss the scenarios with their clinical tutors, who can add their own perspective to the cases, and advise the students on whether their performance is in keeping with the standard expected of their level.

Lastly, the names of the role-play characters are listed under each chapter title in the table of contents. This should assist students in connecting theoretical concepts with a patient's narrative, as well as underscoring that psychiatry is ultimately a specialty about individual people.

David J Castle
Darryl Bassett
Joel King
Andrew Gleason

Part 1

Chapter 1

A HISTORY OF PSYCHOLOGICAL MEDICINE

SHERYLEE BASSETT

Mental illness is no modern invention, nor is it a product of our way of life. From prehistoric times right up until today the mentally ill have been singled out and often mistreated because of their 'otherness'. They have been killed, hidden away, confined in pits, cages, animal stalls, chained to stakes, beaten, humiliated and ridiculed. However, running parallel to this mistreatment has been the search by some for cures to alleviate their suffering.

Table 1.1 offers a brief review of references to mental illness in written works dating from as early as 3000 BC. It considers the buildings used to house the insane, the physicians and thinkers who have influenced the practice of psychiatry, and some of the treatments and medications available in the past up until today.

Table 1.1

Brief review of references to mental illness

Period	Place/beliefs & practices	Details
10,000 BC	**Europe** Trepanation	Around 10,000 BC prehistoric peoples practised trepanation (drilling a hole into the skull without penetrating the dura). We can only speculate why such a drastic procedure came into use.
3000 BC	**Egypt** Magic Demons	One of the oldest medical writings we have is the 20-metre long Egyptian Ebers papyrus, dating to the ninth year of the reign of Amenhotep I (around 1534 BC). The papyrus incorporates earlier texts as well, some dating back to around 3000 BC. It contains many remedies for common ailments, but also magical formulae and incantations for repelling demons bearing disease. Along with discussion of general medical conditions, a number of paragraphs deal with mental disorders that would now be termed depression and dementia.
1100 BC	**India** Madness comes from a divine curse or an imbalance of humours	The *Atharvaveda* is a Hindu sacred text, most of which dates from 1100–900 BC. It attributes *unmada* (insanity) to divine curses or an imbalance of humours. Depressive and anxiety disorders are described in the *Ramayana* and *Mahabharata*, also ancient Hindu sacred texts. The symptoms are ascribed to mythological characters, but the descriptions are clear. The *Ramayana* dates from 400–300 BC, but was added to until about 100 BC. The *Mahabharata* contains references to events from around 800–700 BC, but did not reach its final written form until around AD 400.
490 BC	**China** Chinese medicine Illness comes from an imbalance of yin and yang	In China, *Yellow Emperor's Inner Canon*, an influential medical text regarded as fundamental to Chinese medicine, dates to 400 BC. It attributes illness to natural causes rather than demons, in particular an imbalance of yin and yang, or the five elements. It contains descriptions of epilepsy, dementia and 'madness'.

Continued

Table 1.1

Brief review of references to mental illness—cont'd

Period	Place/beliefs & practices	Details
469 BC	**Greece** Madness is sent by the gods Hippocrates Madness is an imbalance of humours: • blood • yellow bile • black bile • phlegm Melancholia in autumn and spring	Early Greek works, such as Homer's *Iliad* and *Odyssey*, and the plays of Aeschylus, Sophocles and Euripides, explained madness and other mental states as having been imposed from outside the self by a god. Ideas had begun to change by the time of Hippocrates (469–399 BC), a physician from the Greek island of Cos. Although many Greek medical texts are attributed to Hippocrates, he cannot be confidently linked to any of them. The Hippocratic corpus attempted to explain disease in rational terms, as having been caused by an imbalance of humours (blood, yellow bile, black bile and phlegm). Different works describe a range of mental illnesses including melancholia (caused by an excess of black bile), mania, hysteria, anxiety and dementia. Melancholia was observed to be more prominent in autumn and spring. It was also sometimes associated with mania, although no cyclical connection was made. *The Characters* is a work by Theophrastus (c.372–288 BC), the successor of Aristotle at the Lyceum, in which he describes 30 different undesirable personality types.
AD 100	**Ephesus, Turkey** Melancholics and their desire for wine and sex Soranus Mixed states of mania and depression	Rufus of Ephesus (active c. AD 100) worked as a physician in what was then regarded as a centre of excellence for medicine. He had studied at Alexandria and visited Cos and Caria. His work, *On Melancholy*, survives only in Greek, Latin and Arabic fragments. Galen wrote that Rufus's text was 'the best work' on the subject. One of Rufus's conclusions was that desires for sex and wine characterised melancholics, and that the provision of both helped to improve their symptoms. This work was highly regarded and influential right up until the Renaissance.

Table 1.1

Brief review of references to mental illness—cont'd

Period	Place/beliefs & practices	Details
		The Greek physician, Soranus of Ephesus (AD 98–138), appears to have documented the occurrence of mixed states of mania and depression. His work, *On Acute and Chronic Diseases*, survives only in the 5th century Latin translation by the Roman physician Caelius Aurelianus of Sicca in Numidia.
129	**Rome** Galen Aretaeus of Cappadocia Bipolarity	Galen of Pergamum (129–c.199) was originally a gladiator physician in Asia Minor, but rose to become court physician to Marcus Aurelius in Rome. He was greatly influenced by the Hippocratic works, building upon and refining their conclusions. A contemporary of Galen's was Aretaeus of Cappadocia (c.150–200), an author of medical texts who wrote in the Ionic form of Ancient Greek, imitating Hippocrates. He described epilepsy, melancholia, mania and bipolarity.
410	**The sack of Rome** European Middle Ages Mental illness comes from possession by demons or witchcraft	The decline of the Roman empire marked the end of the period commonly referred to as Classical Antiquity and the beginning of the period known as the European Middle Ages. Many classical texts were lost to the West at this time, but were preserved by scholars in Byzantium and the Islamic world. In Middle Ages Europe mental illness was explained in terms of possession by demons or witchcraft.
490	**Middle East** Hospitals for the mentally ill in: • Jerusalem • Baghdad • Fes • Cairo	A hospital dedicated to the treatment of the mentally ill is claimed to have existed in Jerusalem around 490. The first dedicated psychiatric hospitals in Islamic countries were founded in Baghdad in 705, followed not long after by Fes and then Cairo in 872.

Continued

Table 1.1

Brief review of references to mental illness—cont'd

Period	Place/beliefs & practices	Details
980	**Persia** Avicenna Pulse rate measures arousal	The Persian polymath, known in Europe as Avicenna (c.980–1037), wrote the *Al-Qanum fi al-Tibb (Canon of Medicine)*, which developed a system of medicine based upon the principles of Galen. It included Avicenna's observations and descriptions of a number of mental illnesses. Up until around the 17th century this work was used as a medical textbook in both Muslim and European universities (the latter through Latin versions). Avicenna proposed using variations in pulse rate to judge the level of a person's emotional arousal, thus giving an indication of their inner feelings.
1330	**England** Bedlam	A priory for the Order of the Star of Bethlehem was established in England in 1247. In 1330 it became a hospital, admitting its first psychiatric patients in the 1350s. Over time, the hospital became a centre for the care of the insane and its name was gradually corrupted into 'Bedlam'. The site of the hospital has changed and it has been rebuilt a number of times. The City of London became custodian in 1547 and it is now part of the South London and Maudsley NHS Foundation Trust.
1398	**Florence, Italy** The Renaissance Scientific method The printing press	The Renaissance, which began in Florence in the 14th century, saw a resurgence of interest in learning from Classical sources and in educational reform. The Scientific method flourished, focusing on the gathering of empirical and measurable evidence. The invention of the printing press by Gutenberg in the 15th century allowed books to be published more quickly and disseminated more widely than ever before. Likewise, the gradual displacement of classical languages by the vernacular led to the rapid spread of new learning.

Table 1.1
Brief review of references to mental illness—cont'd

Period	Place/beliefs & practices	Details
1518	**England** Royal College of Physicians is formed	The College of Physicians was founded by royal charter of King Henry VIII in 1518. It was modelled upon colleges already established in Europe. Thomas Linacre, the classical scholar and physician, was its first president. The main role of the college was to license those it deemed qualified to practise medicine, and punish the unqualified and those it considered guilty of malpractice. It became known as the Royal College of Physicians of London in 1674.
1567	**Mexico** Hospital for the insane opened	Bernardino Alvarez, a Spanish soldier and later a member of the Religious Order of Saint Hyppolitus, opened the Hospital y Asilo de Convalescientes de San Hipólito (Saint Hyppolitus's Hospital and Convalescent Asylum) in Mexico in 1567. Its original aim was to care for poor convalescents, the insane, the elderly, and even to teach illiterate children. Over time, new hospitals were opened with the aid of donations and the wealth Alvarez had accumulated, and the original hospital was used purely for the care of the insane.
1586	**England** First book in English on melancholy	*A Treatise of Melancholie* was written by Timothy Bright (1551–1615).
1591	**China** Bipolar disorder described	Gao Lian describes bipolar disorder in his work, *Eight Treatises on the Nurturing of Life*.
1621	**England** *The Anatomy of Melancholy* published Melancholia is a humour	Robert Burton (1577–1640) was an Oxford don who suffered from depression. Although presented as a medical textbook, *The Anatomy of Melancholy* is in fact a broad compendium which discourses on subjects as wide-ranging as navigation, digestion, goblins, military discipline and the morality of dancing schools.

Continued

Table 1.1

Brief review of references to mental illness—cont'd

Period	Place/beliefs & practices	Details
		It also incorporates passages copied from many other authors, from Ancient Greeks right up to the latest works of the 17th century. Burton defined melancholy as a humour which lingers in the body and rises up at every opportunity, whether because of a sad event or as the result of fear or grief. The first part of the work deals with causes and symptoms of 'common' melancholies, the second with cures and the third investigated melancholies of a more complex kind, such as those provoked by religion or love.
1637	**Dutch Republic** René Descartes Cogito ergo sum	René Descartes (1596–1650), the French philosopher and writer, lived in the Dutch Republic for much of his life. His *Discourse de la Methode*, written in 1637, included the Latin statement for which he is best known: 'cogito ergo sum' ('I think therefore I am').
1650–1950	**England** The Asylum Era The Industrial Revolution	This was a time when it was considered best practice for the mentally ill to be confined to asylums, where they could be cared for in humane conditions, within a calm environment, with regular routines and daily activities. In part, this was a consequence of the Industrial Revolution (c.1790–1860), which caused an upheaval of traditional ways of living and led to people flocking from farms and villages in the countryside, into cities and to work in factories. Grouping the insane into asylums meant that for the first time asylum owners and doctors gained an understanding of and experience in caring for large numbers of people with a wide variety of mental illnesses.

Table 1.1

Brief review of references to mental illness—cont'd

Period	Place/beliefs & practices	Details
1660	**England** The Royal Society founded The term 'neurology' first used Theories of epilepsy and psychology First English treatise on psychology	Thomas Willis (1621-1675) was an English doctor and founding member of the Royal Society, who performed early research into the anatomy of the brain, nervous system and muscles. He discovered the area of the brain named after him – the Circle of Willis. In 1664 he published *Cerebri anatome*, a detailed work in collaboration with the anatomists Thomas Millington and Richard Lower, with drawings by Christopher Wren. The term 'neurology' came into use as a result of this text. The *Pathologicae cerebri, et nervosa generis specimen* was published in 1667, contributing to knowledge of the pathology and neurophysiology of the brain. This work included Willis's theories on the cause of epilepsy and psychological illness. He published the first treatise in English on the subject of psychology in 1672, *Two Discourses concerning the Soul of Brutes, Which is that of the Vital and Sensitive of Man*.
1758	**England** Asylums are therapeutic Royal College of Physicians appoints a psychiatrist as president	In his 1758 *Treatise on Madness*, William Battie (1703-1776) argued that confining the insane in asylums had therapeutic value in itself. He was the founding doctor of St Luke's Hospital in London, an asylum, and was the owner of two large private madhouses. In 1764 he became president of the Royal College of Physicians – the only psychiatrist ever to hold this position.
1765	**England** King George III is insane! Can mental illness be cured? The Regency Period	King George III (1738-1820) became ill, probably in 1765, with a relapsing mental illness that is commonly thought to have been a symptom of porphyria. However, a 2005 analysis of hair samples revealed high levels of arsenic. The spontaneous recovery from these episodes of madness led to the popular belief that mental illness could be cured.

Continued

Table 1.1

Brief review of references to mental illness—cont'd

Period	Place/beliefs & practices	Details
		In 1811 George III finally accepted that his illness was permanent and assented to his son acting as Regent. George III lived out the rest of his life in seclusion at Windsor Castle, suffering dementia, blindness and increasing deafness.
1773	**America** First American psychiatric hospital built Benjamin Rush First American textbook of psychiatry	In America, the first dedicated psychiatric hospital was constructed in Williamsburg, Virginia in 1773. Benjamin Rush (1746–1813), regarded as the father of American psychiatry, campaigned successfully in 1792 for the establishment of a separate mental ward in the Pennsylvania Hospital. There, he argued, patients could be housed in more humane conditions, without chains. Rush published *Medical Inquiries and Observations upon the Diseases of the Mind*, the first American textbook on the subject, in 1812. In it he attempted to classify the different forms of mental illness. He believed that many of these disorders were caused by problems with blood circulation, which led him to employ treatments such as a restraining chair and a spinning board, intended to improve blood circulation to the brain.
1793	**Florence, Italy** Humane treatment The importance of hope	The Italian Vincenzo Chiarugi (1759–1820) argued for the humane treatment of people with psychiatric disorders and introduced his theories at the Bonifazio Asylum in Florence. In 1793 he emphasised the importance of instilling hope in patients suffering from depression.
1795	**Germany** Reil The term 'Psychiatry' first used Insanity is a medical condition First lectures in psychiatry	In 1795 German physician, physiologist, anatomist and psychiatrist, Johann Reil (1759–1813), established the first journal of psychology, the *Archiv für die Physiologie*. The poet Goethe visited him between 1802 and 1805 to discuss matters of scientific interest, such as psychiatry.

Table 1.1

Brief review of references to mental illness—cont'd

Period	Place/beliefs & practices	Details
		Reil was also the first to coin the term 'psychiatry' in an 1808 journal article. He argued forcefully that the mentally ill should be treated by physicians and that psychiatry should be recognised as a new specialty of medicine. He suggested that illness could not be broken up into physical, chemical and mental diseases, but there was always an interaction between the three. Reil is also regarded as one of the founders of neurology. In 1810 the University of Halle became the first university worldwide to offer lectures in psychiatry.
1796	**York, England** Tuke	William Tuke (1732–1822) was an English tea merchant and Quaker who founded a private asylum in 1796 for local members of the Quaker movement suffering from a mental illness. He stressed the need for calm and gentleness in the treatment of these patients. The policies for the treatment of the insane were developed over 2 years in discussions with the local Quaker group, but the York Retreat had a medical superintendent.
1801	**France** Pinel Sympathy and kindness best for the insane	Philippe Pinel (1745–1826) published a medical textbook arguing that asylums should offer psychological therapy, using the experience of containment to modify behaviour. He had become interested in mental illness following the suicide of a friend. His theories developed while working at the hospices Bicêtre (for men) and the Salpêtrière (for women). At the time Pinel became Physician of the Infirmeries, Bicêtre held some 4000 men, only about 200 of whom had a mental illness. These 200 were housed in a separate ward under the care of Jean-Baptiste Pussin and his wife Marguerite Jubline, who looked after them using sympathy and kindness mixed with authoritarianism.

Continued

Table 1.1
Brief review of references to mental illness—cont'd

Period	Place/beliefs & practices	Details
1811	**New South Wales, Australia** First Australian mental hospital at Castle Hill Tarban Creek Gladesville	Contrary to popular belief, Pinel was not the first to release psychiatric patients from their chains, although he was certainly among the first to do so. The patients were put into straightjackets instead. Following the establishment in 1788 of New South Wales, Governor Phillip initiated plans for the care of the Colony's insane by 1805. By 1810 a board had been set up to assess the mentally ill. The first mental hospital in Australia was built in 1811 at Castle Hill, about 30 km from Sydney Cove. The mentally ill were moved there from the town jail at Parramatta, where they had been housed to that time. Manacles were used at Castle Hill, but the conditions were regarded as superior to those of the jail, leading to at least one convict feigning madness in a bid to be transferred. In 1825 Castle Hill housed 27 male and 8 female patients. Due to a failed water supply and the poor condition of the buildings at Castle Hill, the Court House at Liverpool was converted for use as an asylum between 1825 and 1838. Later a purpose-built asylum was constructed at Tarban Creek to meet the needs of the growing Colony. The Governor wrote to England requesting that a married couple, who could act as keeper and matron, be sent out, and they arrived in mid-1838, with the first patients admitted in 1839. The Tarban Creek Lunatic Asylum was renamed The Hospital for the Insane, Gladesville in 1869 and grew in size. It was modernised and in 1915 became known as the Gladesville Mental Hospital. It became the Gladesville Macquarie Hospital in 1993, with the final inpatients being discharged in 1997.

Table 1.1

Brief review of references to mental illness—cont'd

Period	Place/beliefs & practices	Details
1818	**Germany** Heinroth First professor of Mental Medicine The term 'Psychosomatic' first used	Johann Heinroth (1773–1843), a German physician and the first professor of 'Mental Medicine' at a German university, argued that many illnesses, including mental illness, were caused by the soul. He considered that mental illness was a manifestation of sin accumulated over years. In his 1818 textbook, *Lehrbuch der Störungen des Seelenlebens* (*Textbook on the Disorders of the Soul*), he classified mental disorders into three categories (hyperthymias, asthenias and hypo-asthenias) and coined the term 'psychosomatic'.
1832	**England** British Medical Association founded No restraints to be used in England	John Conolly (1794–1866) was an English doctor who founded the Provincial Medical and Surgical Association in 1832, along with Charles Hastings and John Forbes. Their aim was to improve the standard of medical practice in rural areas. The association later became known as the British Medical Association. From 1839 to 1844 Conolly was resident physician at the Middlesex County Asylum in Hanwell (now known as St Bernard's Hospital). During his time there he insisted that the insane be freed from all forms of restraint. Although the concept had been introduced earlier, it was not until it was enforced at Hanwell that it became accepted practice in England.
1841	**England** Royal College of Psychiatrists founded	The Association of Medical Officers of Asylums and Hospitals for the Insane was founded in 1841. After several name changes it became known as the Royal College of Psychiatrists in 1971.

Continued

Table 1.1

Brief review of references to mental illness—cont'd

Period	Place/beliefs & practices	Details
1844	**United States** American Psychiatric Association founded	In 1844 the Association of Medical Superintendents of American Institutions for the Insane was formed in Philadelphia. Among the founding fathers was Thomas Kirkbride (1809–1883), who established the asylum model used throughout the United States (US). In 1921 the association became known as the American Psychiatric Association.
1845	**England** Lunacy Commission established	The House of Commons passed bills in June 1845, proposed by the reformer Lord Ashley, to establish a permanent Lunacy Commission to oversee the care of both private and pauper lunatics. By 1900 English asylums held about 100,000 patients.
1852	**France** Morel	Bénédict Morel (1809–1873) was a French physician born in Vienna, who used the term *démence precoce* (dementia praecox) in writings dated to 1852 and 1860 to describe groups of young male and female patients suffering from a sub-type of melancholia. He considered that the condition was reversible.
1858	**England** Maudsley Maudsley Hospital First 'first episode psychosis' unit?	Henry Maudsley (1835–1918) wished to work in the East India medical services but, finding that he had to have prior experience with psychiatric patients, accepted a position at an asylum in West Yorkshire in 1858. Maudsley became disillusioned with his specialty and resigned from the Medico-Psychological Association. Nevertheless, he donated £30,000 towards the establishment of a new mental hospital in 1907. The purpose of Maudsley Hospital, which opened in 1915, was to treat patients in the early stages of illness, acute admissions and outpatients.

Table 1.1

Brief review of references to mental illness—cont'd

Period	Place/beliefs & practices	Details
1863	**Germany** Kahlbaum Hecker Dysthymia Cyclothymia Catatonia Paranoia Hebephrenia Schizophrenia	Die Gruppierung der psychischen Krankheiten (The Classification of Psychiatric Diseases) was published in 1863 by Karl Kahlbaum (1828–1899). He categorised mental illnesses according to their typical forms, believing that they progressed through a clearly defined degenerative process, ending with dementia. Kahlbaum became director of a private psychiatric clinic in Görlitz in 1866. His assistant, Ewald Hecker (1843–1909), accompanied him. Through their research they were the first to describe dysthymia, cyclothymia, catatonia, paranoia and hebephrenia (disorganised schizophrenia). Hecker's 1871 article gave the first clinical description of schizophrenia as a distinct disease, using Kahlbaum's classification.
1865	**Berlin, Germany** Griesinger Insanity is a disease of the brain	Wilhelm Griesinger (1817–1868) became professor of psychiatry at Charité Hospital in Berlin in 1865. He established the first university department of psychiatry with interests in teaching and research as opposed to the traditional confining of patients in an asylum. He had come to believe that mental illness was a disease of the brain (although the term he used was 'nerve disease'), and that diagnosis could be made only by close observation of the patient and the course of the illness.
1883	**Heidelberg, Germany** Kraepelin Dementia praecox Classification	In 1890 Emil Kraepelin (1856–1926) became professor of psychiatry at Heidelberg University, where he began the practice of keeping notes on the history and progress of each of his patients over a period of years. Rather than publishing in journals, Kraepelin published updated editions of his textbook, Psychiatrie, first published in 1883.

Continued

Table 1.1

Brief review of references to mental illness—cont'd

Period	Place/beliefs & practices	Details
		In the influential 1893 edition, he described dementia praecox as a distinct disorder, seemingly unaware of Morel's earlier work. The sixth edition of 1899 saw Kraepelin's ideas expressed in their clearest form. He proposed dividing psychiatric illness into 13 groups. The most significant of these groups were dementia praecox and manic-depressive psychosis. It is this work which formed the foundation for the *Diagnostic and Statistical Manual of Mental Disorders* and the International Classification of Diseases.
1887	**Berlin, Germany** First amphetamine synthesised	The first racemic amphetamine, known as 'phenylisopropylamine' was synthesised in Berlin in 1887. It was marketed for use as a bronchodilator from 1932. Awareness of the stimulant effects of dextroamphetamine grew, and in 1937 Smith, Kline and French marketed tablets using the trade name Dexedrine. The United States approved Dexedrine for the treatment of narcolepsy, attention disorders, depression and obesity. In 1937 stimulants were found to improve concentration in children with behavioural and neurological problems.
1888	**Europe** Psychosurgery Leucotomy Moniz awarded Nobel Prize Lobotomy	Psychosurgery on humans in modern times is said to have begun with the Swiss psychiatrist, Johann Burckhardt (1836–1907). At Préfargier Asylum in December 1888 he cut a piece of cerebral cortex out of the brains of six patients. One patient died shortly after the operation. Burckhardt presented his results at the Berlin Medical Congress and published a report, but due to the hostile reception he received, he performed no further operations.

Table 1.1

Brief review of references to mental illness—cont'd

Period	Place/beliefs & practices	Details
		The term 'psychosurgery' was first used by the Portuguese neurologist António Moniz (1874–1955). He theorised that those suffering from mental illnesses had a disorder of the synapses, which led to the continuous circulation of unhealthy thoughts through their brains. In 1935 the operation was refined, using an instrument called a leucotome, and became known as leucotomy, or the cutting of white matter. Moniz was awarded the Nobel Prize for Physiology or Medicine in 1949. US neurologist Walter Freeman and neurosurgeon James Watts adapted Moniz's operation from 1936. They cut the connections between the prefrontal lobes and the deeper structures of the brain in a procedure they called a lobotomy.
1890	**Russia** Conditioned reflex	Ivan Pavlov (1849–1936) was appointed to the Department of Physiology at the Institute of Experimental Medicine and began researching the gastric function of dogs, and later children, in the 1890s. In 1901 he and his assistant, Ivan Filippovitch Tolochinov discovered that using external stimuli (a bell, electric shock, whistle, metronome, tuning fork) before offering food eventually caused the subject to salivate simply on hearing or experiencing the stimulus. This research was fundamental to the development of behaviour therapy.
1893	**Chicago, United States** Bertillon ICD	The International Statistical Institute conference in Chicago in 1893 saw the French physician, Jacques Bertillon (1851–1922), introduce his *Bertillon Classification of Causes of Death*.

Continued

Table 1.1

Brief review of references to mental illness—cont'd

Period	Place/beliefs & practices	Details
		Many countries began to use this system of classification, which distinguished between systemic diseases and those located in one organ. In 1900 the *International Classification of Causes of Death* was revised by an international conference, and it was decided that the classification system should be revised every 10 years. The title was changed to *International Statistical Classification of Diseases, Injuries and Causes of Death* (ICD) with the 6th edition published in 1949. With the publication of the 7th edition in 1957, the World Health Organization became responsible for its revision and publication.
1897	**Europe** Freud Jung	Sigmund Freud (1856–1939) was a Viennese neurologist who, in around 1897, developed the theory that repressed fantasies of incest in childhood led to hysteria in his adult female patients. Early psychoanalysis was characterised by the quest for such sexual origins to explain mental illness. Carl Jung (1875–1961) became a psychiatrist in 1900. His research into psychotherapy, influenced in part by his own early life experiences, led him to conceive the notions of introversion and extraversion and the concept of the collective unconscious. Jung's ideas developed into a new school of psychotherapy, referred to as analytical psychology.
1908	**Germany** Bleuler Schizophrenia	In 1908, and in his classic book of 1911, *Dementia Praecox, or the Group of Schizophrenias*, Eugen Bleuler (1857–1939) built upon Kraepelin's work, arguing that a number of seemingly separate psychotic states could be grouped together, based on their core symptoms, into one diagnosis, to become known as schizophrenia.

Table 1.1

Brief review of references to mental illness—cont'd

Period	Place/beliefs & practices	Details
		He believed that there were important 'splits' between thought and affect in these patients and that schizophrenia was a disease caused probably by some toxin or defect of metabolism.
1921	**Switzerland** Deep Sleep Therapy	The Swiss psychiatrist, Jakob Klaesi-Blumer (1883–1980) introduced Deep Sleep Therapy in 1921. He used a barbiturate, Somnifen, to induce sleep lasting for long periods.
1923	**Russia** Lie detector Neuropsychology	The first lie detector machine was developed by Alexander Luria (1902–1977), the Russian neuropsychologist and developmental psychologist. Luria studied aphasia in the 1930s, looking at the relationship between language, thought and cortical functions. Of particular interest to him was the way the brain compensated for the aphasia. During the Second World War Luria worked at an army hospital and led a team researching patients with brain lesions. His aim was to find ways of compensating for the psychological dysfunctions in these patients. This work led to the development of the field of neuropsychology.
1927	**Vienna, Austria** Sakel Insulin shock therapy	Insulin shock therapy (or Insulin Coma Therapy) was developed by Manfred Sakel (1900–1957) in 1927, as a young doctor working in Vienna. It was used mainly to treat people with schizophrenia up to the 1950s, when it was replaced by neuroleptic medications. The treatment usually involved injections of insulin 6 days a week for approximately 2 months. The dose of insulin was gradually increased until a coma was induced, and then the dose was kept static. The coma lasted for as long as an hour and was terminated by intravenous glucose.

Continued

Table 1.1

Brief review of references to mental illness—cont'd

Period	Place/beliefs & practices	Details
		Following the induction of between 50 and 60 comas, the dose of insulin was reduced quickly and treatment was stopped. Courses of treatment lasting up to 2 years have been recorded.
1933	**Moscow, Russia** First day hospital 'work therapy'	A lack of funding and beds led to the opening of the first recorded day hospital in Moscow in 1933. About 80 patients undertook a course of treatment consisting of 'work therapy'. The average length of stay was 2 months. The Allen Memorial Institute of Psychiatry in Montreal, Canada opened a day hospital in 1947. It aimed to imitate ordinary life by limiting treatment to normal working hours. In 1948 a day hospital for recently discharged psychiatric patients was opened in London, England. The first US day hospital was opened at the Menninger Clinic in Topeka, Kansas, in 1949.
1938	**Italy** Cerletti discovers ECT	Electroconvulsive therapy (ECT) was discovered as a treatment modality by an Italian neurologist, Ugo Cerletti (1877–1963). It was thought at the time that people with epilepsy could not also have schizophrenia. Cerletti believed that ECT could therefore be used to cure schizophrenia. He first used ECT on a patient in 1938.
1939	**Germany** Euthanasia of mentally ill	In October 1939 Adolf Hitler authorised the deaths of the mentally ill and handicapped, on the grounds that this was mercy killing.
1946	**Antipodes** RANZCP formed	The Australasian Association of Psychiatrists was formed in 1946. It became the Royal Australian and New Zealand College of Psychiatrists in 1978. Currently the college has more than 3000 fellows and as many as 1000 trainees.

Table 1.1
Brief review of references to mental illness—cont'd

Period	Place/beliefs & practices	Details
1948–	**Russia**	Hundreds or perhaps thousands of political prisoners were detained in psychiatric hospitals in the Soviet Union as a way of discrediting their views and breaking them mentally and physically. This political abuse of psychiatry continued until the fall of the Soviet Union, but even in modern Russia dissidents have faced threats of being diagnosed with a psychiatric illness in an attempt to suppress opposition.
1948	**Australia** Cade Lithium is a mood stabiliser	John Cade (1912–1980) spent much of his early life living in the grounds of Australian mental hospitals, where his father was medical superintendent. He became a psychiatrist and discovered, in 1948, that lithium carbonate was an effective mood stabiliser for those suffering from manic depression. Dr Cade took lithium himself first, to check that it was safe for human consumption. His discovery made lithium the first effective medication used to treat a major mental disorder.
1950	**France** Chlorpromazine	Chlorpromazine (Largactil or Thorazine), synthesised in 1950, was the first drug to have a specific antipsychotic action. It was discovered as a result of a French search for a tranquilliser to use in conjunction with ether anaesthetic. They built upon the discovery of phenothiazines during the development of the German dye industry at the end of the 19th century. Chlorpromazine has been hailed as the greatest single advance in psychiatric care, directly leading to significant improvement in the prognosis for psychiatric patients and to the deinstitutionalisation of these patients. The impact is illustrated dramatically by the number of inpatients in American psychiatric hospitals. In 1955 there were 558,922, but by 1990 the figure had dropped to a maximum of 120,000.

Continued

Table 1.1

Brief review of references to mental illness—cont'd

Period	Place/beliefs & practices	Details
1951	**United States and France** MAOIs	Isoniazid and Iproniazid, originally intended to treat tuberculosis, were found to improve the mood of patients. N-isopropyl was added to the more potent Iproniazid, and was approved for use as an antidepressant in 1958. It was the first Monoamine Oxidase Inhibitor (MAOI), a class of drug that works particularly well with atypical depression. It interacts adversely with sympathomimetic drugs and foods which contain tyramine. It was found that there are in fact 2 MAO enzymes, MAO-A and MAO-B. Moclobemide was the first reversible inhibitor of MAO-A, discovered in Switzerland in 1972.
1952	**United States** First edition of DSM	The first edition of *Diagnostic and Statistical Manual of Mental Disorders* (DSM), was published by the American Psychiatric Association in 1952.
1957	**Switzerland** First tricyclic antidepressant	Imipramine was the first tricyclic antidepressant developed. Roland Kuhn was trying to improve the effectiveness of chlorpromazine and found that compound G22355 improved depression that was accompanied by mental and motor retardation. It was originally intended to be used as an antipsychotic, but worked better as an antidepressant.
1960s	**United States** Beck Depression Inventory Cognitive-behaviour therapy	Aaron Beck (1921–) developed a number of questionnaires for assessing depression and anxiety; the best known is the Beck Depression Inventory. Beck, who had previously practised as a psychoanalyst, developed cognitive-behaviour therapy in the early 1960s in response to his conclusion that psychoanalytic concepts of depression were invalid. His research demonstrated that depressed patients were subject to spontaneously occurring negative thoughts, which he termed 'automatic thoughts', and distorted thinking. By helping patients to identify and reflect upon these negative thoughts and distorted core beliefs, Beck found that patients felt better and became more functional.

Table 1.1

Brief review of references to mental illness—cont'd

Period	Place/beliefs & practices	Details
1962	**Australia** Deep Sleep Therapy	Between 1962 and 1979 Harry Bailey (1922–1985) and a small number of other psychiatrists practised Deep Sleep Therapy at Chelmsford Private Hospital in Sydney. Patients were given barbiturates and kept unconscious for long periods of time. The treatment was prescribed for conditions such as schizophrenia, depression, obesity, pre-menstral syndrome (PMS) and addiction. By the 1970s 26 patients had died. Dr Bailey committed suicide in 1985.
1971	**England** Hounsfield builds the first CT scanner	The electrical engineer Godfrey Hounsfield (1919–2004) shared the 1979 Nobel Prize for Physiology or Medicine (with Allan Cormack) for his contribution to the development of the diagnostic technique of X-ray computed tomography (CT).
1971	**Worldwide** First SSRI patented Dopamine is a neurotransmitter	Early psychiatric drugs were lethal when taken in overdose. Research interest focused on a search for safer medications. The first selective serotonin reuptake inhibitor (SSRI) antidepressant was Zimelidine, patented in 1971 by the Swedish scientist, Arvid Carlsson (1923–). It is now banned worldwide because of side effects. Carlsson was awarded the Nobel Prize in Physiology or Medicine in 2000 (along with Eric Kandel and Paul Greengard) for his work in demonstrating that dopamine was a neurotransmitter in the brain.
1973	**United States** Dissociative identity disorder	The book *Sybil* was published in 1973, giving a fictionalised account of Dr Cornelia Wilbur's treatment of Shirley Ardell Mason for multiple personality disorder (now dissociative identity disorder). The treatment, augmented with amobarbital and hypnosis, began in 1954 and continued for 11 years. Eventually 16 different personalities were identified.

Continued

Table 1.1

Brief review of references to mental illness—cont'd

Period	Place/beliefs & practices	Details
1973	**United States** The Rosenhan experiment	The book became a best seller, and the diagnosis of dissociative identity disorder flourished. Not everyone was convinced, however, and when the audiotaped recordings of sessions were later examined, it was decided that Dr Wilbur had led or encouraged the patient to fabricate the personalities. The case remains controversial, and this disorder is now rarely diagnosed. The psychologist David Rosenhan (1929–2012) conducted an experiment to test the validity of psychiatric diagnoses and published his findings as 'On being sane in insane places' in the journal *Science*. There were two parts to the experiment. In the first part, pseudopatients simulated auditory hallucinations to engineer admission to 12 different psychiatric hospitals in the United States. All were diagnosed with psychiatric disorders. The pseudopatients acted normally after admission, but staff continued to believe that they remained psychiatrically unwell. A number of the pseudopatients were detained for months and all were compelled to admit to having a mental illness and to agree to take antipsychotic medications as a condition of discharge. The second part of the experiment took place when a psychiatric hospital challenged Rosenhan to send pseudopatients to its facility, with the conviction that these impostors would be detected. Rosenhan agreed to the challenge. Of the 193 new patients, staff identified 41 as potential pseudopatients, but Rosenhan had not sent anyone.

Table 1.1
Brief review of references to mental illness—cont'd

Period	Place/beliefs & practices	Details
		This study was critically important in demonstrating the dangers of dehumanising and labelling patients in psychiatric hospitals. It recommended that community mental health facilities be used for the treatment of the mentally ill and that mental health workers be made more aware of the social psychology of institutions.
1977	**United States** Biopsychosocial model	The psychiatrist George L Engel (1913–1999) published an article in *Science* in 1977 arguing for the need for a new medical model to treat illness. His biopsychosocial model proposes that the traditional medical model is too narrow and that biological, psychological and social factors should be considered when making diagnoses.
1980	**Worldwide** Psychotherapies flourish	By 1980 there were 250 different forms of psychotherapy in use, and by 1996 there were more than 450 forms. (See Chapter 16 for a detailed discussion of the major psychotherapies.)
1980	**Worldwide** DSM-III DSM-IV-TR ICD-10 2nd edn	The *Diagnostic and Statistical Manual of Mental Disorders, Third Edition* (DSM-III) was published in 1980. Part of the aim of the editors of DSM-III was to bring the over-diagnosis of mental illness that had developed in the United States, back into line with psychiatry in the rest of the world, and to make it consistent with ICD-9. DSM-IV was published in 1994, DSM-IV-TR in 2000 and ICD-10 2nd edn in 2004.
2012	**Worldwide** Community care	Management in the community is now regarded as best practice for all but the most severely ill patients. Advances in psychiatric medications and psychotherapies have allowed asylums to close in large numbers and day hospitals and half-way houses have thrived.

Chapter 2

ETHICS AND PSYCHIATRY

KATINKA MORTON & ROBERT ADLER

Ethics have been described as being about 'How we ought to live. What makes our actions the right, rather than the wrong, thing to do? What should our goals be?' Medical ethics examine those dilemmas within the practice of medicine.

Many of these ethical dilemmas are secondary to the power imbalance inherent in all doctor–patient relationships. This *power imbalance* results from the patient's dependence upon the doctor for healthcare and the differing levels of knowledge and expertise about health between doctor and patient. This power imbalance is heightened in psychiatry by four factors, shown in Box 2.1.

The vulnerability and dependence of mental health patients upon their doctor means that ethical dilemmas within psychiatry are of particular importance.

Ethical decision-making

Ethical theories offer guidance when assessing the best answer to an ethical dilemma. These theories evaluate ethical dilemmas by prioritising different philosophical frameworks.

- *Deontology* or *Kantianism* assesses actions as right or wrong in and of themselves.
- *Consequentialism* values the rightness or wrongness of an action according to the consequences of that action. *Utilitarianism*, one form of consequentialism, prioritises the greatest good for the greatest number as the outcome which should guide decision-making.

Box 2.1

Factors heightening the power imbalance in psychiatry

- Psychiatric illnesses and their effects upon *mental state* have implications for the patient's autonomy, and may render them particularly vulnerable.
- The *social consequences* of many psychiatric illnesses, including stigma and socioeconomic disadvantage, further heighten the vulnerability of patients by reducing the supports and healthcare alternatives available to them.
- Psychiatric *treatments*, such as involuntary care and psychotropic medication, may promote and even enforce increased dependence.
- The often highly *personal information* disclosed during history-taking and psychotherapeutic treatments results in another form of power imbalance between doctor and patient. In psychotherapy, *transference* may further heighten the vulnerability of the patient to influence by the doctor.

Box 2.2

The Four Principles Framework of Beauchamp and Childress

According to this framework, ethical decision-making should proceed, based upon an attempt to optimise:

- the *autonomy* of individuals concerned
- *beneficence*, contributing to the 'welfare' of individuals involved
- *non-maleficence*, the 'obligation not to inflict harm on others'
- *justice*, or 'fair, equitable and appropriate treatment in light of what is due or owed to persons'.

- *Virtue ethics* evaluates the rightness or wrongness of an action by the underlying motive of the agent acting.
- *Principle-based ethics* specify a number of principles to guide moral actions. The Four Principles Framework of Beauchamp and Childress is the best known of these (see Box 2.2).

Professional codes offer more specific guidance about ethical issues specific to professions, as well as representing that profession's values within the community. All Australian doctors and medical students are bound by the principles set out in Australian Health Practitioner's Regulatory Agency's *Good Medical Practice*.

Autonomy

Autonomy is a particularly complex concept in psychiatry, with psychiatric illnesses having the potential to challenge autonomy. Promoting autonomous decision-making is a key principle of psychiatric care, but ethical clinical practice requires an ability to evaluate and understand when the capacity for autonomous choice is undermined by illness to the extent that some substituted decision-making is required.

Box 2.3

Decisional capacity

The patient must be able to:

- acknowledge their medical condition, and the potential consequences of the available treatment options, including not having treatment. In psychiatry, this means that the individual must understand that their symptoms are abnormal, and due to mental illness
- understand information relevant to making healthcare choices
- process this information, comparing the potential consequences of healthcare choices
- communicate their choice to their treating team.

Consent

The 1947 Nuremberg Trials, which documented atrocities perpetrated by German doctors during the Second World War, led to recognition that there was a historical lack of ethical standards guiding medical experimentation with human subjects. The Nuremberg Code was subsequently developed, with ten standards for ethical medical research. One of these standards was the 'voluntary consent of the human subject'.

Consent is essential in clinical practice, as well as in research. There are three requirements for consent to be valid: decisional capacity; freedom from coercion, or voluntariness; and disclosure of information.

Decisional capacity

To have decisional capacity, the patient or potential research participant must meet the criteria listed in Box 2.3.

Decisional capacity may be undermined by the effects of illness (such as psychosis or dementia) or pre-existing conditions (such as intellectual disability), which undermine the ability to comprehend information. When decisional capacity is undermined, substituted decision-making may be required in the form of involuntary care under the Mental Health Act or guardianship.

Freedom from coercion or voluntariness

Valid consent must occur with the patient or potential research participant free from the undue influence of others. This does not mean that the decision must be made in the absence of any influence from others. The opinions of family and friends will often be important for individuals making complex healthcare decisions. The involvement of significant others does not compromise consent unless it is coercive and contrary to the autonomous preferences of the patient or potential research participant.

Disclosure of information

Valid consent requires disclosure of information about the potential consequences of the research project or medical procedure (see Box 2.4).

Box 2.4
Young's criteria for disclosure

For a medical procedure, the disclosure must include:
- the nature of the procedure
- the risks of the procedure
- the alternatives, if any, to the procedure
- the benefits of the procedure.

The standard of information that should be disclosed has changed in response to community expectations and legal precedents:

- The Professional Practice Standard – This standard, prominent in Australia until 1985, requires the doctor to disclose information such that they 'have acted in accordance with the practice accepted as proper by a "reasonable body of medical men"'.
- The Reasonable Person Standard – This standard requires the doctor to disclose information based upon the expectations of 'a reasonable person'.
- The Subjective Standard – The case of *Rogers v. Whitaker* (see Case example 1) set a major legal precedent within Australian law, establishing a new standard of information required for disclosure by the doctor.

Case example 1

In 1983, 47-year-old Maree Lynette Whitaker, who was legally blind in her right eye, consequent to a childhood injury, consulted an eye surgeon, Mr Christopher Rogers, regarding the appearance of her eye. Mr Rogers advised Ms Whitaker that surgery on her right eye may not only improve its appearance but could also restore significant sight in that eye. On the basis of this information, Ms Whitaker proceeded with surgery.

Subsequent to the surgery, Ms Whitaker's right eye did not improve, and her left eye developed a condition called sympathetic ophthalmia. This resulted in a loss of sight in Ms Whitaker's left, previously normal, eye. Ms Whitaker subsequently sued Mr Rogers in the Supreme Court of New South Wales for damages relating to negligence. Mr Rogers was found liable in that he had failed to warn Ms Whitaker of the potential for sympathetic ophthalmia, and ordered to pay $808,564. Mr Rogers appealed to the High Court of Australia.

Evidence before the High Court was that sympathetic ophthalmia occurred with an incidence of one in approximately 14,000 similar procedures. The High Court upheld the decision on the basis that Ms Whitaker had particularly expressed concern about potential harm to her 'good' eye.

The finding was that the doctor must disclose information that an individual patient may require to make an informed consent, even if that patient does not ask specific questions seeking this information. Although the likelihood of sympathetic ophthalmia was extremely low, this had particular relevance for Ms Whitaker, given its serious consequences; and she had requested 'relevant' information.

Confidentiality

'Whatsoever I shall see or hear in the course of my profession ... if it be what should not be published abroad, I will never divulge, holding such things to be holy secrets.'

Hippocratic Oath

Patients disclose extremely private information to doctors to enable their healthcare. For patients to be willing to disclose this information, they must be confident that it will be treated as confidential. The principle of confidentiality is fundamental to all healthcare, but is particularly important in psychiatry, when information may be particularly personal and the consequences of disclosure heightened.

Despite its importance, confidentiality is not an absolute obligation, and there exist three situations in which breach of confidentiality may be appropriate or even necessary. These are shown in Box 2.5.

Case example 2

In 1969 Prosenjit Poddar was an international postgraduate student at the University of California. He was seeing psychologist Dr Lawrence Moore after becoming distressed when rejected by another student, Tatiana Tarasoff. Mr Poddar disclosed to his psychologist that he intended to kill Ms Tarasoff, and that he had a gun. Dr Moore communicated with university campus police, both verbally and in writing. Dr Moore asked that they apprehend Mr Poddar, on the basis that he (Dr Moore) was going to arrange for civil commitment under a 72-hour emergency provision of the local Mental Health Act.

Mr Poddar was released by campus police after they interviewed him and he promised not to contact Ms Tarasoff. Mr Poddar then ceased all mental healthcare. He subsequently killed Ms Tarasoff. Ms Tarasoff's parents brought a civil suit against the Regents of the University of California, the campus police, and Dr Moore, claiming damages for a 'failure to warn of a dangerous patient'. This suit was dismissed on the grounds that the professional's duty was to the patient, and not to other third parties. The Tarasoffs appealed to the Californian Supreme Court. The first ruling that resulted is known as Tarasoff I (1974). This ruling stated that the health professional was obliged to avert foreseeable danger arising from the patient's mental state by warning the threatened person. This ruling is also described as the Duty to Warn. In response to Tarasoff I, Dr Moore and several other interested parties, including the American Psychiatric Association, petitioned for a rehearing. The result was Tarasoff II (1976), which stated 'When a therapist determines, or pursuant to the standards of his profession should determine, that his patient presents a serious danger of violence to another, he incurs an obligation to use reasonable care to protect the intended victim against such danger. The discharge of this duty may require the therapist to take one or more of various steps. Thus, it may call for him to warn the intended victim, to notify the police, or to take whatever steps are reasonably necessary under the circumstances'. Tarasoff II has consequently been known as the Duty to Protect.

Box 2.5
Situations in which confidentiality may be breached

- with the express or implied consent of the patient; or
- when the doctor is required to breach confidentiality by mandatory reporting laws, or if subpoenaed; or
- when there is an overriding duty to a third party because of concerns for their safety, as exemplified by the Tarasoff Rulings (see Case example 2).

According to Tarasoff, a breach of confidentiality to protect a third party is *mandated* when a foreseeable harm may be anticipated to an identifiable third party that is serious and probable. Although Tarasoff is not binding in Australia, this legal precedent does offer important guidance for all doctors.

Conflicts of interest

A conflict of interest may be defined as:

- According to Thompson, 'A set of conditions in which professional judgement concerning a primary interest (such as patients' welfare or the validity of research) tends to be unduly influenced by a secondary interest (such as a financial gain).' or
- According to Olowski and Wateska, 'A discrepancy between the personal interests and the professional responsibilities of a person in a position of trust.'

Conflicts of interest may be classified according to:

- What is being influenced – for example, patient care or research outcomes, or
- How the influence occurs – financial or non-financial; examples of *non-financial conflicts* include the 'allegiance effect' on psychotherapy research effect size, or the political commitments of psychiatrists. *Financial conflicts of interest* include relationships with pharmaceutical companies and other healthcare industry relationships.

Relationships with pharmaceutical companies

The relationship between doctors and pharmaceutical companies has been the subject of considerable adverse community interest in recent years. Consequently, there has been increased regulation of these relationships, with restrictions on doctors in terms of the financial incentives they may receive from pharmaceutical companies. Pharmaceutical companies have consequently increasingly engaged with doctors in education. Relationships between doctors and pharmaceutical companies are of interest to the community because of the way that influence within these relationships may impact upon patient care, research findings, and the public's perception of the medical profession as trustworthy.

The Medical Board of Australia's *Good Medical Practice* states that good medical practice involves 'Recognising that pharmaceutical and other medical marketing influences doctors, and being aware of ways in which (your) practice may be being influenced'. Healthcare services that employ doctors, in addition to specialty colleges responsible for accrediting doctors, and medical organisations representing doctors, increasingly have their own guidelines regarding relationships with pharmaceutical companies.

Other conflicts of interest

There are other examples of conflicts of interest pertinent to psychiatry. For example, there are 'negative conflicts of interest': public hospitals that place restrictions upon prescribing because of cost; pressure to avoid admissions due to limited resources, and pressures to avoid expensive practices because of responsibility for budget decisions. These are often overlooked as 'practical decisions' but are truly conflicts of interest between the politically driven funding organisations (e.g. government) and patient need. Some doctors receive benefits from private hospitals with the potential for bias in admitting practices. Team-based practice makes referral to other professionals more likely to occur, even when the need is minimal and the patient's treatment could be provided just as easily by less expensive means. It is difficult for some members of the team to be left out when management is being planned. This occurs in many settings, public and private, but is not recognised as a conflict between membership of the team and the optimal provision of an expensive service.

Professional boundaries

'Whatever houses I may visit, I will come for the benefit of the sick, remaining free of all intentional injustice, of all mischief and in particular of sexual relationships with both male and female persons, be they free or slaves.'

                                                                        Hippocratic Oath

A professional boundary has been described by Gutheil as 'the edge of appropriate, professional behaviour'. The Medical Board of Australia's *Good Medical Practice* states that 'Professional boundaries are integral to a good doctor–patient relationship'; this means 'Never using your professional position to establish or pursue a sexual, exploitative or other inappropriate relationship with anybody under your care'.

The Health Practitioner Regulation National Law Act requires Australian health practitioners, including doctors, to notify the National Board if, in the course of practising their profession, they form a reasonable belief that another registered health practitioner has behaved in a way that constitutes 'notifiable conduct', as shown in Box 2.6.

Box 2.6

Australian Commonwealth Government rules regarding notifiable conduct of a doctor

The doctor has:

- practised the profession while *intoxicated* by alcohol or drugs; or
- engaged in *sexual misconduct* in connection with their profession; or
- placed the public at risk of substantial harm in their practice because they have an *impairment*; or
- placed the public at risk of harm during their practise because of a significant *departure from professional standards.*

Professional boundaries include appropriately defined limits of role, timing, place and space, money, clothing, language, self-disclosure, physical contact and gifts. According to Gutheil and Gabbard, these boundaries 'create an atmosphere of safety and predictability within which the treatment can thrive'. They are particularly important given the nature of psychiatric illnesses, and treatments.

There is now a well-described 'slippery slope' phenomenon in which boundaries are progressively transgressed with minor deviations from standard care, gradually escalating as Gabbard states 'to major violations that are damaging to the patient'. Doctors are expected to monitor and reflect upon their conduct with patients to avoid such escalations. Boundary violations are classified as sexual or non-sexual in nature. *Non-sexual boundary violations* include employment of a patient by a doctor, or engaging a patient in a business relationship. *Sexual boundary violations* include any sexual behaviour between a doctor and their patient, including verbal comments.

REFERENCES AND FURTHER READINGS

Australian Commonwealth Government, 2010. Health Practitioner Regulation National Law Act 2009 Queensland.

Beauchamp, T.L., Childress, J.F., 2001. Principles of biomedical ethics, fifth ed. Oxford University Press, New York.

Bloch, S., Green, S.A., 2009. Psychiatric ethics, fourth ed. Oxford University Press, New York.

Breen, K., Plueckhahn, V., Cordner, S., 1997. Ethics, law and medical practice. Allen and Unwin, St Leonards.

Chadda, T., Slonim, R., 1998. Boundary transgressions in the psychotherapeutic framework: who is the injured party? American Journal of Psychotherapy 52, 489–500.

Edelstein, L., 1989. The Hippocratic oath: text, translation and interpretation. In: Veatch, R.M. (Ed.), Cross Cultural Perspectives in Medical Ethics: Readings. Jones and Bartlett, Boston, pp. 6–24.

Gabbard, G.O., 1996. Lessons to be learned from the study of sexual boundary violations. American Journal of Psychotherapy 50 (3), 311–322.

Gutheil, T.G., 2005. Boundary issues and personality disorders. Journal of Psychiatric Practice 11 (2), 88–96.

Gutheil, T.G., Gabbard, G.O., 1998. Misuses and misunderstandings of boundary theory in clinical and regulatory settings. American Journal of Psychiatry 155 (3), 409–414.

Heres, S., Davis, J., Maino, K., et al., 2006. Why Olanzapine beats Risperidone, Risperidone beats Quetiapine, and Quetiapine beats Olanzapine: An exploratory analysis of head-to-head comparison studies of second-generation antipsychotics. American Journal of Psychiatry 163, 185–194.

McCormick, B., et al., 2001. Effect of restricting contact between pharmaceutical company representatives and internal medicine residents on post training attitudes and behaviours. Journal of the American Medical Association 286, 1994–1999.

Medical Board of Australia, 2009. Good Medical Practice: A Code of Conduct for Doctors in Australia, pp. 1–19.

Orlowski, J., Wateska, L., 1992. The effects of pharmaceutical firm enticements on physician prescribing patterns. There's no such thing as a free lunch. Chest 102, 270–273.

Perlis, R., et al., 2005. Industry sponsorship and financial conflict of interest in the reporting of clinical trials in psychiatry. American Journal of Psychiatry 162, 1957–1960.

Rogers v Whitaker, 1992. HCA 58, April 28, November 19 Edition. Canberra, High Court of Australia.

Singer, P. (Ed.), 1994. Ethics. Oxford University Press, Oxford.

Spingarn, R., Berlin, J., Strom, B., 1996. When Pharmaceutical manufacturers' employees present grand rounds, what do residents remember? Academic Medicine 71, 86–88.

Steinman, M.A., Shlipak, M.G., McPhee, S.J., 2001. Of principles and pens: Attitudes and practices of medicine and housestaff toward pharmaceutical industry promotions. American Journal of Medicine 110, 551–557.

Thompson, D., 1993. Understanding financial conflicts of interest. New England Journal of Medicine 329 (8), 573–576.

Young, R., 2002. Informed consent and patient autonomy. In: Kuhse, H., Singer, P. (Eds.), A companion to bioethics, third ed. Blackwell Publishing, Carlton South, pp. 441–451.

Ziegler, M., Lew, P., Singer, B., 1995. The accuracy of drug information from pharmaceutical sales representatives. Journal of the American Medical Association 273, 1296–1298.

Part 2

THE TOOLS OF PSYCHIATRY

Chapter 3

THE PSYCHIATRIC INTERVIEW AND MENTAL STATE EXAMINATION

DAVID J CASTLE & DARRYL BASSETT

The key to psychiatric assessment is a comprehensive history and mental state examination. The *history* needs to cover the history of the presenting complaint, past psychiatric history and a longitudinal perspective of the patient, with important 'milestones' and events highlighted. A family history is also important.

The *mental state* is similar to the physical examination in general medicine, and provides a comprehensive cross-sectional assessment of signs and symptoms.

Any relevant *physical examination and laboratory tests* need to be performed to cover treatable 'organic' causes and contributors to the psychiatric presentation. This is covered in Chapter 4 of this book.

Finally, one should arrive at a *formulation*, working diagnosis and differential diagnosis. The formulation essentially brings together in a succinct yet comprehensive way all the factors relevant to the patient presenting in a particular way at a particular time.

The framework presented here is largely taken from the 'Maudsley' approach, named after the famous London psychiatric hospital. For a more detailed explanation, see the 'References and further reading' at the end of this chapter. This schema is for use in adults: adaptations for children and adolescents, and the elderly are provided in Chapters 18 and

19, respectively. Special considerations for people with an intellectual disability are given in Chapter 21.

The history

Taking a thorough psychiatric history requires patience and skill. The initial phase of the interview is used to establish rapport with the patient, to put both yourself and the patient at ease, and to set the agenda for the interview. Always introduce yourself, say why you are there, the sort of areas you want to cover, and the approximate time frame. It is better to start with a general and non-threatening topic (e.g. one would not immediately ask about child sexual abuse).

A suitable opening phrase might be:

> *I am Dr Jones, and I am a registrar here at the hospital. I want to spend 30 minutes or so with you to try to understand a bit more about why you have come to hospital, and try to work out a plan as to how best we can help. Is that okay?*

Reassuring the patient that your interview is confidential, but that you work as part of a team and do share information with them, sets the parameters nicely.

It is useful to employ a combination of *open* and *closed* questions: the open questions allow the patient to bring to the conversation what they prioritise and to express things in their own way without being directed by the interviewer, while closed questions ensure that the interviewer covers all the necessary ground in a reasonable time period. Examples of open questions are: 'Tell me about what happened.'; 'How did you end up in hospital?'; 'How do you feel about that?'; closed questions include: 'Can you tell me what medications you are on?'; 'Who is living with you?' and so forth.

Reflecting back and *empathic listening* are useful techniques. For example, 'From what you have told me, it sounds like you have been under a very great deal of stress'; 'It sounds like you have been doing it really tough lately'.

The main areas covered in the history are shown in Box 3.1. Of course, there is some flexibility about the sequence of questions, but ensure you cover the major areas. Generally, starting with non-directive, open questions is recommended, later honing in on specific issues with more focused questioning. Certain issues, such as suicidality, must always be thoroughly assessed (see Chapter 17 for a suggested approach).

Identification

Present basic issues here. For example:

> *Mr Smith is a 42-year-old unmarried man on a disability pension, living by himself in a boarding house. He has a longstanding history of schizophrenia and also has a number of cardiovascular risk factors, including diabetes.*

History of presenting complaint

This is an account of the circumstances leading up to the current presentation. It should detail the relevant recent events in the person's life, the sequence of their responses to

Box 3.1

Overview of the psychiatric history

The psychiatric history should cover:

- identification
- history of presenting complaint
- a quick review of psychiatric symptoms not covered under 'presenting complaint'
- past psychiatric history, including past and current treatments
- past medical history, including past and present treatments, allergies and so forth
- family history
- personal history
- drug and alcohol history
- forensic history
- current life situation
- hobbies
- premorbid personality.

these circumstances, and the main presenting symptoms. Some detail should be provided of the major symptoms and behaviours with which the patient presents, relevant to why and how they are presenting for help at this time in this way. Details of help-seeking behaviour, including recent interventions and treatments, should be assessed.

Other psychiatric symptoms

This is an opportunity to go through a quick checklist of psychiatric symptoms and behaviours other than those elicited under 'presenting complaint'. Positives and salient negatives should be enumerated. For example, in a patient presenting with social anxiety disorder, other anxiety symptoms, the presence of panic attacks, mood state and use of drugs or alcohol are relevant. In the patient with an exacerbation of psychotic symptoms, comorbid depression is important to elicit, especially if linked to suicidality.

Past psychiatric history

Full details are needed of past psychiatric illnesses, including the first manifestation of psychiatric symptoms, first contact with a health professional for a mental health problem, and the longitudinal course of psychiatric problems, including any hospitalisations; self-harm and suicide attempts should be asked about specifically. An overview is required of treatments received (psychological, medication and electroconvulsive therapy (ECT)); engagement with and adherence to such treatments; treatment response and any adverse effects experienced. A list of current medications should be obtained.

Past medical history

An overview is required of any relevant medical conditions, injuries and times spent in hospital for medical conditions. Longstanding, expressly debilitating and painful medical conditions are especially important, given their impact on quality of life and on psychiatric symptoms. *Treatments* should be reviewed, with particular attention paid to those with psychiatric side effects, such as beta-blockers (depression) or dopaminergic agents (psychotic symptoms). Allergies, medication sensitivities and current medications should be documented.

Family history

The family history should encompass any history of psychiatric or physical health problems. This should include established or suspected diagnoses, and treatments received. It is useful to draw a genogram, which is often best done with the patient. Collateral history from another family member greatly enhances accuracy of the family history.

Personal history

The personal history is best mapped in a longitudinal manner.
- Pregnancy and birth – Was the pregnancy planned/wanted? Were there any complications during the pregnancy or the birth?
- Early milestones – Include motor, verbal and social milestones. Preschool: What sort of child were they? Did they adapt easily to change? Were they anxious and clingy? What was the family situation like? Gently broach issues of possible physical or sexual abuse.
- School – Ask about primary and secondary schooling, covering: academic endeavours (including best and worst subjects, grades achieved); sporting prowess; engagement with peers; being teased or bullied; attitudes to authority (e.g. teachers); periods of non-attendance at school; and drug or alcohol use.
- Studies/occupational – Ask about the highest level of educational attainment achieved; first paid employment; pattern of subsequent jobs; longest job held; and current job.
- Psychosexual – Ask about age of onset and attitude to puberty; sexuality; sexual abuse; first intimate relationship; subsequent pattern of relationships; first 'serious'/enduring relationship; longest relationship; marriage, pregnancies and children; and current relationship.

Drug and alcohol history

People are often averse to discussing drug and alcohol problems, and can become evasive. It is, however, critical to assess this in anyone presenting with psychiatric symptoms. A reasonably non-threatening screening instrument is the CAGE, which was initially developed for alcohol abuse, but can be adapted for other drugs. Ask:
- Have you thought about Cutting down your alcohol/drug use?
- Have you become Angry or Annoyed at others criticising your drinking/drug use?
- Have you felt Guilty about the extent of your alcohol/drug use?
- Have you found you need an Eye-opener in the mornings after heavy drinking or have you had to use a drug to settle you down?

Any two positive responses should prompt a full alcohol/drug history. This should include assessment of the longitudinal course, including first exposure, first regular usage, first problematic usage, periods of abstinence, and periods of heavy use. Treatments, successful and unsuccessful, should be recorded. A typical drinking/drug use day should be mapped, with a view to eliciting elements of the dependence syndrome, such as narrowing of the drinking repertoire, and salience (see also Chapter 22). Current use, including quantity and type of substance and route of administration (e.g. intravenous), should be recorded.

The impact of alcohol/drug use on the person's life should be explored. For example, the impact on relationships, work and studies, physical health and finances. An assessment of the person's 'stage of change' can be helpful in planning treatment (see Chapter 22).

Forensic history

Ask about the person's forensic history, but in a non-threatening way. For example, 'Have you ever been in trouble with the law?'. If the answer is in the affirmative, explore patterns of misdemeanours and consequences, especially convictions and imprisonments.

Current life situation

This covers current work and social arrangements. Include details of: housing; finances; friendship networks; and relationships with family, spouse and children.

Hobbies

Ascertain what the person does for enjoyment, and how often they manage to engage in such activities.

Premorbid personality

The assessment of personality is difficult, and cross-sectional interviews are suboptimal for this task, especially in the setting of an Axis I disorder (see Chapter 14). However, one can get a sense of the person's inner world, and their way of reacting to others and to the world around them, from the personal history elicited above. At the end of the interview it is instructive to ask: 'So, what sort of words would you use to describe the 'real you'?'. Another approach is: 'How do you think people who know you well would describe the person you really are?'. A few adjectives can provide a flavour of the person's view of themself.

The mental state examination

The mental state examination aims to provide a comprehensive cross-sectional appraisal of the patient's current mental state. Current symptoms, and salient symptoms that have been asked about but which are not present, should be reported. The structure shown in Box 3.2 is preferred.

Appearance and behaviour

The idea here is to describe the patient in sufficient detail that a colleague could pick that patient out of a waiting room full of people. Gender, apparent age and ethnicity are all

Box 3.2
Overview of the mental state examination

The mental state examination should cover:

- appearance and behaviour
- speech
- affect and mood
- thought content
- perceptions
- insight
- judgement
- cognition.

relevant. Clothing should be described, especially if it provides a clinical clue to the working diagnosis, such as flamboyant colours in hypomania, or ill-kempt, smelly clothing with numerous layers, in chronic schizophrenia. Florid, gaudy make-up can also signal a manic or hypomanic mood state.

Behaviours should be described in terms that are understandable and easily identifiable by a third party. Examples include withdrawal, apathy and avoidance of eye contact in depression or severe anxiety; tearfulness in depression; histrionic, overfamiliar and seductive behaviour in the patient with borderline personality disorder; and arousal, pacing and threatening behaviour in the patient with paranoid psychosis.

Certain specific behaviours should be commented on, as positives or salient negatives: for example, a Parkinsonian facies, tardive dyskinesia, or stereotypies and mannerisms in chronic schizophrenia; responding to external stimuli, such as hallucinations, may also be apparent.

Speech

A careful description of the form of the patient's speech gives a window into the *form* of their thoughts. This has nothing to do with content of thought, which is described separately (see below). A useful analogy is of a river flowing from the mountains (A) to the sea (B):

- *Route taken.* The route may be direct from A to B, such as in clear goal-directed speech, or meandering and taking a long and convoluted path but eventually getting to B (circumstantiality, or being circumlocutory). This is seen in anxious people, in obsessionality and in mild schizophrenic thought disorder. In more severely disordered thought form, the river runs off at a tangent (tangentiality), or unexpectedly jumps its banks and starts on a completely unconnected route (derailment or knight's move). In extreme forms, the river gets nowhere at all, meanders around disconnectedly and ends up in a series of eddies (sometimes referred to as 'word salad').
- *Amount and speed of flow.* The amount of water in the river can be miniscule (paucity of content – seen in both negative symptom schizophrenia and severe depression) and

a slow trickle (e.g. short unembellished answers to questions); or a torrent delivered at high speed (pressure of speech – classically, in mania).

* *Amount of surface variation on the river (prosody) and volume.* The water can be still and languid, with no waves (little variation in prosody – monotonous and dull, with a soft voice, as in depression); show the usual lilt of spontaneous speech; or have excessive variation and be too loud, as in mania.

Affect and mood

Affect is the external expression of internal emotion. It is assessed by observing the patient's facial expression throughout the interview. Affect occurs on a spectrum from normal reactivity through restricted affect (e.g. in depression or severe anxiety) to flat to blunted affect (almost no affective expression, as in negative symptom schizophrenia). Remember that restriction of affect can also occur in Parkinson's disease, or in the Parkinsonian syndrome seen with some antipsychotic drugs. Affect can also present as *incongruent* (e.g. smiling inanely while talking about something sad, which is usually a sign of schizophrenia or schizotypy).

Mood is assessed by both patient report and through objective observation. Assessment of *objective mood* uses features noted under 'appearance and behaviour' above. *Subjective mood* can be gauged in response to what the patient volunteers and/or responses to direct questions, such as: 'How do you feel in terms of your mood? How happy or sad are you feeling?'. Mood can be anxious, depressed, irritable or euphoric.

Thought content

This describes the predominant themes of the patient's account of themselves. It is useful to present this in the context of the whole clinical picture. For example, depressive themes are emphasised in patients with a mood disorder. Overvalued ideas and delusional beliefs, where present, provide excellent keys to the formulation, and should be presented in some detail.

Perceptions

Any abnormal perceptions are presented here. These include hallucinations in any of the sensory modalities, namely: auditory (hearing); visual (seeing); olfactory (smell); tactile (touch); gustatory (taste); and somatic (bodily sensation).

Insight

This is a multifaceted construct, encompassing insight into:

* whether the *symptoms* experienced are 'real' or part of an illness
* whether they are suffering from a *mental illness*, and
* the fact that they will benefit from *treatment*.

Interestingly, there can be an inconsistency across these parameters (e.g. a patient who absolutely denies having schizophrenia, but agrees that the voices he hears may be 'abnormal' and takes antipsychotic medication to help alleviate them). It is also important to understand the cultural background of the individual, and the attitudes towards mental illness and treatment in that culture.

Box 3.3
Brief cognitive screen

- *Orientation.* Does the patient know where they are, what day and time it is, and who the people around them are?
- *Attention and concentration.* Can the patient attend to you and your questions? Can they perform serial sevens, or count the months backwards?
- *Registration and recall.* Did they register your name when you introduced yourself, and can they recall it later; if in doubt, ask them to register and recall three objects, or a name and address.
- *Memory.* Evaluate short-term memory (e.g. can they remember what they had for breakfast? and can they tell you what has been happening in the news recently?). Also evaluate long-term memory (e.g. do they give a good account of their past; can they remember dates of events such as the Second World War?).
- *Praxis and constructional ability.* Use the established figure in the MMSE, or simply ask the patient to draw a clock face showing a specified time.
- *Rate of thought processing (verbal fluency).* Ask the patient to list as many words as possible beginning with the letter F, in 1 minute (expect at least 10 words).
- *Reasoning.* Ask something like: 'If you were visiting friends in a city you had never been in before, and you had lost their address and telephone number, how would you find them?'.

Judgement

This is generally an indication of how well the patient can make balanced appraisals of life circumstances, and act accordingly.

Cognition

It is always required that a brief cognitive screen is performed in patients presenting with psychiatric symptoms, as delirium and dementia can often be missed in their milder forms, and may help explain the rest of the mental state. The use of the full mini-mental state examination (MMSE – see 'References and further reading') has virtue in it being a well-established instrument and a useful screen for dementia, but in some ways individual item scores are more instructive than the total score; nor are all items required in all patients. It is suggested that the items shown in Box 3.3 are a useful brief screen in patients who are not suspected of having a predominant cognitive element to their illness.

A specific area to cover in patients with suspected schizophrenia is that of *concreteness of thinking*. Ask about similarities and differences (e.g. a wall and a fence) and interpretation of sayings or proverbs (e.g. 'a rolling stone gathers no moss'); a very literal response suggests concrete thinking (e.g. 'if a stone rolls down a hill it won't have any moss growing on it').

	Biological	Psychological	Social
Predisposing factors			
Precipitating factors			
Perpetuating factors			
Protective factors			

Figure 3.1 **Matrix for structured formulation**

The formulation

The formulation serves to bring all the information elicited in the history and mental state examination together in a concise, comprehensive and plausible way. It is useful to present this in terms of:

- *Predisposing factors* – e.g. is there a family history of a mental illness, child sexual abuse or a difficult relationship with a violent alcoholic father while growing up?
- *Precipitating factors* – e.g. has the person experienced death of a loved one, loss of employment, intercession of a physical illness, a traumatic event or an anniversary?
- *Perpetuating factors* – e.g. is there ongoing alcohol or drug abuse, social isolation, unemployment or financial worries?
- *Protective factors* – e.g. does the person have a stable marital relationship?

It can be helpful to follow the matrix shown in Figure 3.1 to ensure coverage of all aspects of the formulation.

The formulation ends with a working diagnosis and a list of differential diagnoses. The American Psychiatric Association's *Diagnostic and Statistical Manual of Mental Disorders* (DSM) multiaxial approach can be helpful (see Box 3.4).

Box 3.4
The DSM multiaxial structure

- *Axis I*. This axis Includes mental disorders (e.g. schizophrenia) or 'V-code' (conditions requiring attention, but not severe enough to attract a diagnostic label (e.g. marital problems)).
- *Axis II*. This includes developmental (e.g. attention-deficit hyperactivity disorder (ADHD)) and personality disorders (e.g. borderline).
- *Axis III*. This includes physical conditions (e.g. hypothyroidism).
- *Axis IV*. This includes psychosocial stressors over the previous year (e.g. death of a spouse). Severity should be rated from 1 (none) to 6 (catastrophic).
- *Axis V*. This covers functioning over the past year and is the so-called Global Assessment of Functioning (GAF) Scale, which considers psychological, social and occupational functioning on a continuum from 0 (worst) to 100 (excellent; no impairment).

REFERENCES AND FURTHER READING

American Psychiatric Association, 2000. Diagnostic and statistical manual of mental disorders, fourth ed rev. American Psychiatric Association, Washington DC.

Fish, F., 1967. Clinical psychopathology. Wrights, Bristol.

Folstein, M., Folstein, S., McHugh, P., 1975. The mini mental state: a practical method for grading of cognitive state of patients for the clinician. Journal of Psychiatric Research 12, 189–198.

Goldberg, D., Murray, R.M., 2006. Maudsley handbook of practical psychiatry, fifth ed. Oxford University Press, Oxford.

Mullen, P.E., 2008. The mental state and states of mind. In: Murray, R.M., Kendler, K.S., McGuffin, P., Wessely, S., Castle, D.J. (Eds.), Essential psychiatry, fourth ed. Cambridge University Press, Cambridge, pp. 1–38.

Sims, A., 1988. Symptoms in the mind. Balliere Tyndall, London.

CHAPTER 3

A MAN NAMED JAKE
CASE-BASED LEARNING

JOEL KING & ANDREW GLEASON

The following role-play requires two participants: one to play a general practice (GP) registrar (candidate) and the other to play a patient named Jake Kirk (actor).

OSCE Station Instructions

(Reading time: 2 minutes)

You are a GP registrar working in a country practice. Your next patient is Mr Jake Kirk, a 34-year-old man with schizophrenia. He takes olanzapine 10 mg BD. Last week he complained of a mole on his left arm that had become darker and grown larger over the preceding months. He was otherwise in good health. You asked him to come back today so that you can do a punch biopsy on the mole.

Task (10 minutes)

Obtain informed consent for the punch biopsy.

Actor role: Jake Kirk

You are 34 years old. You live with your parents, who are in their late sixties and are healthy. You get on well with them. You have no siblings. You have been on a disability pension for schizophrenia for ten years. You manage your own finances. You are otherwise well, and do not use drugs or alcohol. You have a few friends in town and you enjoy playing football or watching movies with them.

SCHIZOPHRENIA

Prior to your first psychotic episode, you were working as a mechanic at the local auto shop and had a good circle of friends. You dropped out of school at age 16 and became an apprentice mechanic. You enjoyed going to the pub for drinks and played football on the weekend in a local club. You had a few girlfriends but none that lasted more than a year.

Your first psychotic episode occurred at age 21. You experienced delusions that the government was listening to your conversations and had bugged your house because you had been chosen by God to be his special agent. You had some auditory hallucinations at the time, telling you that people were after you. Your parents managed to get you to the local hospital and you were transferred to a psychiatry ward in the larger town of Harrisville. You had four admissions there in total. The first was as an involuntary patient, and the longest lasted two months. You have not been admitted to hospital since age 27.

You are not currently under the Mental Health Act. You take your olanzapine every day because it keeps you well and out of hospital. It stops your thoughts becoming muddled and keeps the voices from coming back. You see a mental health case manager and psychiatrist at Harrisville every two months. They have no concerns about your health at present, but are unaware that you are worried about the mole.

CURRENT MENTAL STATE

You have no active psychotic features. You may appear slightly withdrawn, but you are otherwise cooperative, polite and articulate. You have no psychomotor abnormalities.

TIMELINE OF THE MOLE

You first noticed a mole on your left arm four months ago, while in the shower. Since then, you think that it has been growing bigger. You think it might have become darker, but you're not too sure. It has never been painful and you have noticed no other symptoms. You wondered whether it might be cancer and went to the GP. You are hoping that the GP will do a test and tell you that it is not cancer.

INSIGHT INTO SURGERY

When you saw the doctor last time, they explained the punch biopsy procedure to you. You have also done some research on the internet. You have excellent insight into what your mole might be and the procedure proposed. The doctor should ask about your understanding of the reason for the biopsy and should ask you to explain the procedure.

In simple terms, you should explain that the doctor will draw around the mole and disinfect the area first with a solution, before injecting the skin with a local anaesthetic so you don't feel any pain. You should explain that the doctor will use a small device that will cut a hole into the skin and remove the mole and some of the surrounding tissue. The doctor will then suture the wound. You will come back to the clinic in a week for the suture removal. You will be left with a very small scar. The biopsy will be sent to a pathologist who will examine it and tell the GP whether it is cancer or not.

The doctor should ask about the risks of the procedure. You should describe that the risks are minimal, but include bleeding and infection. Occasionally, inadequate amounts of tissue are obtained, requiring further biopsies.

You are aware that the mole may be cancerous or may be some other disease and not having the biopsy might lead to the disease progressing unchecked. You are quite worried that if it is cancer, it may spread if not removed promptly. The doctor should ask you whether you have any questions. You may ask anything you want.

Model Answer

This station focuses on assessment of the capacity to make informed consent in a patient with a mental illness.

The first part of this task is to assess the patient's current mental state (see pages 40–43), particularly for active psychotic symptoms that may impact on his ability to give informed consent. An example of a symptom that might impact this ability is a delusion that if the mole was removed he would definitely die. On the other hand, mental illness does not by default equate to lack of capacity to consent. Informed consent is specific and contemporary to a particular decision. Consequently, a patient who is actively hallucinating could potentially retain the capacity to consent, provided their symptoms were not impacting on their decision-making ability.

When seeking psychotic symptoms it can be helpful to gain a sense of the patient's current functioning by opening with questions about demographic details. The candidate could then use the station introduction, or other information volunteered by the patient, as a springboard into assessing their understanding of their illness. One could ask, 'I see that you're taking a medication called olanzapine. What do you take that for?'. A patient who says, 'I take it for schizophrenia' would have a higher degree of insight into their illness than a patient who takes it because their doctor tells them to but does not understand what it is for.

Obtaining a picture of the patient's conceptualisation of their condition allows the candidate to use the patient's own words to assess for the presence of psychotic symptoms, such as auditory hallucinations, particularly of a command nature, passivity phenomena, thought disorder, and delusions. If these are elicited, the candidate should determine if they affect the patient's understanding of the nature of their illness and the proposed treatment (see Chapter 7, pages 93–95).

In this case, Mr. Kirk does not currently have positive symptoms. He has not been admitted for seven years, is being treated in a voluntary capacity, and is compliant with his medication. These facts suggest that Mr. Kirk's schizophrenia is unlikely to impact on his capacity to make informed consent.

The next part of the task is to ask about the procedure. Patients should be able to demonstrate an understanding of the nature of the proposed treatment, the likely outcome, the benefits and risks, the consequences of not undertaking the proposed treatment, and other treatment alternatives (see Appelbaum 2007). Mr. Kirk can demonstrate all of this adequately and thus can make informed consent to this procedure at this time.

If there are doubts about the capacity to make informed consent in a patient with a mental illness, one should seek guidance from a psychiatrist.

REFERENCE

Appelbaum, P.S., 2007. Assessment of patients' competence to consent to treatment. New England Journal of Medicine 357, 1834–1840.

Chapter 4

PHYSICAL EXAMINATION AND SPECIAL TESTS

DARRYL BASSETT & DAVID J CASTLE

This chapter provides a brief overview of the physical examination in psychiatry, as well as pointing to special investigations that might be pertinent in the psychiatric setting. Of course, the extent of special investigations depends upon the clinical presentation and findings on physical examination, but as a general guide the investigations listed in Box 4.1 are recommended in most cases.

Why a physical examination?

Many psychological disorders are provoked, amplified or complicated by general physical illness. In addition, some patients present with psychological symptoms due entirely to general physical illness (see Chapter 6). It is appropriate to ensure that a comprehensive history and physical examination is included in the management of most patients presenting with psychological disorders. Exceptions to this include patients whose medical history is already well known or who choose to decline such examination (the potential consequences must be explained to the patient and documented). Nevertheless, a physical examination should be a routine element when assessing any patient that presents with psychological symptoms or signs. Sometimes the examination will need to be postponed until the patient is capable of informed consent. Capacity for consent may be impaired

Box 4.1

Summary of common investigations for first presentation of psychological disorders

- Full blood count
- Electrolytes
- Liver function tests
- Renal function tests
- Fasting vitamin B12 and red cell folate levels
- Thyroid function tests
- Serum calcium and phosphate
- CT scan of head
- Urine screen for substances.

by factors such as psychosis associated with fear of contact; or a history of sexual abuse may provoke anxiety about an examination.

Who performs the examination?

A physical examination is a vital component of any psychiatric examination, whoever performs it. While psychiatrists should remain competent in physical examination skills, some patients may prefer that someone other than a psychiatrist has physical contact with them and this requires sensitive negotiation.

Context of examination

A thorough mental state examination (see Chapter 3) will help focus the physical examination, but a brief review of all systems is essential. A good motto is 'when in doubt, think organic'. Review all physical findings, as some general medical disorders may present with psychological symptoms (see Chapter 6).

The physical examination

The physical examination should follow the usual clinical principles, but certain elements are particularly important in the psychiatric context.

Observation

- Facial expression (e.g. tearfulness, injected conjunctivae from substance abuse, dystonia and dyskinesia with medications, fixed gaze or grimacing in schizophrenia, mask-like expression, suggesting Parkinson's disease or parkinsonism).
- Posture (e.g. bizarre posturing in schizophrenia), unusual movements (e.g. tremor, dystonia, dyskinesia, choreoathetosis, stereotypy).

- Bruising, needle marks, mutilation (e.g. lacerations, scratching, burns), unusual hair loss (e.g. trichotillomania, hypothyroidism), altered appearance of skin (e.g. jaundice, pallor, pigmentation suggestive of Addison's disease) or nails (altered shape from nutritional deficiency or metabolic disorder).
- Truncal obesity with striae (possible Cushing's syndrome) or severe weight loss with lanugo hair (possible anorexia nervosa).
- Gait (ataxia, bradykinesia, peculiar gait suggestive of conversion disorder).
- Facies: consider dysmorphic facial features (e.g. Down's syndrome, Fragile-X syndrome, velo-cardio-facial syndrome).

Palpation

- Altered tone (e.g. medication effects).
- Enlarged thyroid gland (e.g. hypothyroidism).
- Enlarged and/or tender liver (e.g. alcohol abuse).
- Pulse examination (e.g. anxiety disorders).

Mensuration

Blood pressure measurement (e.g. medication effects).

Waist circumference

- Males = > 94 cm moderate risk, > 102 cm high risk
- Females = > 80 cm moderate risk, > 88 cm high risk
of cardiovascular disease and/or diabetes mellitus (type 2).

Body weight and height measurement

For calculation of the body mass index or BMI:
  weight in kilograms divided by height in metres squared
  > 25 = overweight
  > 30 = obese

Other neurological features

- Pupillary changes (e.g. Argyll Robertson pupils, signs of raised intracranial pressure).
- Fundal examination (e.g. papilloedema, hypertensive or diabetic changes).
- Oculomotor functions (useful screen of the 'horizontal' axis of the brain).
- Visual fields to confrontation (raising suspicion of intracranial pathology).
- Primitive reflexes (raising suspicion of frontal lobe pathology).

Blood and urine tests

(The focus is upon those of particular psychiatric importance.)

Baseline measures are invaluable with all relevant investigations, and the frequency of certain tests thereafter will vary with clinical variables, such as medication use, substance abuse and the progression of illness.

Complete blood examination

This is essential as a general screening test. White cell counts are particularly important with medications such as clozapine, where agranulocytosis may occur. Platelet counts are relevant, particularly with medications such as sodium valproate and carbamazepine. Note that macrocytosis can be associated with alcohol abuse.

Electrolytes

This includes serum sodium, potassium, chloride and bicarbonate estimations. Note that lithium levels are altered by fluctuations in sodium levels, and several medications (e.g. SSRIs and SNRIs) can provoke hyponatraemia, particularly in the elderly. Hypokalaemia promotes delayed cardiac conduction and therefore the QT interval. This is very significant when using medications that have similar effects. Low magnesium levels may affect mental state.

Renal function

This includes serum urea, creatinine and calculated GFR estimations. It should be noted that several medications (e.g. lithium, amisulpride) are predominantly or significantly excreted through the kidneys and renal dysfunction can significantly alter their blood levels. Lithium can rarely cause kidney damage and, very rarely, renal failure.

Liver function

Includes serum bilirubin, ALP, GGT, ALT, AST, total protein, albumin and globulin estimations. Most psychotropic medications are metabolised in the liver and liver dysfunction can significantly alter the blood levels of these medications. Alcohol and several psychotropic medications can cause liver damage (e.g. chlorpromazine, sodium valproate, etc.) and monitoring can be invaluable. Intravenous substance use may provoke significant liver dysfunction through infection with viruses.

Endocrine functions

- *Thyroid function tests* (includes serum TSH, T4 and T3) are particularly important in a variety of psychological disorders (e.g. anxiety disorders, depressive disorders, cognitive disorders, etc.). Thyroid monitoring is particularly important in the use of lithium, which can cause thyroid damage: annual monitoring is usually sufficient unless clinical factors suggest a higher risk.
- *Fasting blood glucose* (after 3 months and then 6-monthly unless a particularly high-risk patient) is particularly important with some antipsychotic medications (e.g. clozapine, olanzapine, quetiapine, risperidone) and sometimes with other medications associated with weight gain (e.g. lithium, mirtazapine). Concurrent monitoring of waist circumference and body weight (with BMI) at each visit is helpful.

- *Calcium* (adjusted for albumin levels) and phosphate levels may be important in depressive disorders or as a consequence of treatment with lithium.
- *Prolactin levels* are relevant for medications that promote increased release of prolactin, such as amisulpride, risperidone and paliperidone. This is usually indicated by the development of gynaecomastia and/or lactation (outside pregnancy), but should be considered if breast cancer is diagnosed. Hyperprolactinaemia can promote osteoporosis, menstrual irregularity and loss of libido.
- *Oestrogen and gonadotrophin levels* may be relevant if a perimenopausal state is clinically significant (e.g. depressive disorders).
- *Testosterone levels* (best measured as an 'androgen ratio') may be useful in males with mid-life depressive symptoms and prominent amotivation. However, gonadotrophin, luteinising hormone and testosterone levels tend to fall during depressive disorders and recover with treatment. Supplementary testosterone is rarely required to effectively treat depressive disorders. They may also be relevant in females with persistent loss of libido.
- *Other endocrine tests* are usually reserved for less common clinical situations (e.g. 24-hour urinary cortisol for adrenocortical disorders, noradrenaline and serotonin levels in adrenomedullary disorders).

Lipids

Fasting cholesterol and triglyceride levels are very important when prescribing several antipsychotic medications (e.g. clozapine, olanzapine, quetiapine, risperidone). Monitoring after 3 months of commencement of the agent, and thereafter every 6 to 12 months (depending on levels and risk profile) is recommended.

Medication blood levels

Lithium

The low therapeutic index of lithium makes close monitoring of blood levels very important. Blood should be taken between 10 and 12 hours after ingestion of lithium, close to the expected end of the 'distribution phase', to allow meaningful comparison with other patients. Persistent monitoring should be performed every 3 months and at times of suspected toxicity (note: toxicity can occur even when the blood level is within the accepted range).

Levels of other medications, such as antidepressants, anticonvulsants and antipsychotic medications, can be appropriate in certain clinical situations.

Blood should be sampled at the expected 'trough' level of the medication.

Serology

Hepatitis B and hepatitis C are relevant if there is a history of risk behaviours such as intravenous substance use.

Human Acquired Immunodeficiency Virus (HIV): HIV/AIDS is seen in excess in a number of psychiatric disorders, and infection has a myriad of psychological presentations. It is ethically appropriate to ask the patient's permission for these tests and to be attentive to appropriate counselling.

Syphilis serology may be performed, as the illness can imitate a number of psychiatric and neuropsychiatric disorders.

Vitamin assays

These are performed mostly in depressive disorders, delirium, and dementias, and in the setting of chronic substance use and/or malnutrition. They include assays of vitamin B12, red cell folate, thiamine and vitamin D.

Urine drug screens

Screening for substance use is particularly useful for patients with a history of substance abuse, those with psychosis and those in whom substance use might contribute to complications in treatment. Dilution of urine, for example, by drinking copious amounts of water or directly adding water, may lead to false negative results. The urine creatinine level is measured and reported to allow recognition of this. Optimally, the urine sampling should be supervised.

Initial urine screening is usually performed using radioimmunoassay techniques. High pressure chromatography with mass spectrometry, is used to establish the precise nature of a substance detected by initial screening.

Electroencephalography (EEG)

EEG examinations are particularly useful in psychiatric disorders as a screening examination for 'organic' brain disorders, such as encephalopathies, epilepsy and a range of other neurological disorders. Indications include clinical presentations suggestive of epilepsy or other neurological disorders that might be evident on EEG (e.g. encephalopathies, unusual psychotic symptoms or signs, recent significant changes in behaviour or personality).

Neuroimaging

Computed Tomography (CT)

This is a very useful investigation to exclude major brain pathology and the indications are similar to those for an EEG . When there is some suspicion of possible intracranial pathology prior to ECT, a CT scan prior to treatment is essential.

Magnetic Resonance Imaging (MRI)

This is useful to exclude major neurological pathology which might be suspected. Subtle signs such as sub-cortical hyperintensities can be relevant in mood disorders. While CT scanning is more readily available, MRI scans provide much more information for assessment of brain disease.

Single Photon Emission Computerised Tomography (SPECT)

SPECT is an imaging technique that uses a single photon source injected into the bloodstream to provide scans indicating metabolic activity (and hence blood flow) throughout the brain. It is predominantly a research tool in psychiatry but can be useful to detect relevant cerebrovascular disease, early degenerative diseases (e.g. dementias in younger patients) or sometimes to offer possible options in psychopathology. While false negative findings are common in clinical practice, the presence of significant alterations in function (see Chapters 7, 8, 9, 10 and 11) can help support the presence of major mood disorders, schizophrenia and major anxiety disorders.

Positron Emission tomography (PET)

PET is an imaging technique similar to SPECT that uses dual photon sources (at 180° to each other) and provides a higher level of resolution than SPECT. This remains only a research tool in psychiatry but may have clinical applications in the future.

REFERENCES AND FURTHER READING

Hurley, R., Taber, K. (Eds.), 2008. Windows to the brain. American Psychiatric Publishing, Washington DC.
Levenson, J., Lyketsos, C., Trzepacz, P. (Eds.), 2002. Psychiatry in the medically ill. The Psychiatric Clinics of North America, 25(1) B. Saunders, Philadelphia.
Sadock, B., Sadock, V. (Eds.), 2009. Kaplan and Sadock's concise textbook of clinical psychiatry. Lippincott Williams and Wilkins, Philadelphia.

CHAPTER 4

JAKE RETURNS
CASE-BASED LEARNING

ANDREW GLEASON & JOEL KING

The following role-play requires two participants: one to play a
general practice registrar (candidate) and the other to play the role
of a patient named Jake Kirk (actor).

OSCE Station Instructions

(Reading time: 2 minutes)

You are a GP registrar working in a country practice. Your next patient is Mr Jake
Kirk, a 34-year-old man with schizophrenia, for which he takes olanzapine 10 mg
BD. You last saw Mr Kirk four months ago for a mole on his left arm. You performed
a punch biopsy, which came back benign. This relieved Mr Kirk greatly.

He has come to your clinic for his annual physical examination. This morning, you
spoke to his psychiatrist, who stated that Mr Kirk has no positive psychotic
symptoms at this time.

Task (10 minutes)

Perform a physical examination on Mr Kirk.

Actor role: Jake Kirk

Please refer to the role description in Chapter 3.

You are happy that this doctor is interested in your physical health. You are a bit withdrawn and don't say much, but are agreeable to any reasonable examination suggested by the doctor.

Model Answer

The life expectancy of people with schizophrenia is about twenty years less than that of the general population. The majority of this increase in mortality is due to the same conditions that cause death in the general population, and is in part explained by disparities in healthcare provision. Patients with pronounced negative symptoms are also less likely to seek care for physical symptoms compared to the general population. Physical symptoms are often falsely attributed to mental illness by clinicians. Good general medical screening, including regular physical examination, is an essential part of care for people with schizophrenia.

A physical examination on a patient with a chronic psychotic illness should include the same components as a screening physical examination in other populations, with an increased focus on identifying modifiable risk factors, such as obesity and hypertension. Additionally, the physical examination may provide evidence of adverse effects of treatment or an organic cause for psychiatric symptoms, and in doing so will direct ongoing investigations and treatment.

The physical examination should follow a good history and system review. These, of course, guide the physical examination. In this example, we focus on Mr Kirk's general health and potential side effects of treatment. A student would not be expected to look for all of the signs listed here in a ten minute examination. These are included to stimulate reflection on the myriad, and often subtle, stigmata of organic causes of psychosis and comorbid conditions that can occur in people with schizophrenia. As a minimum, a medical student doing this station should perform a good multi-system screening examination (including neurological, cardiovascular, respiratory, gastrointestinal, and endocrine systems), mention that they are looking for organic causes of psychotic symptoms (listing a few examples of signs of relevant conditions), and examine for signs of antipsychotic side effects, such as the metabolic syndrome and tardive dyskinesia. A good bedside manner is, of course, essential!

INTRODUCTION

Consider the need for a chaperone. Obtain consent from Mr Kirk and explain what you are going to do. Wash your hands.

Observation

Be sure to ask Mr Kirk to undress appropriately. The authors have seen several cases of major life-threatening conditions being missed in patients with schizophrenia because of failure to have the patient undress.

Note Mr Kirk's general cleanliness, which will help provide information about his self-care ability. Obesity may be a side effect of treatment or a consequence of a sedentary lifestyle. Cachexia may indicate a malignancy. Comorbid malignancies may go undetected in patients with schizophrenia, and can also rarely cause psychotic symptoms via paraneoplastic effects on the central nervous system. Look for stigmata of a neurodevelopmental condition associated with schizophrenia such as velo-cardio-facial syndrome (22q11.2 deletion syndrome). Other signs of systemic illness, such as jaundice or pallor, may be present.

Observe for motor restlessness, which might indicate akathisia. Abnormal movements, such as choreoathetosis, dyskinesia, tremor or myoclonus, may represent drug side effects or an underlying organic cause of psychosis, such as Huntington's disease.

Vital signs and BMI

Some psychotropics can cause hypertension, and others cause orthostatic hypotension. Autonomic instability occurs in neuroleptic malignant syndrome (NMS). Other signs of NMS include pyrexia, rigidity, and altered sensorium (see Chapter 15, pages 238–239). Tachycardia can occur in myocarditis – a rare complication of clozapine therapy.

It is essential to measure weight, height, and waist circumference, and to calculate body mass index in people on antipsychotics as they are at increased risk of the metabolic syndrome.

Hands

Mr Kirk's hands may show signs of systemic disease, such as muscle wasting (which could indicate malignancy or malnutrition), koilonychia (due to iron deficiency), leukonychia (from hepatic disease), or clubbing. There may be evidence of substance use, such as tobacco stains and Dupuytren's contractures. The arms may show signs of systemic disease, self-harm, or drug use, such as bruising, scratch marks or track marks.

Head

It is important to examine the dentition of people with chronic psychotic conditions, as poor dental hygiene is common, and Mr Kirk may need a referral to a dentist. There may be evidence of malnutrition, such as glossitis. Some antipsychotics can cause sialorrhoea. Mouth ulcers may reflect myelosuppression, a rare side effect of some antipsychotics.

Neck

The JVP may be raised in myocarditis, in which case other signs of heart failure might be seen. Tracheal deviation or lymphadenopathy could suggest a malignancy. The thyroid should be examined. Schizophrenia is associated with an increased risk of Graves' disease (and also of other autoimmune conditions such as psoriasis and pernicious anaemia). Thyroid disease can also cause psychotic symptoms.

Chest

Gynaecomastia and galactorrhoea can occur as a side effect of antipsychotics or from endocrine disease. Mr Kirk should have a comprehensive cardiovascular and respiratory examination. People with schizophrenia frequently smoke, putting them at risk of chronic obstructive pulmonary disease, ischaemic heart disease, and malignancy.

Abdomen

Mr Kirk should also have a thorough abdominal examination. Antipsychotics can cause liver dysfunction and constipation. Hepatitis and substance misuse are not uncommon in people with schizophrenia.

Legs

Pay special attention to Mr Kirk's feet. Negative symptoms of schizophrenia can contribute to poor foot care requiring podiatry. Examine for signs of peripheral vascular disease (such as weak peripheral pulses) or diabetes (such as a peripheral neuropathy).

Neurological

A thorough neurological examination is essential.

Spontaneous facial or mouth and lip movements, such as the bon-bon sign, occur in tardive dyskinesia, which is associated with long-term exposure to typical antipsychotics. Signs of parkinsonism, such as rigidity, which can be a side effect of antipsychotics, should be sought. Cataracts can be caused by some older antipsychotics.

There may be evidence for an underlying organic aetiology. An Argyll Robertson pupil would suggest syphilis. Niemann-Pick disease type C is a rare metabolic disorder that can present with schizophrenia-like symptoms and is associated with impairment of vertical saccadic eye movements. Cortical release signs, such as the grasp, palmomental, rooting, snout, and pout reflexes, can occur in some psychiatric and neurological conditions. An abnormal gait may indicate an organic cause, substance misuse, or a comorbid neurological condition.

Remember to examine the site where Mr Kirk had the punch biopsy performed, looking for signs of recurrence.

Thank Mr Kirk for his cooperation. Wash your hands.

Investigations

Consider investigations, such as an ECG (for prolonged QTc, which may occur with some antipsychotics), fasting blood glucose (to screen for diabetes mellitus) and fasting lipids. Additionally, patients prescribed antipsychotics should also have other investigations depending on clinical need, such as a regular full blood count, urea and electrolytes, liver function tests, thyroid function tests, and also serum prolactin if there are symptoms suggestive of hyperprolactinaemia.

Part 3

THE SYNDROMES OF PSYCHIATRY

Chapter 5

CLASSIFICATION

DAVID J CASTLE & DARRYL BASSETT

The classification of psychiatric disorders has been subject to substantial changes over the decades. The two most well-accepted and widely used current systems are the World Health Organization's *International Classification of Diseases*, 10th edn (ICD–10), and the American Psychiatric Association's *Diagnostic and Statistical Manual of Mental Disorders*, 4th edn, revised (DSM–IV–TR). These two classification systems differ in a number of important ways (see Table 5.1), but in terms of the psychiatric disorders they describe, there is rather more congruence than dissonance. It should be noted that a new (5th) edition of the DSM is due for publication in 2013. There will be a number of changes from DSM–IV–TR, but these have not been finalised at the time of writing. Where relevant, mention is made throughout this book to those changes that are most likely to be promulgated.

One feature of both the ICD and DSM systems is that they provide operational criteria that rule diagnosis (ICD–10 applies operational criteria only in its research version). *Operational criteria* essentially provide a checklist of symptoms and signs, a proportion of which need to be endorsed for the subject to be considered a 'case'; there are also usually some exclusionary items, such as a clear organic cause for the signs and symptoms. There is a downside to this approach as to some extent it eschews clinical intuition and judgement, possibly lulling one into a false sense of security regarding whether they describe valid entities. Indeed, none of the disorders in the nosologies are necessarily 'true' or *valid* entities, and the boundaries of many are permeable. Also, there is a danger of labelling of

Table 5.1

Differences between DSM–IV–TR and ICD–10

DSM–IV–TR	ICD–10
US-based, published by the American Psychiatric Association, but has wide acceptance around the world	Published by the World Health Organization; international perspective, and encompasses a diversity of opinion, including from a developing country perspective
Not part of a general medical classification system	Part of a general medical classification system
One version only	Clinical and research versions
Atheoretical	Groupings ('blocks') on the basis of presumed shared aetiologies
Multiaxial, with personality disorders on a separate axis (Axis II)	Personality disorders and intellectual disability (mental retardation) not on a separate axis
Global functioning assessed using Global Assessment of Functioning (GAF) Scale	*Disability* assessed using the Disability Assessment Schedule (WHO-DAS)

individuals according to their diagnosis, with all the associated downsides. Arguably, the psychiatric formulation is a much more satisfactory approach to understanding the individual and why they are presenting with certain symptoms at a specific time (see Chapter 3).

However, operational criteria are, in the main, fairly *reliable*, at least in terms of inter-rater reliability. There is also the major advantage that they ease communication between mental health professionals (and others), such that one can at least be assured different people mean much the same thing when they apply a diagnostic label.

The approach taken in this book is a pragmatic one, with both ICD–10 and DSM–IV–TR criteria being outlined for each of the major disorders. The grouping of disorders, as described here, is largely congruent with both ICD–10 and DSM–IV–TR, but also reflects the influential 'hierarchical' model espoused by Graham Foulds.

The pragmatic classification system

Figure 5.1 provides a schematic representation of the major psychiatric disorders in adults. A number of general issues should be noted:

- There is an implied hierarchy, such that one 'drills down' from top to bottom of the pyramid, eliciting pertinent signs and symptoms in turn. Of course, this is not always compatible with clinical interviewing practice, and more often than not clinicians will hone in on the major presenting symptom set first and then turn to the others. Also, simply making a diagnosis of, for example, schizophrenia should not stop enquiry about mood and anxiety and other symptoms: indeed, such comorbidities are common in psychiatry. There is a danger, for example, in making a diagnosis of schizophrenia and then interpreting social withdrawal behaviour as a manifestation of negative

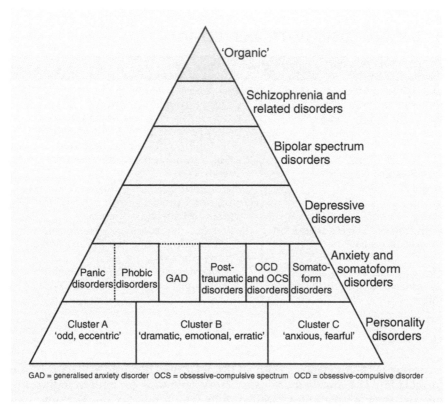

Figure 5.1 Overview of psychiatric disorders (adult)

symptoms of that illness, when it might actually be due to social anxiety disorder, with very different treatment implications.

- 'Organic' disorders are at the top of the pyramid. This reinforces the importance of always asking oneself whether a set of presenting symptoms could potentially be either caused by, precipitated by, or perpetuated by, an organic condition (see Chapters 4 and 6). Again, this is crucial as organic disorders require specific treatments, and can be dangerous if not adequately dealt with.

- The lines between sets of disorders are presented as solid, and this implies a level of delineation that is far from reality. Indeed, many of the boundaries are very fuzzy indeed, and patients often present with symptoms of two adjoining sets. For example, schizoaffective disorder is a rather loose quasi-category spanning schizophrenia and bipolar disorder (and perhaps unipolar depression), while many of the anxiety disorders have substantial depressive comorbidity.

- The sizes of each section of the pyramid can roughly be seen to represent the population prevalence of each disorder. Thus, schizophrenia and related disorders afflict some 0.5–1.0% of the population; bipolar spectrum disorders 2.0–4.0%; depressive disorders 10–15%; and anxiety and somatoform disorders over 20%.

- The 'base' of the pyramid represents personality disorders. This is more compatible with the ICD–10 conceptualisation than DSM–IV–TR, as the latter places personality disorders on a separate axis (Axis II). However, the point is made that personality predispositions and vulnerabilities both flavour and underpin many Axis I disorders, and arguably a personality disorder diagnosis should not be made without exclusion of active Axis I pathology (see Chapter 14).

It should also be noted that this schematic applies to adult psychopathology, and child and adolescent psychiatry adopts a somewhat different approach (see Chapter 18). Finally, the schematic does not explicitly include the addictive disorders (see Chapter 22), though they can be subsumed under the 'organic' rubric.

Organic disorders

In clinical practice, it is vital to examine each patient physically, and to perform laboratory tests where indicated (see Chapter 4).

One can consider organic factors as:

- *causal*. The factor is sufficient to cause the psychiatric symptoms (e.g. a temporal lobe tumour presenting as a post-ictal psychosis).
- *precipitating*. For example, cannabis can precipitate a panic attack in vulnerable individuals, in part at least because of its propensity to induce tachycardia.
- *perpetuating*. For example, thyrotoxicosis can contribute to ongoing anxiety symptoms.

The organic disorders can themselves be classified, as shown in Box 5.1. See Chapter 6 for more details.

Schizophrenia and related disorders

Schizophrenia itself is at the core of this group. As discussed in Chapter 7, it is a disorder characterised by sets of symptoms in three main domains – namely, positive (delusions and hallucinations), negative (apathy, withdrawal, restriction of affect) and disorganisation (disorganised thoughts and actions; inappropriate affect). Cognitive impairment is also often part of the illness. DSM–IV–TR requires a 6-month duration of symptoms (2 weeks of which should be 'positive' symptoms), while ICD–10 has an overall 1-month duration requirement.

For disorders characterised by features of schizophrenia (see Box 5.2), but of briefer duration, various terms are applied, including *schizophreniform psychosis* (DSM–IV–TR), *brief reactive psychosis* (Scandinavia) and *bouffée delirante* (France).

Box 5.1
Broad classification of organic factors

Organic disorders can be classified as:

- *exogenous* (e.g. imbibed amphetamines producing a manic syndrome), and
- *endogenous*, either inside the central nervous system (e.g. temporal lobe tumour presenting with psychotic symptoms) or outside the central nervous system (somatic) (e.g. myxoedema presenting with psychosis).

Box 5.2

Schizophrenia and related disorders

The disorders are:

- schizophrenia
- schizophreniform psychosis
- delusional disorder
- schizoaffective disorder (on the border between schizophrenia and the affective disorders).

Box 5.3

Bipolar spectrum disorders

Disorders include:

- bipolar I: mania +/- depression
- bipolar II: hypomania +/- depression
- bipolar III: mania/hypomania in setting of antidepressant exposure
- cyclothymia: mood swings (up and down) not severe enough to meet the criteria for bipolar disorder.

Delusional disorders are characterised by psychotic symptoms, which are to some extent 'understandable' and not bizarre (e.g. of marital infidelity; or of illness – monosymptomatic hypochondriacal delusions, or delusional disorder, somatic subtype).

On the border between schizophrenia and the affective disorders lies *schizoaffective disorder*, with an admixture of features of both sets of disorders. In DSM–IV–TR, by definition, the features need to occur separate from each other, but other conceptualisations are less stringent and in clinical practice a schizoaffective label is often applied when patients have an admixture of mood and psychotic symptoms that do not lend themselves readily to either a schizophrenia or mood disorder label. This includes mood disorders with 'mood incongruent' delusions (i.e. the delusions are not explicable in terms of the current mood state).

Bipolar spectrum disorders

Bipolar disorder was originally delineated along with unipolar mania, as distinct from unipolar depression. Nowadays, unipolar mania has been subsumed under the bipolar label. Thus, bipolar disorder, as detailed in Chapter 9, is characterised by episodes of mania (bipolar I) or hypomania (bipolar II). Mania is a more severe form of hypomania, by definition requiring psychiatric treatment. More often than not, sufferers also experience depressive episodes, which often are severe and prolonged, and carry significant morbidity and mortality (see Box 5.3).

There is some debate about the nosological status of patients who manifest manic or hypomanic symptoms only on exposure to antidepressant drugs or ECT. They have been

Box 5.4
Depressive disorders

Disorders include:

- *major depressive disorder*: at least 2 weeks of pervasive depressed mood and/or loss of pleasure
- *dysthymia*: chronic low mood most days for at least 2 years, and
- *depression 'not otherwise specified'*: for example:
  - premenstrual dysphoric disorder (PMDD): recurrent low mood in late luteal phase of the menstrual cycle
  - minor depressive disorder: symptoms > 2 weeks, but milder than major depression
  - recurrent brief depressive disorder: recurrent symptoms of less than 2 weeks duration and not menstrual-related
  - depression in the setting of a medical illness or substance use, where primacy is not clear
  - depression in the context of another active psychiatric illness, such as schizophrenia, or in the post-psychotic period.

labelled bipolar III by some authors. Presumably, such individuals carry a bipolar predisposition, but only manifest the illness with a suitable stimulus.

Cyclothymia used to be considered a personality disorder, but sufferers appear to respond to mood stabilising drugs; hence, it has been moved from Axis II to Axis I in DSM–IV–TR.

Depressive disorders

No entirely satisfactory classification of the depressive disorders has yet been arrived at (see Box 5.4). For so-called *major depressive disorder* (MDD), DSM–IV–TR stipulates a 2-week illness duration with features that must include pervasive low mood and/or loss of interest/pleasure. *Dysthymia* is a term reserved for those patients who have a chronic low-grade depression present on more days than not, for at least 2 years. Superimposed major depressive episodes in people with dysthymia is sometimes referred to as *double depression*.

It is likely that PMDD will be given 'full' rather that residual status, in DSM-5. Various descriptors of a major depressive episode are allowed – namely mild, moderate or severe. Also, melancholic features and the presence of 'mood congruent' psychotic symptoms should be stipulated; 'mood incongruent' symptoms suggest a diagnosis of schizoaffective disorder, or schizophrenia with a mood disorder.

Anxiety and somatoform disorders

The anxiety and somatoform disorders are divided here in a pragmatic manner, with a view to treatment implications (see Box 5.5). Further details can be found in Chapters 10, 11, 12 and 13.

Box 5.5

Anxiety and somatoform disorders

Disorders include:

- panic disorder
- phobic disorders:
  - agoraphobia
  - social anxiety disorder
  - specific phobias
  - blood-injury phobia
- generalised anxiety disorder
- post-traumatic syndromes:
  - acute stress disorder
  - post-traumatic stress disorder
- obsessive-compulsive spectrum disorders:
  - obsessive-compulsive disorder
  - bodily preoccupation (e.g. body dysmorphic disorder, anorexia nervosa)
  - neurological (e.g. Tourette's syndrome)
  - impulse control (habit) disorders (e.g. trichotillomania), and
- somatoform disorders:
  - somatoform pain disorder
  - somatisation disorder
  - hypochondriasis.

Panic disorder is characterised by repeated panic attacks, at least half of which occur 'out of the blue'. Once panics are linked to specific situations (e.g. crowds in agoraphobia, social situations in social phobia) or things (e.g. spiders or snakes in specific phobias, see also Chapter 10, page 150), and there is consequent avoidance of those situations or things to a degree to which functioning is impaired, they can be considered *phobic disorders*. DSM–IV–TR links panic with agoraphobia in particular, but panics can occur in any of the phobic disorders.

Generalised anxiety disorder is something of a residual category with very high comorbidity with depression: some authorities believe it should be subsumed under the depressive disorders.

Post-traumatic syndromes in DSM–IV–TR include an acute stress disorder (less than 1 month), and a more enduring (greater than 1 month) post-traumatic stress disorder. Symptoms are similar in each (see Box 5.6), but dissociation is given particular prominence in acute stress disorder. ICD–10 does not formally distinguish acute from more prolonged stress reactions.

The nature of the stressor in the post-traumatic syndromes has been subject to debate: currently, DSM–IV–TR stipulates the stressor should be such that it is a perceived threat to the life or physical integrity of the individual, their family, or those around them.

The obsessive-compulsive spectrum disorders are discussed in some detail in Chapter 11. Suffice to say here that there is a current vogue for grouping together a number of

Box 5.6

Symptoms of post-traumatic stress disorder (PTSD)

Symptoms include:

- reliving experiences (e.g. dreams and nightmares)
- hyperarousal, including an exaggerated startle response
- avoidance behaviours (of situations or things that serve as reminders of the traumatic event) and emotional numbing.

Box 5.7

Pragmatic grouping of personality disorders, as in DSM–IV–TR

The clusters are:

- cluster A ('odd, eccentric'): paranoid, schizoid and schizotypal personality disorders
- cluster B ('dramatic, emotional, erratic'): borderline, histrionic, narcissistic and antisocial personality disorders
- cluster C ('anxious, fearful'): avoidant, dependant and obsessive-compulsive personality disorders.

disorders into a so-called obsessive-compulsive spectrum (OCS), on the basis of shared symptomatology and treatment response. In fact, the veracity of the putative spectrum has been challenged, but for ease of discussion we can consider three main groupings, as shown in Box 5.7. *Obsessive-compulsive disorder* (OCD) itself sits at the centre of this grouping. It is characterised by intrusive thoughts (obsessions) and associated compulsive acts aimed at reducing the anxiety associated with the thoughts. As outlined in Chapter 11, OCD is arguably itself a heterogeneous group of conditions, rather than an entity; certainly, hoarding does not sit easily under this label.

Somatoform disorders are a highly contentious and unsatisfactory grouping of disorders that ostensibly have somatisation at their core. They are discussed further in Chapter 13. DSM–IV–TR includes body dysmorphic disorder (BDD) here, but this approach has little to support it, and we have placed it in the OCD spectrum. It is likely that BDD will be removed from the somatoform disorders in DSM-5.

Personality disorders

The definition and classification of the personality disorders is particularly problematic. One reason for this is that the presence of another psychiatric disorder (an Axis I disorder in DSM–IV–TR) can flavour the way the patient presents and lead to erroneous judge-ments being made about their personality. Also, personality disorders have often been seen as 'untreatable' (this is not in fact the case: see Chapters 14 and 16) and the label often carries pejorative and unhelpful connotations. Furthermore, there is little empirical support for any of the proposed subtypologies, and much overlap between putative sub-types, such that patients more often that not fulfil criteria for a number of personality disorders at the same time. Finally, a number of personality disorders appear to be *formes frustes* of Axis I disorders: schizotypal personality disorder and schizophrenia being obvious examples (see Chapter 7).

DSM–IV–TR has taken a pragmatic approach to the problem. The establishment of a separate axis for personality disorders has its detractors, but has served to focus research attention on this group of maladies. A clustering of the personality disorders, as shown in Box 5.7, has little research validity, but can be of clinical utility.

The personality disorder category is likely to change substantially in DSM-5, with the introduction of dimensional constructs to supplement the categories.

REFERENCES AND FURTHER READING

American Psychiatric Association, 2000. Diagnostic and statistical manual of mental disorders, fourth ed rev. American Psychiatric Association, Washington DC.

Berrios, G.E., 1999. Classifications in psychiatry: a conceptual history. Australian and New Zealand Journal of Psychiatry 33, 145–160.

Castle, D.J., Jablensky, A.V., 2012. Diagnosis and classification in psychiatry. In: Wright, P., Stern, J., Phelan, M. (Eds.), Core psychiatry, third ed. Saunders, London, pp. 511–520.

Cloninger, C.R., 1999. A new conceptual paradigm from genetics and psychobiology for the science of mental health. Australian and New Zealand Journal of Psychiatry 33, 174–186.

Foulds, G.A., 1976. Hierarchical nature of personal illness. Academic Press, London.

Kendell, R., Jablensky, A., 2003. Distinguishing between validity and utility of psychiatric diagnoses. American Journal of Psychiatry 160, 4–12.

Robins, L., Guze, S.B., 1970. Establishment of diagnostic validity in psychiatric illness: its application to schizophrenia. American Journal of Psychiatry 126, 983–987.

World Health Organization, 1992. The ICD-10 classification of mental and behavioural disorders: clinical descriptions and diagnostic guidelines. World Health Organization, Geneva.

Chapter 6

ORGANIC PSYCHIATRY

DARRYL BASSETT & DAVID J CASTLE

General medical conditions are associated with psychological disorders in several ways. This chapter is not meant to be comprehensive, but rather to bring attention to important links between psychological function and other body functions. The presence of psychological illness does not exclude the presence of general medical illness and *vice versa*, even if the diagnosis explains all of the symptoms.

The presence of relevant general medical disorders ('organic disorders') must be considered with any presentation of psychological illness, particularly when it is severe or resistant to treatment. The interaction between general medical disorders and psychological disorders is complex and requires careful consideration. This chapter considers a variety of general medical or organic disorders that can cause significant psychological illness. Box 6.1 presents some of the more common associations between psychological symptoms and general medical disorders.

Psychiatric disorders secondary to medical disorders

Delirium

Delirium is a syndrome characterised by concurrent disturbances of consciousness and attention, perception, thinking, memory, psychomotor behaviour, emotion and the sleep-wake cycle. Typical symptoms are shown in Box 6.2.

There are multiple causes (see Box 6.3) and differential diagnoses include dementia, depressive disorders and schizophrenia. Delirium is particularly common in the elderly

Box 6.1

Common psychological disorders and potential contributing general medical disorders

Depressive disorders

- High or low thyroid hormones, high or low adrenal cortical hormones (endogenous and exogenous), high or low calcium levels, vitamin deficiencies.
- Acquired brain injuries (including post-concussional syndrome), cerebrovascular diseases, or a variety of infections, neoplasia, demyelinating diseases, autoimmune diseases, various toxins.
- Delirium may be followed by depression.
- Dementias are commonly associated with depression.

Anxiety disorders

Cardiovascular diseases (e.g. supraventricular tachycardia), delirium, dementias, acquired brain injuries, high or low thyroid hormones, high or low calcium levels, high adrenal medullary hormones, a variety of infections, neoplasia, demyelinating diseases, autoimmune diseases, various toxins.

Schizophreniform psychosis

Delirium, dementias, acquired brain injuries, cerebrovascular diseases, a variety of infections (notably viral), demyelinating diseases, autoimmune diseases, severe hypothyroidism, low calcium levels, exogenous corticosteroids.

Box 6.2

Typical symptoms of delirium

- Diffuse cognitive deficits (including attention, orientation, memory, visuoconstruction and executive functions)
- An acute onset
- Psychotic symptoms (including perceptual abnormalities, delusions and thought disorder)
- Sleep/wakefulness disturbances including possible sleep cycle reversal
- Alterations in psychomotor behaviour
- Impairment of language
- Abnormal affect (labile, irritable, apathetic and/or incongruous)
- Arousal may be increased (most commonly) or reduced.

where urinary tract and respiratory infections are particularly common causes, although many other forms of pathology may be responsible.

Management ultimately requires identification and appropriate treatment of the underlying cause. Management of immediate symptoms and reducing distress for the individual encompasses adequate lighting (to minimise misinterpretation of visual

Box 6.3

Common causes of delirium

- Toxins:
  - Prescribed medications, e.g. anticholinergic medications, corticosteroids
  - Drugs of abuse, e.g. alcohol intoxication and withdrawal, opiates, stimulants
  - Poisons, e.g. solvents, petroleum, carbon monoxide, pesticides.
- Metabolic disorders:
  - Electrolyte disturbances
  - Hypothermia and hyperthermia
  - Respiratory failure
  - Cardiac failure
  - Liver failure
  - Renal failure
  - Vitamin deficiencies such as B12, thiamine, folic acid, niacin
  - Dehydration and/or malnutrition
  - Anaemia.
- Infections:
  - Systemic infections
  - CNS infections.
- Endocrine disorders:
  - Hyperthyroidism or hypothyroidism
  - Hyperparathyroidism
  - Adrenal insufficiency.
- Cerebrovascular disorders:
  - Reduced cerebral blood flow
  - Hypertensive encephalopathy
  - Focal haemorrhage or ischaemia (notably parietal lobes and thalamus).
- Autoimmune disorders:
  - CNS vasculitis of various kinds
  - Systemic lupus erythematosus.
- Seizure related disorders:
  - Non-convulsive status epilepticus
  - Prolonged post-ictal states.
- Neoplastic disorders:
  - Diffuse cerebral metastases
  - Carcinomatous meningitis
  - Gliomatosis cerebri (diffuse cerebral neoplastic spread).

information), minimal noise, a calm, positive and reassuring approach, and a secure environment to maintain safety of self and others. Antipsychotic medications (see Box 6.4) can be helpful for the heightened arousal, anxiety and florid psychotic symptoms, but the response to treatment is often disappointing until the basic cause has been relieved.

Box 6.4

Medications for the management of delirium

- Haloperidol can be helpful for the agitation or aggression which may accompany delirium, depending upon circumstances. Usually 1 to 2 mg given intramuscularly or intravenously will be sufficient, and may be repeated half-hourly if needed. If oral administration is satisfactory, doses of 2 to 5 mg are appropriate. The total dose required may reach 20 mg per day in some individuals. Monitor for extrapyramidal side effects.

- Risperidone 0.5 to 2 mg orally (particularly in rapid dispersal form) is very useful and preferable to haloperidol because of greater tolerance.

- Olanzapine and quetiapine can also be used.

- Benzodiazepines such as lorazepam can be used as adjunctive treatment to antipsychotic medication, because of their tranquillising effect. However, care should be exercised to use minimal doses, as there is an increased risk of confusion and falls. Parenteral midazolam (see Chapter 15) may be necessary at times of crisis. Benzodiazepines (notably diazepam) are particularly useful in alcohol and other substance withdrawal states, partly because of their anticonvulsant and tranquillising effects. They are also useful in the management of anticholinergic delirium. Paradoxical aggravation of delirium and aggression can occur (particularly with diazepam) and care should be exercised in their use. Respiratory suppression is another potential risk, particularly with parenteral midazolam.

Dementia

Dementia (see Chapter 19) is a syndrome secondary to brain disease, which is progressive in nature and accompanied by a disorder of multiple higher cortical functions, including memory, thinking, orientation, comprehension, calculation, learning capacity, language and judgement. It is usually accompanied by deterioration in emotional regulation, social behaviour and/or motivation. It may occur at any age but is most common in later life. Some forms are reversible, but many are not: common reversible and irreversible types of dementia are shown in Box 6.5.

Huntington's disease

Huntington's is an inherited progressive neurodegenerative psychiatric disease. Degeneration of striatum occurs with progression of the disease and more widespread cerebral degeneration follows. Inheritance is via an autosomal dominant gene; hence, 50% of offspring will be at risk of developing this disease. The gene is on chromosome 4, with an unstable CAG trinucleotide repeat sequence of increased length. Relevant nucleotide sequences can be identified, allowing early determination of risk.

Clinical features

Onset of the clinical syndrome can occur in adolescence but is most commonly observed in the fifth decade. Cognitive dysfunction occurs early in the progression of the disease and may include impairment of memory (declarative and non-declarative), impairment

Box 6.5
Selected causes of dementia

Reversible causes of dementia

- Hypothyroidism
- Vitamin deficiencies (see below)
- Normal/low pressure hydrocephalus
- Autoimmune vasculitis
- Infection (see below); notably HIV/AIDS (limited), neurosyphilis
- Intracranial haemorrhage/sub-dural haematoma
- Neoplasia
- Diabetes mellitus; poorly controlled
- Anaemia; chronic, untreated
- Delirium; apathetic presentation.

Currently irreversible causes of dementia

- Alzheimer's disease
- Vascular dementia
- Mixed Alzheimer's disease and cerebrovascular disease
- Parkinson's disease/Lewy body disease dementias
- Huntington's disease (see above)
- Alcohol-related dementia
- Dementia secondary to multiple sclerosis and other demyelinating diseases
- Other dementias (other degenerative neurological disorders).

of executive cognitive functions (e.g. verbal fluency, planning, sequential activities) and visuospatial skills. Abnormal movements are characteristic of the disease and include chorea and choreoathetosis, as well as impaired oculomotor functions, coordination of movement, dysphagia and dysarthria. Rigidity, bradykinesia, myoclonus/epilepsy, bruxism and dystonia may also arise. Apathy, irritability/aggression, dysphoria, generalised anxiety and obsessive compulsive disorder arise commonly. Major mood disorders (major depressive disorder or bipolar disorder) and schizophreniform psychosis are seen in many patients with Huntington's disease. The risk of suicide is very high once the diagnosis has been made.

Management

Supportive psychotherapy is essential when the diagnosis is established. Family support is often required. Huntington's disease cannot be retarded in progress by any current means, but the chorea can often be reduced using tetrabenazine (25 mg twice daily, increasing to a maximum of 200 mg daily; side effects can include sedation, depression, insomnia, dysphagia, Parkinsonism), or antipsychotic medications (see Chapter 15).

Box 6.6

Post-concussional syndrome

- Somatic symptoms:
  - Headache, dizziness, fatigue, insomnia.
- Cognitive symptoms:
  - Memory impairment, impaired concentration.
- Perceptual symptoms:
  - Tinnitus, hyperacusia, photophobia.
- Emotional symptoms:
  - Depression, anxiety, irritability.

Psychosis is treated using antipsychotic medications (see Chapter 15). Myoclonus and epilepsy can be helped with anticonvulsants, and botulinum toxin has been employed for bruxism and dystonia. Depression and anxiety disorders require antidepressants.

Acquired brain injury

Post-concussional syndrome and mild traumatic brain injury (TBI)

Mild TBI is defined as a closed head injury which is associated with brief loss of consciousness (<20 minutes) or none, and anterograde amnesia of less than 24 hours. This may be accompanied by a 'post-concussional syndrome' (see Box 6.6).

Symptoms of post-concussional syndrome and mild TBI usually resolve themselves within 6 months, but occasionally they become more persistent. The pathophysiology appears to be related to chemical changes in some neurones in response to injury, which then leads to mostly reversible axonal degeneration. More severe rotational injury can lead to profound cognitive and other impairment. Psychological vulnerability (as described for anxiety, mood and personality disorders), current psychosocial stresses (including specific psychological disorders, problems with employment, legal matters and relationships) and lack of supports, contribute significantly. Psychological trauma surrounding the physical trauma (including acute stress disorder, post-traumatic stress disorder or major loss such as bereavement) also contribute to the severity and persistence of post-concussional syndrome. The prognosis is therefore variable and the contributing factors multi-factorial.

Post-traumatic amnesia

Memory loss following trauma includes retrograde amnesia (loss of recall before the injury) and anterograde amnesia (loss of recall after the injury). *Retrograde amnesia* is heavily determined by psychological as well as organic factors, and tends to 'shrink' to some extent with recovery from the injury. *Anterograde amnesia* is more sensitive to the severity of the trauma and more indicative of the likely prognosis.

Psychosis

Psychotic illness may develop following trauma and can take the form of a schizophreniform psychosis, a bipolar affective disorder or a delusional disorder with paranoid features.

Box 6.7
Frontal lobe syndrome

- Impaired volition with lack of spontaneity and motivation.
- Psychomotor disorder with retardation and/or restlessness.
- Alteration in mood/affect with fatuousness, euphoria and/or irritability.
- Reduced awareness and concern for social appropriateness in behaviour, including reduced concern for the consequences of behaviour; disinhibited behaviour, including sexual promiscuity, inappropriateness (e.g. propositioning a stranger) or perversity (e.g. child sexual abuse); rude or boorish behaviour.
- Impaired judgement in a variety of life decisions (e.g. financial).

Frontal lobe syndrome and personality disorder

Injury to the frontal lobe carries many effects, but the 'frontal lobe syndrome' refers to a cluster of symptoms and signs associated particularly with damage to the supra-orbital prefrontal cortex (see Box 6.7).

Cognitive impairment

A range of cognitive impairments can result from acquired brain injury. These include, *inter alia*, problems with:

- executive function: impaired judgement; difficulty with multiple cognitive tasking, abstract thinking, changing case, verbal fluency, rapid changes in motor tasks, etc.
- memory: declarative and non-declarative; short and long term.
- visuospatial functions, calculations, right/left discrimination, etc.
- language: grammar, syntax, semantics, etc.

Psychological reactions, such as grief, loss of confidence, altered sense of identity, and anxiety about performance in tasks can occur in the setting of brain injury. Some people become behaviourally disturbed and aggressive after brain injury. Management is as outlined in Chapter 17.

The introduction of *legal matters* into the experience and management of organic psychiatric disorders complicates and distorts the perceptions, responses and treatment that accompany these disorders. Complete fabrication of symptoms is rare and symptoms are *not* 'cured by verdict', except in exceptional cases of fraud. Financial settlement of a claim is psychologically rewarding because it offers 'validation' of the person's injury, financial benefit (usually at a time of financial loss) and a perception of 'closure' of the injury experience which promotes rehabilitation.

Chronic traumatic encephalopathy is a syndrome that follows long-term repetitive head injury, often without loss of consciousness or obvious acute brain trauma. This syndrome has been observed in athletes whose sports include repetitive head trauma, such as boxing, football of various codes, hockey and wrestling. Clinically the syndrome presents with a variety of forms of amnesia, behavioural and personality changes (including apathy, irritability, and impulsiveness), Parkinsonism, speech difficulties and abnormal gait. The pathology includes atrophy of the cerebral hemispheres, medial temporal lobe, thalamus,

Table 6.1

Sites of cerebrovascular disease

Psychological disorder	Site of lesion (any pathology)
Depressive disorders	Frontal lobe and basal ganglia, particularly after cerebrovascular accidents and particularly left-sided lesions Lesions in the parietal and occipital lobes, particularly left-sided, can also be associated with depression, but less often and less severely
Mania	Right frontal and temporal lobe lesions; particularly orbitofrontal and basal temporal regions
Bipolar affective disorder	Basal ganglia and thalamic lesions; particularly right-sided
Anxiety disorders	Cortical lesions; particularly left-sided and left dorsolateral frontal lobe
Delusions and hallucinations	Temporo-parietal-occipital region; particularly right-sided
Apathy	Posterior internal capsule

mammillary bodies and brain stem, with ventricular dilatation. Tau protein deposition, neurofibrillary tangles, β-amyloid deposition and inflammatory changes are observed microscopically. Depressive disorders are a common complication, the risk of suicide significant, and paranoid psychosis may develop.

Cerebrovascular disease

Cerebrovascular disease in particular brain regions can provoke psychological illness, but in clinical practice the presentations are often less distinct (see Table 6.1). Cerebrovascular accidents (strokes) are sometimes followed by depressive episodes which may be persistent. Treatment with antidepressant medications is usually effective, but SSRIs can enhance the risk of stroke in the elderly because their serotonergic effect reduces platelet adhesiveness. Mania or delusional disorders may follow stroke, but are less common than depressive disorders. Atherosclerosis of arterioles, or other diseases of vascular endothelium in the brain (small vessel disease most commonly), increase the risk of depressive disorders. Diffuse gliosis secondary to multiple vascular injuries in the brain (secondary to haemorrhage or thromboembolism) may contribute to dementia.

Infectious diseases

Human Acquired Immunodeficiency Syndrome: This virus often causes severe damage to neurological structures with cognitive deficits (including possible dementia), motor dysfunctions (including paralysis, hypertonia, tremor, abnormal movements), a variety of affective disorders (including anxiety disorders, depression, mania), or psychosis. Opportunistic infections, cerebrovascular disease and neoplasia are significant complications.

Box 6.8

Wernicke-Korsakoff syndrome

- *Wernicke's encephalopathy*: syndrome of confusion, ataxia, nystagmus, and diplopia from ophthalmoplegia; pathology develops from thiamine (vitamin B1) deficiency and includes damage to anterior/medial thalamus, mammillary bodies, cerebellar vermis, periaqueductal grey and dorsal nucleus of vagus; *may be reversed by prompt thiamine 100 mg IV.*

- Thiamine should be given before carbohydrates if thiamine deficiency is suspected or Wernicke's encephalopathy may be precipitated.

- Prolonged Wernicke's encephalopathy can result in Korsakoff's syndrome, through permanent damage to the regions above (particularly mammillary bodies) the basal forebrain and dorsal raphe nuclei.

- *Korsakoff's syndrome*: irreversible syndrome of severe anterograde amnesia (immediate memory is usually spared), apathy, poor insight and confabulation (creation of answers to questions from imagination, with conviction of their truth). Cognitive functions may be more broadly affected.

- Other forms of brain injury can produce Korsakoff's syndrome, including carbon monoxide poisoning, heavy metal poisoning and acquired brain injury.

Neurosyphilis is relatively rare in most developed countries, but used to be the 'great mimicker' of numerous neurological and neuropsychiatric disorders. Other infective causes of neuropsychiatric symptoms include cytomegalovirus, herpes simplex (cerebral), Lyme disease, toxoplasmosis, malaria (cerebral) and tuberculosis.

Neoplasia

Raised intracranial pressure can present with unusual symptoms, including atypical behaviour and unexplained headache. Sometimes the tumour itself can produce neuropsychiatric symptoms, akin to those for cerebrovascular lesions (see Table 6.1).

Paraneoplastic syndromes encompass a variety of disorders and can develop distant from the primary neoplasm and not be related to metastases (e.g. via hormone secretion). Manifestations include memory impairment, delirium, dementia, anxiety, depression and a variety of neurological syndromes.

Demyelinating diseases

Multiple sclerosis and other demyelinating diseases may present with multiple neurological deficits, including cognitive impairment of various kinds, disorders of affect (anxiety, depression, mania, incongruity of affect, blunting of affect) or psychosis in various forms.

Autoimmune diseases

Systemic lupus erythematosus and several other autoimmune diseases may present with a wide variety of clinical syndromes, similar to those seen with demyelinating diseases.

Epilepsy

The core clinical feature of epilepsy is the stereotypic and repetitive nature of its symptoms and signs, which cascade along a regular sequence. Distinguishing some forms of epilepsy from psychological disorders can be difficult, particularly when both are present. Seizures can be divided into those that are limited to one region (partial or focal seizures) or involve the entire brain. Partial seizures may (complex partial seizures) or may not (simple seizures) be associated with loss of conscious awareness, while generalised seizures are always associated with loss of consciousness. Sometimes partial seizures are followed by a generalised seizure, when the electrical excitation spreads more extensively. Partial and complex partial seizures may be associated with psychological symptoms or signs, but these are most prominent with complex partial seizures.

In the case of complex partial seizures, there is usually an aura which may include:

- experiences of *déja vu* (perception that current events have been experienced previously)
- *jamais vu* (perception that the current experience of repetition of a previous event appears unfamiliar)
- intense anxiety
- euphoria
- depersonalisation
- visceral symptoms, such as rising epigastric sensations
- altered perception of actual objects (e.g. appearing unusually small or large)
- hallucinations potentially of any modality (visual, auditory, gustatory, olfactory, tactile).

Complex partial seizures may arise from any lobe of the brain, but most commonly they arise from the mesial temporal lobe (particularly the amygdalae, hippocampi and neocortical regions). Often these are associated with mesial temporal sclerosis. Once there is loss of consciousness, stereotyped complex movements may arise, known as automatisms (e.g. lip smacking, swallowing or other repetitive movements). The patient is amnesic regarding those automatisms.

Toxic disorders

Intoxication with heavy metals, carbon monoxide, insecticides, and other substances can present with a variable range of psychological symptoms (e.g. mood disorders, cognitive impairment, personality changes) with neurological symptoms and signs.

Endocrine and metabolic disorders

Thyroid disease

Hypothyroidism can present with depression, anxiety, cognitive impairment, psychomotor retardation and (rarely) psychosis. *Hyperthyroidism* can present as anxiety, depression, cognitive impairment and (rarely) psychosis including mania.

Adrenal cortical disease

Cushing's syndrome is commonly associated with depression, but can also be accompanied by anxiety, cognitive impairment and psychosis. Addison's disease can be associated with cognitive impairment, and rarely with depression, anxiety and psychosis, including delirium.

Exogenous corticosteroids

These may cause or precipitate mania, depression, irritability and psychosis including delirium.

Adrenal medullary disease

Rare tumours secreting adrenaline and noradrenaline can present with severe and unpredictable episodes of anxiety accompanied by tachycardia and often other physical symptoms.

Parathyroid disease

Anxiety may be prominent in hypocalcaemia; both hypocalcaemia and hypercalcaemia can be accompanied by depression as well as cognitive impairment. Severe hypocalcaemia can promote schizophreniform psychosis.

Diabetes mellitus

This carries a significant risk of cognitive impairment and depressive disorders, while hypoglycaemia and hyperglycaemia can be accompanied by mood disorders, unusual behaviours and cognitive impairment.

Vitamin deficiencies

Thiamine deficiency can precipitate Wernicke/Korsakoff's encephalopathy (see Box 6.8).

All B group vitamin deficiencies can be associated with depressive symptoms, encephalopathy and dementia, except perhaps for riboflavin.

Speech and language disorders

Speech and language disorders are complex phenomena and can be simplified as disorders of *reception* (hearing/comprehension of auditory information), *processing* (to and from the auditory cortex) and *expression* (speech, components of language and non-verbal behaviours related to communication). Psychological disorders are strongly connected with all aspects of speech and language, and these links are discussed in other chapters. However, general medical disorders which affect the functioning of speech and language areas of the brain need to be identified and the interaction with psychological processes understood. The details of these are well beyond the scope of this book, but a few basic elements are important.

- The prime language areas of the brain include Broca's area (frontal operculum) and Wernicke's area (posterior region of superior temporal gyrus), which are linked together by the arcuate fasciculus, and with other relevant brain regions.
- Disease in Broca's area causes disruption of the production of speech and is associated with abnormal verbal fluency (words are produced but are poorly linked together). Language comprehension may also be impaired.

- Disease in Wernicke's area causes disruption of the comprehension of language, but language expression may also be impaired.
- The assessment of disordered language requires the differentiation of disordered speech production (dysarthria), disordered aspects of language (aphasia) and disordered thought form or content (see Chapter 3).
- Most patients with dysarthria or aphasia are aware (good insight) of their difficulties and will indicate this clearly. It will also be evident that they are trying to correct their disability.
- The majority of patients with disordered thought content (e.g. delusions) or thought form (for example, thought disintegration in schizophrenia), do not recognise their disorder as abnormal (poor insight) and do not try to correct their errors. In addition, such thought disorder is often in the form of highly disjointed themes rather than inappropriate use of words.

Sleep disorders

The process of sleep serves a 'homeostatic' function, which includes maintenance of brain health through neuronal repair and neurogenesis, the processing of memories, the production of hormones from the pituitary gland and elsewhere, relaxation and repair of skeletal muscle, and the relaxation of stress upon numerous other body parts. Sleep mechanisms include changes in brain arousal and the distribution of that arousal, with the progression through five recognised 'stages' of brain activity (see Box 6.9).

The other aspect of the sleep process is the rhythm it follows, which is largely connected to the day/night cycle and known as the '*circadian rhythm*'. It is vitally important in the physiological coordination of a myriad of processes, including hormone secretion from the pituitary gland (see Box 6.10).

Box 6.9
Stages of sleep

- Stage I   Barely asleep and very easily woken. Some slow waves and occasional 'spikes' on EEG.
- Stage II   Clearly asleep and slow to waken. Slow waves are evident on EEG but of low amplitude, and are punctuated by large spike complexes ('sleep spindles and K complexes').
- Stage III   Deeply asleep and very slow to waken. Prominent slow waves of large amplitude.
- Stage IV   Very deeply asleep and difficult to waken. Slow waves are even more prominent. Neuronal repair, dendritic growth and synaptogenesis, as well as neurogenesis are prominent. Hormone and transmitter synthesis is significant.
- REM   Rapid Eye Movement sleep in which arousal is high. Dreaming occurs. Eyes move rapidly and laterally under eyelids. Includes periods of skeletal muscle paralysis. Memory processing is prominent. Very easily woken.

Box 6.10
Sleep disorders

- *Sleep apnoea*: Disruption of respiration during sleep. Predominantly due to upper airways obstruction. Adverse effects include brain injury from hypoxia (notably cognitive impairment), heart failure and hypertension. Daytime somnolence and depression can also result. *Management* is by reduction in abdominal girth, mandibular splint or positive airways pressure (C PAP device). Central sleep apnoea of neurological origin occurs rarely.

- *Circadian rhythm disruption*: Disturbance of regular sleep rhythm associated with disconnection from day/night cycle, 24-hour period (strictly around 25 hours), and hence multiple physiological processes (e.g. hormone regulation). Contributes to mood disorders, cognitive functions and numerous general medical disorders (e.g. myocardial infarction).

- *Periodic limb movement disorder*: Related to 'restless legs syndrome' and consists of involuntary movement when asleep. Disrupts sleep homeostasis.

- *Chronic pain*: Persistent pain is highly disruptive to sleep homeostasis.

- *Nocturnal epilepsy*: Seizures disrupt sleep homeostasis.

- *Parasomnias*: Disturbing dreams, violent or sexual activity while dreaming, sleep walking (somnambulism) and night terrors (violent distressing dreams; also called 'pavor nocturnus'). All can disrupt sleep quality through disruption of sleep homeostasis and poor sleep quality, as well as adverse effects on others.

- *Traumatic brain injury*: Adversely affects circadian rhythms and sleep homeostasis.

- *Metabolic disorders*: Adversely affects circadian rhythms and sleep homeostasis.

- *Infection*: Adversely affects circadian rhythms and sleep homeostasis.

- *Delirium*: Adversely affects circadian rhythms and sleep homeostasis.

- *Dementia*: Adversely affects circadian rhythms and sleep homeostasis.

Psychological responses to general medical conditions

Living with illness is often highly disruptive and challenging for both the patient and significant others. Understanding and providing assistance with these challenges is invaluable.

These challenges can include:
- grief over loss of health (see Chapter 8)
- guilt if the illness is considered linked to behaviour or lifestyle (e.g. smoking, obesity, substance abuse etc)
- anger (interwoven with grief)
  - the perceived 'unfairness' of being ill, particularly when young
  - blame of others for illness, e.g. work injury
  - failure by health professionals to diagnose early
  - failure to respond to treatment.

- denial of the illness and its implications; often an 'unconscious' process
- 'demoralisation': a combination of:
  - apprehension
  - perceived helplessness
  - perceived hopelessness
  - perceived incompetence and reduced self-esteem
  - perceived isolation and loss of meaning in life.
- Poor adherence to treatment regimens – for many reasons:
  - distractions of everyday life
  - grief
  - guilt
  - anger
  - nuisance of treatment
  - disagreement about the nature of the illness
  - disagreement about the nature of the treatment
  - unwanted effects of treatment ('side effects')
  - stigma of illness and/or treatment.
- Precipitation of psychological illness, including depressive disorders and anxiety disorders through the stress of the medical illness and its meaning to the patient.

Psychological disorders and interaction with general medical conditions

Distortion of diagnosis

Psychological disorders such as depressive disorders, anxiety disorders, schizophrenia, eating disorders and dementia can interfere with a person's capacity to recognise physical symptoms or their significance.

Cardiovascular disorders

Depressive disorders, schizophrenia and prolonged anxiety disorders increase the risk of, and impair recovery from, myocardial infarction and a variety of other cardiac disorders. Panic attacks may also aggravate cardiac dysrhythmias. Personality factors and emotional arousal contribute to hypertension.

Gastrointestinal disorders

Psychological distress from a variety of disorders aggravates a variety of GI tract disorders, including irritable bowel syndrome, inflammatory bowel disorders (e.g. ulcerative colitis) and gastro-oesophageal reflux.

Immune function

Mood disorders (depressive disorders and bipolar disorders) promote significant variations in immune function, extending over a range of elements, including cell mediated immunity, a variety of cytokine levels and variations in acute phase proteins. The full implications and characteristics of these changes are still being investigated, but the implications are partly suggested by the increased rate of neoplasia in mood disorders and possible increases in vulnerability to certain infections. *Infections* are also often followed or accompanied by depressive episodes, suggesting a significant association in both directions. Similar observations have been made with schizophrenia and, again, the implications and details are as yet poorly understood.

Endocrine/metabolic functions

Anxiety and depression can provoke significant changes in blood sugar levels and regulation of sex hormone production. Melancholic depression is associated with reduced hypothalamic response to circulating levels of cortisol, thyroxine/liothyronine and growth hormone. *Anxiety* can reduce release of antidiuretic hormone. Many other endocrine functions are also altered by mental state to a lesser extent. *Bipolar disorders* may be associated with a higher incidence of hypothyroidism, and schizophrenia is associated with a higher incidence of diabetes mellitus and hyperlipidaemia than occurs in the general population.

Chronic pain

The experience of chronic pain is frequently accompanied by depressive disorders. This would appear largely related to the psychological implications of persistent distressing symptoms, but may also be related to the pathophysiology of chronic pain and its involvement of glutamate, amine and other pathways. The experience of chronic pain is also modified by alteration in serotonergic and noradrenergic pathways by antidepressant medications (e.g. amitriptyline and duloxetine). The *management* of chronic pain is greatly enhanced by psychological strategies that alter awareness of pain and alteration in the psychological responses to the pain experience (e.g. thought content and meaning). Structured physical, interpersonal and cognitive activity with an emphasis upon pleasure is also very helpful.

Sleep and sleep disorders

Insomnia is commonly due to a psychological disorder of some form (particularly anxiety disorders and depressive disorders), and psychological distress commonly follows persistent insomnia. Specific sleep disorders, such as periodic limb movement disorder and sleep apnoea, are further aggravated by anxiety and depression. They are also commonly associated with daytime fatigue and impaired cognitive function (often of only mild severity). Parasomnias (disturbing dreams, somnambulism, violent or inappropriate sexual behaviour while asleep) can be due to general medical disorders (such as epilepsy, substance use, hypoxia or infections) or to severe psychological illness (such as post-traumatic stress disorder). Management of any sleep disorder requires attention to the patient's mental state.

Respiratory disorders

Anxiety disorders, particularly generalised anxiety and panic attacks, are common among patients with respiratory disorders. Being unable to breathe normally is extremely anxiety provoking, and persistent or severe anxiety aggravates dyspnoea and can further impede respiratory function.

Case examples: Organic psychiatry

- A 46-year-old woman presented with significant mood swings which lasted several weeks and were interspersed with periods of apparently normal mood and function lasting a week or more. She and her husband reported periods of elevated mood with increased spending, pressured speech, rapid shifting of thought content over multiple topics and a reduced need for sleep. While she regarded these times as entertaining and her husband enjoyed her increased libido, playfulness and more stimulating conversation, they both found the episodes exhausting and increasingly irritating. The periods of elation were interspersed with periods of depressed mood and tearfulness, accompanied by social and personal withdrawal. These times were unpleasant for everyone and very distressing. She had been diagnosed with multiple sclerosis about 5 years earlier and suffered fluctuating sensory changes over her body, intermittent reduction of power in her limbs, which seemed unpredictable, and lapses in memory, which were frustrating. Her behaviour seemed a little disinhibited at times, being overfamiliar with strangers and an inclination to giggle at unusual times. A diagnosis of an organic bipolar affective disorder was made. Management has been predominantly supportive psychotherapy with psychoeducation, but quetiapine gives some extra stability in mental state.

- A 21-year-old woman presented with auditory hallucinations of several voices discussing her every action, delusions that her thoughts were being controlled by 'electric waves' coming from the house next door and the belief that her body was gradually changing in some peculiar fashion, which she found frightening. At times her speech became disordered with tangential thinking and loss of coherence. She was unable to concentrate at work and had to give up her job in a real estate office. Her parents reported that she had changed in personality over the past 6 months and that she had spoken about 'bizarre' thoughts and was not the person she used to be. They said the changes had occurred at a frightening speed and that she 'just changed without any warning'. A diagnosis of acute schizophrenia with disorganised features was made. After several weeks she suffered a generalised seizure and began to deteriorate in self-care and grooming. Her cognitive functions deteriorated further with severely impaired memory, poor judgement and increasing perplexity. An EEG revealed signs of subacute sclerosing pan-encephalitis (a degenerative disorder secondary to measles infection) and a history of severe measles was obtained from her parents. The diagnosis was changed to an organic schizophreniform psychosis. She continued to deteriorate and died 1 month later.

REFERENCES AND FURTHER READING

Clarke, D., Kissane, D., Trauer, T., Smith, G., 2005. Demoralization, anhedonia and grief in patients with severe physical illness. World Psychiatry 4 (2), 96–105.

David A., Fleminger, S., Kopelman, M., Lovestone, S., Mellers, J., 2009. Lishman's organic psychiatry: A textbook of neuropsychiatry. Blackwell Scientific, Oxford.

Kandel, E., Schwartz, J., Jessell, T. (Eds.), 2013 (Kindle edition). Principles of neural science. Elsevier, New York.

Lishman, W., 1998. Organic psychiatry. Blackwell Scientific, Oxford.

Manu, P., Suarez, E., Barnett, B.J., 2006. Handbook of medicine in psychiatry. American Psychiatric Publishing, Washington.

Wellen, M., 2010. Differentiation between demoralization, grief and anhedonic depression. Current Psychiatry Reports 12 (3), 229–233.

Yudofsky, S., Hales, R. (Eds.), 2008. American Psychiatric Publishing textbook of neuropsychiatry and clinical neurosciences. American Psychiatric Association Press, Washington.

CHAPTER 6

A NURSE NAMED SAM

CASE-BASED LEARNING

JOEL KING & ANDREW GLEASON

The following role-play requires two participants: one to play an intern working nights (candidate) and another to play the role of a nurse, Sam (actor).

OSCE Station Instructions

(Reading time: 2 minutes)

You are the intern in a small country hospital. There is no psychiatry ward. You receive a page from Sam, a nurse on the medical ward: 'Please come quickly and see this 82-year-old lady, Mrs Papadakis, who is wandering around the ward and looks like she's crazy. She was admitted earlier this evening and I don't know what to do with her.'

Task (10 minutes)
- Ask Sam focused questions and address Sam's concerns.
- Explain what you think is wrong with Mrs Papadakis.
- Explain your immediate management plan to the nurse.

Actor role: Sam

You are a recently qualified nurse, who has no psychiatric experience apart from your rotation in your final year of your degree. The only other nurse on the ward is currently on break.

You feel stressed by Mrs Papadakis's behaviour. She is an 82-year-old woman from a Greek background. She was admitted earlier this evening because the nursing home could not cope with her wandering into other people's rooms and mumbling in Greek, and shouting angrily when people tried to redirect her.

Mrs Papadakis has continued to behave like this on the ward. She has not been overtly aggressive to anyone, but shouts in Greek at you when you try to redirect her away from parts of the ward where she isn't supposed to be. This has scared you significantly. Occasionally, she stares at the lights and curtains for several minutes, as if transfixed. Currently, Mrs Papadakis is sitting on her bed, mumbling to herself.

If you are asked about Mrs Papadakis's baseline function, you may tell the candidate that the previous nurse informed you that she was moved into the low-level care nursing home because of decreasing mobility secondary to her chronic obstructive pulmonary disease. She normally walks independently, albeit slowly, and speaks fluent English with a Greek accent. She is well-liked by residents and staff at the nursing home. She normally spends most of her time in the nursing home's garden smoking or playing checkers. Her husband died ten years ago from a myocardial infarction. She has a daughter who lives nearby and is the next of kin. There is no prior diagnosis of a cognitive impairment, such as dementia.

MRS PAPADAKIS'S PAST MEDICAL HISTORY

You have read the case notes and found out that Mrs Papadakis has a past medical history which includes the following:

- Chronic obstructive pulmonary disease (COPD): This was diagnosed ten years ago. She is not on home oxygen. She experienced a recent infective exacerbation two weeks ago. Her GP started her on prednisolone and cephalexin.
- Urinary incontinence: This is secondary to detrusor instability and was diagnosed two months ago. Her GP placed her on oxybutynin.
- Depression: Her GP diagnosed her with depression six months ago and started dothiepin 150 mg daily.
- Hypertension: This was diagnosed ten years ago. She takes perindopril.
- Hypercholesterolaemia. This was diagnosed seven years ago. She takes atorvastatin for this.
- There is no drug and alcohol history.

MRS PAPADAKIS'S MEDICATIONS

You received the following medication list from her nursing home. Unfortunately, the admitting doctor forgot to write the drug chart. You should ask the candidate to write the following medications into the drug chart:

- Oxybutynin 5 mg QID
- Prednisolone 50 mg daily
- Cephalexin 500 mg QID
- Dothiepin 150 mg nocte
- Perindopril 2.5 mg mane
- Atorvastatin 40 mg nocte
- Aspirin 100 mg mane.

MRS PAPADAKIS'S EXAMINATION FINDINGS

You should tell the candidate the following examination findings that were elicited by the admitting doctor:
- Speaking only in Greek. Examination difficult due to lack of cooperation. Patient kept getting off bed and wandering aimlessly around the room.
- Vital signs were unremarkable apart from temperature of 37.8°C.
- Chest showed coarse widespread crackles. Otherwise nil.
- Heart sounds dual and nil. Abdomen soft and non-tender. Bowel sounds present. Calves soft and non-tender.
- No focal neurological signs.

HOW TO PLAY THE ROLE

You are very anxious and worried about Mrs Papadakis. You are also angry that the intern took so long in coming here. If the intern pauses for too long, you should suggest very angrily getting the registrar or someone more qualified, or giving the patient some haloperidol: 'You have to do something!'. You really think the patient is psychotic or demented or something, and needs some medication or a transfer to a psychiatric ward: anything to get her out of your ward. If you are specifically asked about a certain piece of history that you have available, you state it without hesitation. If you are asked about any investigations performed, state that a full blood examination (FBE) is still pending.

Model Answer

The candidate should quickly recognise that the nurse is describing a case of delirium. Delirium is very common in the hospital setting and is associated with high rates of mortality. The hallmark of delirium is a disturbance of consciousness, with a reduced ability to focus, sustain, or shift attention. It is accompanied by a change in cognition, such as a memory deficit, disorientation, or language disturbance, or the development of a perceptual disturbance that is not better accounted for by a dementia (see Box 6.2, page 72). Unlike dementia, delirium develops over a short period of time, usually hours to days, and has a fluctuating course over the day. The sleep–wake cycle is often disordered. Psychomotor findings vary from marked agitation or aggression to apathy and inactivity. There should be evidence of an underlying organic cause from history, physical examination and laboratory findings, although a cause is not always found. Further information can be found on pages 71–73.

The student should recognise that the nurse is highly anxious and employ a suitable calm, but confident approach. Asking whether the nurse has ever encountered a similar case will reveal that the nurse is newly qualified and has little experience with delirium. The student should adjust their explanations accordingly.

The student should focus on what exactly is concerning the nurse. This greatly changes the risk profile and management. Wandering patients who are not aggressive can often be contained with environmental measures, such as regular redirection and closing doors. More agitated patients who are bordering on becoming aggressive may require medication, such as haloperidol.

The student should clearly distinguish the time course of the disturbed behaviour. This involves asking about baseline function ('Do you know how Mrs Papadakis normally behaves at the nursing home?') compared to the present. In this case, it is documented in the notes, but this is not always the case and may involve calling the nursing home or a relative as part of the immediate management plan. A past history of cognitive impairment, including dementia, should always be sought out.

One must seek out the cause(s) of delirium so that treatment of the underlying condition can be commenced, through a history, physical examination and investigations. This patient exemplifies some of the most common causes – infection, hypoxia and medication changes, especially anticholinergics. Both oxybutynin and dothiepin, a tricyclic antidepressant that is now used in more treatment-resistant cases of depression and rarely first-line, are anticholinergic in nature. Electrolyte imbalance, pain, cardiac arrhythmia, trauma, acute surgical conditions, post-surgical state, and inflammation are other common causes. Stroke should be excluded, especially given Mrs Papadakis's multiple risk factors, including age, hypertension and hypercholesterolaemia.

As part of the immediate management plan, students should provide an understandable explanation to Sam about delirium and the likely causes. This should also include distinguishing it from dementia and psychosis, which were two of Sam's concerns. Dementia is a progressive decline in cognitive function that is less acute in nature. Psychosis is a state of impaired reality-testing and may involve formal thought disorder, perceptual disturbances such as auditory hallucinations, and delusions, which are not present here, although it is hard to clarify this due to the fact that Mrs Papadakis is not speaking English at present. Psychotic disorders, such as schizophrenia, are unlikely to first present in this age group and usually present in late teens through to early thirties. In most circumstances delirious patients should not be placed under the Mental Health Act, or transferred to a psychiatric ward.

Students should offer to examine the patient to look for signs of infection, impaired cardiorespiratory function, neurological abnormalities, and an acute abdomen. They should tell the nurse that they will chase the full blood examination and order further tests. This might include urea, creatinine and electrolytes, calcium, magnesium, phosphate, liver function tests, troponins, and inflammatory markers such as ESR or CRP. An ECG, chest X-ray, and urinalysis would also be appropriate.

Students should first employ environmental measures to control this patient's wandering to ensure the safety of the patient and others. A Greek interpreter may be useful in helping give the patient instructions. Other measures may involve redirection, improved lighting in the patient's room, moving the patient to a single room, providing orienting cues such as a clock or window, and organising a special nurse or a familiar family member, such as the patient's daughter. If sufficient staffing cannot be achieved on the general ward, a transfer to a high dependency unit may be considered.

Many hospitals have delirium guidelines and these should be mentioned and followed. The student should offer to return to the ward and reassess throughout the night. The student should liaise with their senior colleague, which would be the medical registrar or the consultant, to discuss changing other aspects of medical management. As some patients with COPD rely on a hypoxic, rather than hypercapnic, drive to breathe, increasing the patient's oxygen with nasal prongs or mask should be done with caution. Changing antibiotics and removing offending agents, such as anticholinergics and prednisolone, should be done with caution as well. Some patients become more confused with multiple, rapid medication changes.

Students should warn against mechanical restraint or sedative medication in a patient who is only wandering and redirectable. Mechanical restraint can be very frightening for patients, especially confused patients, and lead to an escalation in agitated behaviour. Furthermore, mechanical restraint can be painful and compromise the patient's ability to breathe. Sedative medication, such as benzodiazepines and antipsychotics, have side effects, increase the risk of falls, and accumulate more rapidly in the elderly. Occasionally, benzodiazepines cause paradoxical disinhibition. Lastly, there should be a plan to communicate this patient's delirium with the morning home team and the need for further collateral history.

Chapter 7

SCHIZOPHRENIA AND RELATED DISORDERS

DAVID J CASTLE & DARRYL BASSETT

Schizophrenia is a disorder that affects roughly one in 200 people, and it can have a profound effect upon the individual and their families. The term schizophrenia refers to a 'splitting of the psychic functions', not, as is commonly believed, to a 'split personality'. Key aspects of the disorder are shown in Box 7.1.

Clinical features

The signs and symptoms of the disorder are most usefully divided into:

- *positive symptoms*: delusions (fixed false beliefs held with tenacity and not understandable in terms of the sociocultural context); and hallucinations (false perceptions that can occur in any sensory modality, but with auditory hallucinations being most common)
- *negative symptoms*: these are symptoms characterised by 'deficit' and include restricted or blunted affect (decreased range of facial expressions); paucity of thought content (manifested by lack of spontaneous conversation); and apathetic social withdrawal (the individual seems to lack the desire to socialise or indeed interact with the world)
- *disorganisation symptoms*: formal thought disorder (disorganised thoughts, manifested by disjointed speech); disorganised behaviour; and inappropriate affect (e.g. smiling when discussing a sad event)
- *cognitive impairment* (see below).

Box 7.1

Key aspects of schizophrenia

- Symptoms can be divided into:
  - positive symptoms (delusions and hallucinations)
  - negative symptoms
  - disorganisation symptoms
  - cognitive impairment.
- Aetiology is multidimensional, with genetic and environmental factors interacting.
- There is an associated range of structural and functional brain abnormalities.
- There is a variable longitudinal course, with about 40% having significant long-term disability.

There is no specific laboratory or radiological test for schizophrenia, and none of the signs or symptoms outlined above are pathognomonic. However, the 'first rank' symptoms elucidated by Schneider (see Box 7.2) have some degree of diagnostic specificity, and are useful to ask for in the clinical interview.

Negative symptoms can sometimes be 'mimicked' by depression, positive symptoms or the extrapyramidal side effects of antipsychotic medication. It is always important to treat the underlying cause, as shown in Table 7.1.

Not all signs and symptoms occur in any one individual at any one time: different patients show different features and these might change over the course of the illness. Table 7.2 shows the cardinal features of schizophrenia according to DSM–IV–TR and ICD–10. It will be noted that there is considerable overlap between these two constructs: the main difference is that DSM–IV–TR requires a 6-month duration: disorders with the characteristic symptoms but shorter duration are labelled *schizophreniform disorder*.

Differential diagnoses

'Organic' psychoses

Schizophrenia cannot be diagnosed if there are clear organic factors causing the symptoms and signs: this is labelled an organic psychosis. Exclusion of reversible organic causes (e.g. brain tumour) is obviously important in clinical practice, but it can be much more difficult to assess the role of illicit substances, which are commonly used by people with schizophrenia.

A label of *drug-induced psychosis* is only appropriate if there is:

- a clear temporal sequence between drug exposure and onset of symptoms
- a resolution of symptoms on cessation of the drug, and
- a relatively short duration of symptoms (certainly under 1 month).

People with established schizophrenia are vulnerable to relapse if they use drugs such as cannabis: the term *drug-precipitated* relapse is a more appropriate term in such cases.

Box 7.2
Schneider's 'first rank' symptoms of schizophrenia

Auditory hallucinatory experiences

These include:

* *third person auditory hallucinations*: two or more voices discussing the individual in the third person (he, she, it); often derogatory/persecutory

* *running commentary*: a voice commenting on the person's actual actions, in the third person

* *audible thoughts (gedankenlaudwerten)*: hearing one's own thoughts out loud.

Delusional perception

There is a normal percept to which an 'un-understandable' delusional attribution is given.

Passivity phenomena

This is a series of phenomena where the person experiences their *will, actions, affect or bodily (somatic) functions* being 'taken over' by some alien influence. It is an 'as if' phenomenon, such as: 'It is as if my actions are controlled by a robot; I feel like a puppet on a string.'

Permeability of ego boundaries

This includes:

* *thought insertion*: not all thoughts in one's mind are one's own; thoughts are being 'put into' the person's mind; there may be secondary elaboration (e.g. 'An intergalactic machine is putting thoughts into my mind.')

* *thought withdrawal*: this is the reverse of thought insertion; it may be experienced as the mind transiently 'going blank'

* *thought broadcast*: a feeling that thoughts dissipate out of the person's mind, and are 'shared' by others; it is more than just feeling others can read their mind.

(Castle & Buckley 2011, with permission)

Table 7.1
Primary and secondary negative symptoms and treatment

		Treatment
Primary		Use atypical antipsychotic; consider adjunctive treatments; if persistent, consider clozapine
Secondary	To depression	Antidepressant medication (SSRI or mirtazapine preferred)
	To positive symptoms	Optimise treatment of positive symptoms: pharmacological and psychosocial approaches should be explored
	To D2 receptor blockade	Consider atypical antipsychotic; if persistent extrapyramidal side effects on atypical antipsychotic, consider adjunctive anticholinergic agent

(Castle & Buckley 2011, with permission)

Table 7.2

DSM–IV–TR and ICD–10 diagnoses of schizophrenia

DSM–IV–TR (synopsis)	ICD–10 (synopsis)
Symptoms (at least 1 month unless successfully treated): • delusions • hallucinations • disorganised speech • disorganised or catatonic behaviour, and • negative symptoms. At least two symptoms required, unless: • delusions are bizarre • hallucinations are third person conversing or running commentary. Social/occupational dysfunction: • work • interpersonal relations, and • self-care. Duration: 6 months at least Exclusions: • schizoaffective disorder • bipolar disorder • general medical condition • substance induced.	Symptoms: • at least one of: thought echo, insertion, withdrawal, broadcast • passivity phenomena or delusional perception • third person conversing or running commentary hallucinations • 'completely impossible' delusions. At least two of: • persistent hallucinations in any modality, with delusions • disorganised speech • catatonia, and negative symptoms (must be 'primary'). Duration: 1 month at least Exclusions: • mood disorder • organic brain disease • alcohol/drug-related intoxication.

(Castle & Buckley 2011, with permission)

Schizoaffective disorder

If there are clear affective and psychotic symptoms that occur at different times over the course of illness, a label of schizoaffective disorder is applied. There is some debate about the validity of this diagnosis and the boundaries are vague.

Delusional disorder

This group of disorders is characterised by well-circumscribed delusions in the absence of prominent hallucinations or negative or disorganisation symptoms. The delusional content is 'understandable', such as beliefs about having a disease (also termed monosymptomatic hypochondriacal delusions or delusional disorder, somatic subtype) or having an unfaithful partner (delusional jealousy, or Othello syndrome).

Box 7.3

DSM–IV–TR and ICD–10 subtypes of schizophrenia

Subtypes include:

- *paranoid*: delusions and hallucinations, but no prominent negative or disorganisation symptoms

- *disorganised (DSM–IV–TR)/hebephrenic (ICD–10)*: prominent disturbance of affect, volition and thought stream; ICD-10 states adolescent/young adults only

- *catatonic*: prominent motor disturbance

- *undifferentiated*: meet schizophrenia diagnostic criteria, but not one of the foregoing subtypes

- *residual*: prominent negative symptoms in absence of prominent positive symptoms, and

- *simple*: slow progression of negative symptoms in the absence of positive symptoms (ICD-10 considers this akin to schizotypal personality disorder).

(Castle & Buckley 2011, with permission)

Pervasive developmental disorders

Pervasive developmental disorders (e.g. autism, Asperger's disorder – see Chapter 18) are characterised by abnormalities in social interactions and restricted and stereotyped range of interests and activities, evident from before 3 years of age.

Axis II disorders

Some of the cluster A DSM–IV–TR Axis II (personality) disorders (see Chapter 14) could be considered *formes frustes* of schizophrenia. The most obvious is schizotypal personality disorder, characterised by longstanding eccentricity, social withdrawal and odd beliefs. It is placed on Axis II in DSM–IV–TR, but is probably genetically linked to schizophrenia, and sometimes evolves into full-blown schizophrenia.

Subtypes of schizophrenia

Many attempts have been made at subtyping schizophrenia, mostly on the basis of phenomenology and/or longitudinal course. DSM–IV–TR and ICD–10 subtypes are shown in Box 7.3. Probably the best validated of these is the paranoid subtype.

Cognitive functioning in schizophrenia

Cognitive deficits are common in schizophrenia. They tend to affect mostly frontal lobe tasks, such as executive function. These deficits tend to antedate the onset of illness, although they might show some progression. They are associated with impairment in work and social functioning. Current antipsychotic medications do not have powerful beneficial effects on cognition.

Comorbidity

Depression is common in people with schizophrenia. Recognition and treatment are critical, as depression is treatable, and if untreated can lead to an extra burden for the individual, and is associated with suicide (which itself is much more common in schizophrenia than the general population). Depression can be difficult to disentangle from negative symptoms and demoralisation. Features that suggest a depressive disorder include vegetative symptoms (e.g. anorexia, insomnia); functional shift symptoms (e.g. mood worse in the morning; early morning waking); guilty feelings; and suicidality. Treatment of depression in schizophrenia follows roughly the same approach as for depression generally (see Chapters 8, 15 and 16).

Of the *anxiety disorders*, panic disorder, generalised anxiety disorder, agoraphobia, social phobia and obsessive-compulsive disorder (OCD) have all been shown to occur in excess in association with schizophrenia. OCD is particularly also associated with the use of atypical antipsychotics, notably clozapine. Anxiety disorder comorbidities can worsen the long-term course of schizophrenia, and need to be screened for and treated on their own m erits. The same psychological and pharmacological treatments that have been proven effective for these disorders when they occur alone, are often also effective when they are comorbid with schizophrenia (see Chapters 10 and 11).

Post-traumatic stress disorder also occurs in excess in people with schizophrenia. This relates in part to increased rates of child sexual abuse and other early disadvantage; the symptoms of psychosis themselves; and the trauma all too often associated with the treatment process (notably restraint and seclusion in acute hospital settings).

Substance abuse is common in schizophrenia (around 40–60%). Alcohol is the most widely used substance, followed by cannabis. The negative impacts of substance use in schizophrenia are shown in Box 7.4.

Treatment of substance use disorder (SUD) in schizophrenia is complex, but an integrated approach, with both problems being addressed at the same time, is preferred.

Physical comorbidity associated with schizophrenia is a major area of concern, and contributes substantially to lower life expectancy. *Cardiovascular risk factors*, which are elevated in schizophrenia, include obesity, hypertension, smoking, diabetes and hyperlipidaemia. These factors are fed, *inter alia*, by sedentary lifestyles, poor diet and some antipsychotic medications (notably clozapine and olanzapine). *Cancer* mortality rates are higher in people with schizophrenia, compared to the general population, notably breast and gastrointestinal malignancies. These cancers are often not screened for adequately nor treated as vigorously as in people without schizophrenia.

Case examples: Schizophrenia and related disorders

First onset schizophrenia

A 17-year-old boy was brought for a medical consultation because he had been behaving oddly. Over the previous 8 months he had been spending most of his time alone in his room, his self-care had been poor, and he had been up all night on the internet. He had been sleeping most of the day and had abandoned his studies. Increasingly, he had been isolating himself and did not want to have anything to do with his friends. More recently, he had been talking to himself and had stopped eating prepared food, saying it was poisoned: he would eat only canned food, which he insisted on opening himself.

Case examples continued

Chronic schizophrenia with negative symptoms

A 45-year-old man lived in a run-down boarding house. He spent most of his time alone, occasionally attending a local drop-in centre and coming for his depot injection at the mental health clinic. He had no particular hobbies or interests and no friends; he occasionally spoke with his mother on the phone, but had no other contact with his family. He presented with restricted affect, gave only short, unembellished answers to direct questions, and was generally evasive. His self-care was poor, he was malodorous, had rotting teeth, and wore many layers of clothing even though the weather was warm. On direct questioning, he said he believed that other people in the boarding house had been talking about him behind his back, and he could hear them even through the brick walls.

Late onset schizophrenia

A 67-year-old woman came to the attention of psychiatric services because her neighbours complained she was abusive towards them and accused them of breaking into her apartment at night. She presented as suspicious and guarded, but eventually allowed the team into her apartment. She stated that her neighbours were plotting against her, that they broke through the window at night (despite it being closed) and left marks on the floor: she pointed to some innocuous-looking stains on the carpet. She said they had been pumping gas through the air conditioning, and that she could smell it at night.

Pathological jealousy (a form of delusional disorder)

A 50-year-old man was charged with assault after manhandling his wife. His wife reported that over the previous months he had become increasingly obsessed that she was having an affair with another man, although she denied this. She said he would check her mobile phone, her handbag, and even her underwear, whenever she had been out by herself. He was not amenable to reassurance, and became increasingly accusatory and threatening towards her, saying he was going to kill her and her 'lover'.

Epidemiology

The World Health Organization (WHO) undertook two influential studies that showed rates of schizophrenia to be similar in a number of developed and developing countries; the incidence rates were between 7 and 14 new cases per 100,000 per year. Also of interest was an overall better outcome in developing countries. Prevalence studies (i.e. reporting the number of cases in a given population at a given point in time–point prevalence; or over a set period–period prevalence) have also been remarkably similar, when they have used appropriate methods, including operational criteria for diagnosis. Modern general population studies from the US, the UK and Australia have all reported prevalence rates of around 0.5–1.5%; the lower figure is more consistent with the total international literature. Another way of expressing these figures is that of lifetime morbid risk—that is, the risk at birth of anyone developing the illness, all else being equal. This is usually rounded to 0.5–1.0%.

Rates of schizophrenia do vary at a city or even neighbourhood level, with a well-established association with *social deprivation*. This is partly due to a 'drift' of vulnerable people down the social strata, and partly to a 'toxic' effect of city upbringing. Also, *migrants* are at greater risk of schizophrenia: black migrants in predominantly white

Box 7.4

Impact of problematic substance use on outcomes in schizophrenia

Mental health issues

Issues include:

- increased psychotic symptoms
- greater relapse rates
- higher hospitalisation rates
- frequent emergency contacts with mental health services
- reduced adherence to treatment
- higher attempted and completed suicide rates.

Violence and crime

There is:

- increased violence
- an elevated crime rate
- an increased rate of incarceration.

Physical health

Impacts include:

- poorer overall healthcare and nutrition
- increased specific physical health risks, including HIV and hepatitis C
- overall increased mortality.

Finances and vocation

There may be:

- financial problems directly and indirectly related to drug use
- instability of work/studies.

Housing and families

There may be:

- unstable accommodation
- homelessness
- increased family conflict.

(Castle & Buckley 2011, with permission)

cultures are particularly at risk (e.g. African-Caribbeans in the UK). Interestingly, this elevated risk also pertains to British-born African-Caribbeans.

Overall, males and females appear roughly equally prone to schizophrenia across the whole lifespan, but males have an overall earlier onset (late teens) compared to females (early 20s, but with later peaks of onset in the 40s and 60s to 70s).

Females also tend to have better overall outcomes in terms of symptoms, recurrences and psychosocial parameters. Postulated reasons for these findings include the potential 'protective' effect of oestrogens, and/or that the sexes are differentially prone to different types of illness, notably males to an early-onset severe illness consequent upon neurodevelopmental deviance.

Outcome

Schizophrenia has a variable long-term course, with roughly a quarter of cases having a single episode before returning to good psychosocial functioning; around a third having an episodic course with reasonably good intermorbid functioning; and 40% tending to have a poor outcome. Certain factors do tend to be associated with a poor outcome in schizophrenia. Some of these are potentially remediable, while others are not (see Box 7.5).

Box 7.5

Factors associated with a poor outcome in schizophrenia

Factors not subject to amelioration

Factors include:

- male gender
- early onset of illness
- strong family loading for schizophrenia
- insidious onset of illness
- long prodrome
- poor premorbid functioning
- lack of affective symptoms at onset
- prominent negative symptoms at onset
- lack of obvious precipitating factors at onset
- neurological soft signs
- significant neurocognitive deficits at onset, and
- structural brain abnormalities (somewhat inconsistent findings).

Factors potentially addressed by optimal clinical care

Factors include:

- long duration of untreated psychosis (debated)
- suboptimal treatment of psychotic symptoms
- suboptimal treatment of comorbid symptoms
- poor medication adherence
- medication side effects (e.g. neuroleptic-induced deficit syndrome)
- substance abuse, and
- high family expressed emotion.

(Castle & Buckley 2011, with permission)

Particular recent interest has been shown in *early intervention*, but whether this ameliorates the long-term course is still unclear.

Family environment can impact the course of the illness, notably those families that exhibit high *expressed emotion* (EE), characterised by hostility, critical comments and/or over-involvement. Such families can benefit from specific family therapy interventions.

Life events are events that occur during the course of a person's life and which might impact on risk of relapse. The individual can be taught useful strategies to deal more effectively with stressful life events, and thus reduce the chances of relapse.

Aetiology

Genetic factors

Genetic causality is well established in schizophrenia, with family studies and adoption studies all confirming an increased risk in biological relatives of people with schizophrenia (rates are roughly 10% in siblings, including dizygotic twins, 50% in monozygotic twins, 15% if one parent affected, and around 50% if both parents are affected). Inheritance is certainly non-Mendelian, and there is no single schizophrenia gene, but rather multiple genes of small effect. Genes that have attracted attention and shown some evidence of linkage in some samples include some associated with neurodevelopment (e.g. dysbindin, dysregulin) and with the metabolism of dopamine, notably catechol-O-methyltransferase (COMT). There is also an excess of multiple copy number variants (CNVs) in people with schizophrenia.

Environmental factors

The fact that monozygotic twins are only 50% concordant for schizophrenia shows that non-genetic or 'environmental' factors must also operate to increase risk. The main putative factors are shown in Box 7.6. It should be stressed that none of these factors independently cause schizophrenia, and that they have only modest effects on risk: presumably they act on individuals who already carry some genetic vulnerability. There is much interest in how genetic and environmental factors interact in the causation of schizophrenia (so called 'gene-environment interaction' or G/E).

Schizophrenia as a brain disease

That some people with schizophrenia show subtle brain structural abnormalities is beyond doubt, with the most common findings of neuroimaging studies shown in Box 7.7. However, there is a great degree of overlap with 'normals' and no single neuroimaging finding is pathognomonic. These structural abnormalities seem to be evident even at the onset of illness, although some progression might occur over the course of the disorder. Of particular interest are findings that show an acceleration of brain changes at the time of 'transition' to the first episode of psychosis.

People with schizophrenia tend to show functional brain abnormalities (e.g. 'hypofrontality' associated with negative symptoms, and increased blood flow to Broca's area during auditory hallucinations). Various eye-tracking abnormalities and neurophysiological deficits (e.g. increased p-300 latency) have been found in both schizophrenics and

Box 7.6

Summary of putative 'environmental' causal factors in schizophrenia

Factors include:

- season of birth (later winter, early spring), but this has been shown in the northern hemisphere only
- exposure to influenza type A during the second trimester of pregnancy; and possibly some other infectious agents such as toxoplasmosis
- maternal starvation during the first trimester of pregnancy
- maternal anaemia and low vitamin D levels
- pregnancy and birth complications
- maternal stress during pregnancy
- urban birth/upbringing
- migration
- ethnic minorities
- substance abuse (notably cannabis)
- advancing paternal age.

(Castle & Buckley 2011, with permission)

Box 7.7

Structural brain abnormalities in schizophrenia

General abnormalities

General abnormalities include:

- enlarged lateral ventricles
- enlarged third ventricle
- reduced overall grey matter volume
- widespread cortical and cerebellar atrophy.

Site-specific abnormalities

Site-specific abnormalities include:

- *frontal lobe*: volume reduction, especially inferior prefrontal cortex
- *temporal lobe*: volume reduction in amygdala, hippocampus and parahippocampal gyrus; it appears more marked on the left side.

(Castle & Buckley 2011, with permission)

their 'unaffected' relatives, suggesting these may be endophenotypic markers for the disorder.

The neurodevelopmental model

The neurodevelopmental model posits that schizophrenia has its roots in aberrant development of the brain, but that positive symptoms only become manifest in late teens/early adulthood when the brain develops the capacity to produce such symptoms. This model is consonant with findings that even in early life people who later develop schizophrenia are at greater risk of delayed motor, verbal and social milestones. The model also gains support from findings that people with schizophrenia are more likely than the general population to have physical abnormalities such as high arched palate, low set ears, widely spaced eyes, and unusual fingerprint patterns. These are thought to reflect early neurodevelopmental deviance.

Neurochemistry

There are a number of theories that address various aspects of schizophrenia in terms of perturbations of neurochemical balance. None of these theories is definitive, nor are they exclusive of each other: indeed, the complexity of the illness speaks to a number of different pathogenetic mechanisms likely to be responsible for the various sets of signs and symptoms.

Dopaminergic mechanisms

The dopamine hypothesis of schizophrenia has its roots in observations that dopaminergic agonists such as amphetamines can cause (positive) psychotic symptoms, and drugs that ameliorate such symptoms block dopamine D2 receptors (in mesolimbic tracts). An expansion of the theory suggests that negative symptoms are caused by dopamine deficit in mesocortical pathways. But the issue is complex, and other neurotransmitter systems have also been implicated.

Serotonergic mechanisms

Serotonergic mechanisms have also been of interest in schizophrenia, in part because the serotonergic agonist lysergic acid diethylamide (LSD) is a hallucinogen, but also because most of the 'atypical' antipsychotic agents block serotonin 5HT-2 receptors (see Chapter 15).

Glutamatergic mechanisms

Phencyclidine (PCP), an antagonist of the N-methyl-D-aspartate (NMDA) subtype of the glutamatergic receptor, can produce a clinical picture that looks much like schizophrenia. Recent findings that a glutamatergic 2/3 agonist has antipsychotic properties have opened up a potential new therapeutic avenue for schizophrenia, albeit that that particular agent has now been withdrawn.

Management

With the worldwide move towards deinstitutionalisation, people with schizophrenia are preferentially treated in the community. Inpatient care is usually reserved for episodes of acute care, when the person is at risk to themselves or others and/or is unable to be safely managed in their own environment. These days very few patients have protracted inpatient stays.

Treatment summary: schizophrenia

- Always consider the patient as a person, not a label.
- Consider the aspirations and goals of the individual in setting management plans.
- Be vigilant about comorbidities, such as depression and anxiety, and treat these effectively.
- Be alert for suicidality, and make appropriate risk management plans.
- Monitor the physical health of the patient, as well as their mental health.
- Monitor and address problematic substance use.
- Engage families and carers as much as feasible.
- Use the resources of the multidisciplinary team to effect comprehensive care.
- Encourage engagement in social activities and hobbies.
- Enhance opportunities for employed work, where appropriate.

To maintain them in the community, people with schizophrenia require a long-term treatment plan that encompasses biological and psychosocial domains. A multidisciplinary team is usually required, with each professional bringing their own expertise, but with a coordinating case manager who can ensure consistency and comprehensiveness of interventions. In those with severe illness and multiple problems, intensive case management, with the capacity to provide a high level of face-to-face contact (up to twice daily if required), can be beneficial and reduce hospitalisations. There is much investment currently in the so-called 'Recovery' framework, working with individuals with schizophrenia to manage their own illness as much as feasible and to build on their innate strengths.

Biological treatments

Antipsychotic medication is the mainstay of the treatment of people with schizophrenia. These drugs are described in Chapter 15. One of the major challenges for clinicians is to ensure patients (who often lack insight into their need for treatment) actually take their medication as prescribed. The provision of adequate information regarding the rationale for and potential side effects of the medication is key in this. Some patients benefit from more structured *adherence therapy*. For those who perennially do not adhere and thus continue to relapse, a long-acting injectable ('depot') form of antipsychotic can be considered.

Not all patients respond fully to the first prescribed antipsychotic. Negative symptoms and cognitive symptoms are often particularly under-responsive. Trialling another agent from a different class or, if that also fails, the use of clozapine, is suggested. Sometimes, use of adjunctive agents (e.g. another antipsychotic, or a mood stabiliser) is of benefit at an individual level, though monotherapy should be the preferred goal.

Psychological treatments

Psychological treatments can benefit some patients. For example, cognitive behavioural techniques can be used to help with persistent delusions and hallucinations that are not responsive to medication. Cognitive remediation techniques, which enhance cognitive capacity in certain domains, can also be helpful, as are programs addressing social skills deficits (social skills training). Lack of opportunity to socialise is a major barrier for many people with schizophrenia. Engagement with local drop-in centres, attending outings and group activities can assist, as can specific programs addressing social skills deficits.

Vocational aspects

Most people with schizophrenia do not have paid employment. In part, this is a consequence of the positive, negative and cognitive symptoms of the illness itself, compounded by medication side effects such as sedation. But workplaces are often 'unfriendly' to people with schizophrenia, and working with potential employers and supporting the patient in the workplace can be helpful. *Supported employment* can be augmented by cognitive remediation, and *social firms* (part-owned by people with a mental illness, and with a specified proportion of employees living with a mental illness) offer particular support structures.

The family in treatment

As outlined above, the family is not to blame for schizophrenia, but can suffer enormously because of the illness in a loved one, not least through stigma. Psychoeducation is vital for family members, and, where feasible and appropriate, they should be active participants in treatment plans. Family support groups can assist family members to cope, and ensure they know they are 'not alone'. Some families benefit from specific family therapy, addressing, *inter alia*, high expressed emotion (see above).

REFERENCES AND FURTHER READING

Castle, D.J., 2012. Schizoaffective disorder. Advances in Psychiatric Treatment 18, 32–33.

Castle, D.J., Buckley, P.F., 2011. Schizophrenia, rev ed. Oxford University Press, Oxford.

Castle, D.J., Copolov, D., Wykes, T., Mueser, K. (Eds.), 2012. Pharmacological and psychosocial treatments in schizophrenia, third ed. Informa Healthcare, London.

Crow, T.J., 1980. Positive and negative symptoms and the role of dopamine in schizophrenia. British Medical Journal 346, 383–386.

Green, A.I., Canusa, C.M., Brenner, M.J., et al., 2003. Recognition and management of comorbidity in patients with schizophrenia. Psychiatric Clinics of North America 26, 115-139.

Harrison, P.J., Weinberger, D.R., 2005. Schizophrenia genes, gene expression and neuropathology: on the matter of their convergence. Molecular Psychiatry 10, 40-68.

Hoenig, J., 1983. The concept of schizophrenia: Kraepelin, Bleuler, Schneider. British Journal of Psychiatry 142, 547–556.

Jablensky, A., Sartorious, N., Ernberg, G., et al., 1992. Schizophrenia: manifestation, incidence and course in different cultures. Psychological Medicine Monograph 20.

Jones, P.B., Buckley, P.F., 2006. Schizophrenia. Elsevier, London.

Liddle, P., Carpenter, W.T., Crow, T., 1994. Syndromes of schizophrenia. British Journal of Psychiatry 165, 721-727.

Lieberman, J., Stroup, T.S., McEvoy, J.P., et al., 2005. Effectiveness of antipsychotic drugs in the treatment of schizophrenia. New England Journal of Medicine 353, 1209-1223.

Murray, R.M., O'Callaghan, E., Castle, D.J., Lewis, S.W., 1992. A neurodevelopmental approach to the classification of schizophrenia. Schizophrenia Bulletin 18, 319-332.

Zubin, J., Spring, B., 1977. Vulnerability: a new view of schizophrenia. Journal of Abnormal Psychology 86, 103-126.

A MOTHER AND DAUGHTER, KAREN AND MELISSA

CASE-BASED LEARNING

JOEL KING & ANDREW GLEASON

The following role-play requires three participants: one to play a general practice registrar (candidate) and two to play a patient, Melissa, and the patient's mother, Karen (actors).

OSCE Station Instructions

(Reading time: 2 minutes)

You are a GP registrar in a suburban clinic. Your next patient is Melissa Chung, an 18-year-old woman who recently had a four week admission to a psychiatric inpatient unit. She was diagnosed with schizophrenia. She receives follow-up from a community mental health clinic on a voluntary basis. Her case manager, Rex, and psychiatrist, Dr Foreman, communicate with you about her care on a regular basis. You last saw her two months ago. At that time, she was taking olanzapine 10 mg nocte and had no positive psychotic symptoms. Her mother, Karen, has brought her in today because she is concerned that Melissa is getting fat. She would like you to fix this.

Task (10 minutes)
- Please address the above concern and propose a short-term management plan to the patient and her mother.
- You do not need to perform a physical examination in this station.

Actor role: Melissa Chung (patient)

You may freely give any of the information in this history if asked, but you should not volunteer it spontaneously.

You are Melissa, an 18-year-old locally born girl of Chinese extraction. You are the eldest of three siblings (Stephen, 16; Sophie, 14). Six months ago you experienced your first episode of psychosis, while doing your first year of a Bachelor of Arts degree. You were admitted into the psychiatry unit at St Christopher's Hospital under the Mental Health Act. At the time, you believed that you had been selected for a special mission by God and Buddha. They had granted you special powers that would help you unite the different religions of the world and bring harmony to war-torn areas such as the Middle East. God and Buddha would often whisper to you, telling you that you had a 'divine purpose', but never told you to do anything.

You also believed that the CIA and the Catholic Church were trying to stop you from uniting the world's religions and had sent spies to monitor you. The spies had sneaked cameras into your house. They looked like normal people but they were so powerful that they had somehow convinced your parents to work for them. At the time you believed the CIA had rigged your television and computer to pick up your brain waves and send them to their receiving devices in Washington DC. You were very scared and couldn't trust anyone.

In hospital, you were started on olanzapine 10 mg in the evening. Over the following four weeks you became less fixated on conspiracies or your religious destiny and the voices stopped. You were discharged as a voluntary patient to a community mental health clinic, where you see your case manager, Rex, on a fortnightly basis, and your psychiatrist, Dr Foreman, every month. You find Rex okay and think Dr Foreman is a bit of a nerd, but he tries really hard and probably means well.

Dr Foreman has told you that you have a disorder called schizophrenia, but you didn't like the sound of that, so he then rephrased it as a psychotic disorder, which you thought sounded better. He has emphasised that you need to keep taking the olanzapine in order to remain well, which you have done, mainly because you're afraid of being re-admitted against your will.

You didn't return to university and now stay at home during the day, playing computer games and watching DVDs. You still like going out with friends at night and play guitar in a Christian rock band every week. This has upset your mother greatly, who thinks that you should have returned to university or sought a job. She berates you for being 'lazy' and 'a disgrace to our family'. She is very angry that you aren't setting a better example for your younger brother and sister. You believe that she is being unfair and this has led to many heated arguments. Your father usually retreats to his study when this happens.

One month ago you started to believe that the neighbours might be spying on you. You weren't sure why they were doing this, but this led you to become more isolated and you stopped going outside, even to go to the local shops. Rex and Dr Foreman came to visit you and increased your dose of olanzapine from 10 mg to 20 mg nocte. Your beliefs about the neighbours decreased and became less distressing for you, but you have been very tired and lethargic for the last month.

It is very difficult to get out of bed in the morning. When you are awake, you find that you are very hungry all the time and spend a lot of time eating potato chips and lollies. You are able to get outside, but you now spend a lot of money ordering take-away junk food.

Today, you were dragged to the clinic by your mother. You just wish she would get off your back. You have no positive psychotic symptoms. You are not suicidal and do not wish to harm anyone. You are not depressed, anxious, or manic. You have no other side effects to olanzapine, such as postural hypotension. You do not have cold intolerance, dry and coarse hair, muscle cramps, changes in bowel habit, dry skin, changes in menses, or changes in concentration.

Your most recent blood tests, including fasting glucose and thyroid, and ECG tests at the psychiatric clinic were normal one month ago.

You deny taking recreational drugs, smoking cigarettes or drinking alcohol. You deny symptoms of any medical condition. You do not have a forensic history. If asked about your family, you must reply, 'Look. I don't want to talk about my family now, except my mum is crazy and I probably get it from her.'

Statements you must make:
(You may improvise around these lines)
- 'Shut up, Mum! It's your fault I got admitted and put on psychiatric drugs.'
- 'If you hadn't stressed me out, Mum, I wouldn't have had a mental breakdown! Have you ever considered that?'
- 'I hate this olanzapine. I wish I wasn't on it. I'm only on it so I don't go back to that stupid hospital where the weirdos are.'
- 'Dr Foreman jacked up my dose of medication last month, because he thought I was getting paranoid or something. I dunno.'
- 'Are you really a doctor? You look really young.'

You are very angry at your mother for bringing you to a doctor and spend most of the session blaming her for making you mentally unwell by being overbearing and critical. You are not very pleasant to be around. However, if the candidate asks to see you on your own, state, 'No, my mum stays. She's the one who wants to talk to you.' If the candidate asks to see your mother on her own, state, 'No, I want to hear what you're saying about me.'

Actor role: Karen Chung (patient's mother)

You are Mrs Karen Chung, a 45-year-old stay-home mother. You are very anxious at the start of the interview and become only slightly less anxious as the interview goes on. You have brought Melissa to the GP clinic today because you have noticed that she is eating stacks of junk food, and has put on a lot of weight over the last month. You are not sure of the exact amount. She is also spending a lot more time in bed and has problems getting up in the morning. (These are new features over the last month, but you should not readily admit this unless specifically asked about the duration.)

You think this has happened because Melissa is lazy. You would like the doctor to prescribe some weight-loss pills. You are very embarrassed about your daughter's eating and her doing nothing around the house, and you worry about her long-term prospects. You are also ashamed of her behaviour in front of the doctor, whom you respect as an educated professional. Your husband is very hands-off and thinks Melissa will grow out of being irresponsible on her own. You feel that he is not very helpful and you are left to do all the parenting.

Although you do not agree on your role in Melissa's mental illness, you agree with her responses on other issues, such as lack of positive psychotic symptoms, good compliance with medications and appointments, lack of medical and forensic history, and no current substance use. You also do not want to go into family history at this stage, stating that you have already been through it with Rex and Dr Foreman. You think very highly of these two professionals.

Statements you must make:
- 'I'm very worried about my daughter. She is getting so fat.'
- 'She just eats and eats all day.'
- 'She is very lazy, Doctor. She is now refusing to get out of bed in the morning.'
- 'Doctor, can't you prescribe her some weight-loss pills?'
- 'I think she should go back to university or get a job. It's not healthy for a girl her age to sit at home and play computer games all day. Don't you agree, Doctor?'

Model Answer

There are three main issues in this station. Firstly, the candidate must manage the interaction between Melissa and her mother. Secondly, it is important to screen for symptoms of schizophrenia. Finally, the presenting complaint of weight gain must be addressed.

It is not uncommon for adolescents and younger adults to be brought to the clinic by their parents. In some cases, the identified patient and their family member may have different opinions on whether there is a problem, the nature of the problem, and what should be done about it. As such, the good student should identify the opinion and agenda of both Melissa and Karen and avoid focusing on only one individual. Pausing and reframing information is often useful in understanding the problem.

The candidate should explain that both Melissa's and Karen's points of view are equally important to prevent them from feeling that sides are being taken. Taking a 'one down' position may facilitate this, where the candidate asks both Melissa and Karen to educate the candidate about their situation, such as, 'I'm trying to understand what this might be like for the both of you, so it would be useful if you could tell me what it's like for you, Melissa, and also what it's like for you, Karen ...'

Seeking points of commonality is also a useful strategy for defusing a tense situation in order to facilitate history-taking. An example might be, 'What I'm hearing is that this is a really stressful time for both of you', or 'It sounds like you both feel that you're being blamed and that must be hard.'

The candidate should screen for current psychotic symptoms in order to ascertain whether the recent increase in olanzapine has had the intended effect (see pages 93–96). The candidate should also screen for depressive symptoms.

Depressive episodes are common after psychotic episodes (see Chapter 8, Depressive disorders). Substance use should be screened for (see pages 367–369).

The crucial element in establishing the cause of Melissa's weight gain is the temporal course, particularly the relationship between the increase in olanzapine dose and the increase in appetite. The good student will ask about changes in activity and should consider possible medical causes, such as hypothyroidism and Cushing's syndrome.

The candidate's short-term management should include liaising with the patient's treating psychiatrist and discussing the risks and benefits of decreasing the olanzapine or changing to another antipsychotic with less potential for weight gain, such as aripriprazole, amisulpride, or ziprasidone. It would be unwise for the GP registrar to make changes to the antipsychotic prior to review by the psychiatrist. Ongoing input from the psychiatrist is essential to minimise the risk of relapse. Both the patient and her family should be involved in this process, which should be based on informed consent of the risks and benefits of proposed management. The candidate should emphasise the risks involved with the discontinuation of antipsychotics.

FOR THE MORE ADVANCED LEARNER

The GP registrar should address the mother's concern about weight gain. Rather than prescribing pills for weight loss, the GP registrar should discuss lifestyle modifications, such as a referral to a dietician and exercise options. The GP registrar should also monitor ongoing metabolic risks, including BMI, waist-to-hip ratio, and regular lipid and glucose tests. This should be part of a shared care arrangement with the mental health clinic.

The candidate should be aware of the high expressed emotion in this scenario and recognise that a family intervention could be helpful, although this would probably best be raised at another time (see Family environment, page 102 and The family in treatment, page 106).

Chapter 8

DEPRESSIVE DISORDERS

DARRYL BASSETT & DAVID J CASTLE

We all know what it means to feel sad and unhappy, and in English we often use the term 'depression' to describe that experience. We use this term to describe many states in which there are features such as unhappy mood, including grief, and those which also involve disruption of other functions, such as thinking, self-esteem, sleep, perception of energy, sexual interest, appetite, the experience of pleasure generally and the ability to interact with other people. While grief is a normal response to significant loss (discussed later in this chapter), the latter states which involve persistent and/or severe disruption of function, are called 'depressive disorders'. Normal grief is clearly linked to the loss, some capacity to experience positive emotion persists (even if fleeting) and the mood is predominantly one of sadness rather than emptiness. Depressive disorders are more common in women (lifetime prevalence about 11%) than men (lifetime prevalence about 6%). Table 8.1 lists the diagnostic criteria for depressive episodes in adults.

Table 8.1

Features of a depressive episode in adults according to DSM-IV-TR and ICD-10 (synopsis)

DSM-IV-TR Major depressive episode	ICD-10 Depressive episode
Five (or more) of the following symptoms (must include either (1) or (2)) on most days, for most of the day, over at least 2 weeks, associated with distress and impairment of functioning: 1 depressed mood 2 markedly diminished interest or pleasure in all or most activities 3 significant weight loss when not dieting 4 insomnia or hypersomnia 5 psychomotor agitation or retardation 6 fatigue or loss of energy 7 feelings of worthlessness or excessive or inappropriate guilt 8 diminished ability to think or concentrate, or indecisiveness 9 recurrent thoughts of death (not just fear of dying), recurrent suicidal ideation, or suicidal plan. Exclusions: 1 Part of mixed mood episode 2 Better accounted for by bereavement 3 Better accounted for by direct effect of a substance 4 Better accounted for by a general medical condition.	Classification into mild, moderate or severe depression is determined by the number of items below that can be identified: 1 depressed mood to a degree that is definitely abnormal for the individual, present for most of the day and almost every day, largely uninfluenced by circumstances, and sustained for at least 2 weeks 2 loss of interest or pleasure in activities that are normally pleasurable 3 decreased energy or increased fatigability. An additional symptom or symptoms from the following list should be present, to give a total of at least four: 1 loss of confidence or self-esteem 2 unreasonable feelings of self-reproach or excessive and inappropriate guilt 3 recurrent thoughts of death or suicide or any suicidal behaviour 4 complaints or evidence of diminished ability to think or concentrate, such as indecisiveness or vacillation 5 change in psychomotor activity, with agitation or retardation (either subjective or objective) 6 sleep disturbance of any type 7 change in appetite (decrease or increase) with corresponding weight change.

Box 8.1

Core elements of depressive disorders

- Mood state best described as emptiness
- Anhedonia
- Restricted reactivity in mood
- Negative thought content
- Poor self-esteem
- Significant disruption of sleep accompanied by fatigue
- Amotivation
- Anergia
- Hopelessness
- Helplessness

Clinical features of depressive disorders

Changes in mood

These are predominantly an experience of emptiness rather than sadness. There is little or no capacity for the experience of pleasure (anhedonia), a core feature of depressive disorders. The unpleasant mood tends to be present almost constantly, often with an exacerbation in the mornings and improvement in the evenings (diurnal mood variation) and is associated with the melancholic or somatic subtype of depressive disorder (see Box 8.2). Diurnal mood variation may also be evident during times of high emotional stress and is not a pathognomonic feature of depressive disorder. People with a depressive disorder tend to exhibit a relative lack of response to events or circumstances (loss of 'reactivity' of mood). Unpleasant arousal (anxiety) and anger are sometimes prominent.

Changes in thinking

Depressive disorders have an effect upon thought content and are often provoked by persistently negative and self-defeating patterns of thought about the self, the past and/or the future. Poor self-esteem is often prominent among these. Excessive guilt about actual or even imagined wrong-doings may develop and suicidal thoughts are common. The capacity to think may be significantly impaired (e.g. concentration, memory and comprehension) and executive cognitive functions (decision-making, abstract thinking, changing set, problem solving, etc) may also be affected. Severe impairment of thought function and physical spontaneity is called 'psychomotor retardation' (see melancholia).

Changes in vegetative functions

Disturbances of basic biological functions may occur. Sleep disruption is common, even when depressive illness is relatively mild. Sleep is restless and unrefreshing. Difficulty initiating sleep is due to heightened arousal and anxiety. Waking spontaneously several

Box 8.2

Melancholic (DSM-IV-TR) or somatic (ICD-10) subtype
of depression

- Meets criteria for major depressive episode or severe depression
- Marked psychomotor disorder; retardation or agitation
- Loss of pleasure in all activities, including libido
- Lack of reactivity to pleasurable stimuli
- Distinct quality of depressed mood; different to grief
- Depression much worse in mornings
- Early morning waking; at least 2 hours earlier than usual
- Severe anorexia and/or weight loss
- Excessive or inappropriate guilt

hours earlier than usual (terminal insomnia or early morning waking) may be indicative of increasing severity in depressive illness, and is usually accompanied by diurnal mood variation. Appetite may be reduced (anorexia) and weight loss is common. Energy is typically impaired (anergia) and motivation reduced (amotivation). Finally there is usually reduced libido (sex drive).

Changes in self-care

Self-care often suffers during depressive disorders. The loss of motivation extends to grooming, personal hygiene and dress. Usually the more severe the depressive disorder, the more extreme the disruption of self-care, and the greater risk of self-injury from self-neglect. When psychosis is present the extent of self-neglect can become profound and life-threatening.

Changes in social interaction

Social interaction is often reduced and the consequent social isolation aggravates the depressive illness. Some individuals may actively avoid contact with others because of self-reproach, lack of motivation or embarrassment because of lack of their usual spontaneity. Box 8.1 lists the core elements of depressive disorders and Box 8.2 the core elements of melancholic depression.

Psychotic depression

In some instances the depressive disorder can become psychotic in intensity, with loss of contact with reality and serious risk of self-injury or neglect. *Delusions* in depressive states are mostly linked to negative and self-critical themes (mood congruent delusions). Guilt and self-criticism may become extreme and distorted, with beliefs of being evil or responsible for tragic world events. There may be distortion of body image with delusions of decay in the sufferer's body or of horrible changes taking place. Sometimes the delusional

Box 8.3
Atypical depression

- Mood remains reactive to events
- High sensitivity to rejection
- 'Leaden' feeling in limbs
- Hypersomnia; 2 hours or more of sleep beyond the normal duration
- Hyperphagia (increased appetite), usually with weight gain

beliefs may not contain links to the other depressive symptoms and involve paranoid themes or bizarre notions about the sufferer or the world (mood-incongruent delusions).

Hallucinations may occur and are often auditory in form. For example, the person may hear a voice making critical and disparaging remarks about them, in either the second or third person. Sometimes the sufferer may experience olfactory hallucinations of their body emitting a foul odour (perhaps as it is perceived to decay). Psychotic depression is a particularly severe and destructive form of depressive illness and carries a high mortality rate from suicide.

Less 'typical' presentations

Not all people who suffer depressive disorders present initially with the features outlined above. This less typical presentation is called *atypical depression* (see Box 8.3) and may have implications for choice of treatment. Depressive disorders may also present with less typical features in specific situations, such as during childhood, adolescence, advanced age, in association with pregnancy, premenstrually, and in association with intellectual disability (see Box 8.4).

Natural history of depression

Most depressive disorders arise slowly (bipolar depression is often an exception; see Chapter 9) and have been present for some time before a person presents for assistance. The earliest reported symptoms are often changes in sleep or energy, with other features accumulating over time. If left untreated, depressive disorders may improve spontaneously, but this may take months to years and the risk of suicide is significant. Many individuals will not improve spontaneously and remain depressed for the rest of their lives, usually with some fluctuations in severity. The toll of depressive illness upon the sufferer is enormous and the consequences may include loss of relationships, careers, general health, as well as suicide. Chronic untreated (or inadequately treated) melancholic depressive disorders often result in loss of brain tissue, which may or may not be reversible with treatment. Those close to a person with a depressive disorder also suffer and are often forgotten.

Different diagnoses

Grief is an entirely healthy response to loss and will include the experience of sadness for that which has been lost. The experience of grief and its expression (mourning) is variable

Box 8.4
Special groups and settings

- *Children* may often present with enuresis, encopresis, school refusal or behavioural problems while suffering from depression.
- *Adolescents* often turn to substance abuse or antisocial behaviour as a way of trying to cope with their experience of depression.
- The *elderly* may present with social withdrawal, constipation, weight loss or anhedonia as their prime concern when depressed.
- Depression arising in *pregnancy or post-partum* is of particular concern as women often feel guilty about becoming depressed at such a 'special' time. Nevertheless, depressive symptoms at these times are not uncommon and must be taken very seriously. The welfare of the foetus or infant must also be considered carefully in management. Infanticide is a very real risk.
- Those with *comorbid intellectual disability* present with depressive disorders, but this may be reflected more in behaviour than in self-report. Information from observers and family will be invaluable, and their involvement in treatment essential (see Chapter 21).
- *Premenstrual dysphoric disorder* is a syndrome of depressive symptoms which arise immediately before the menses (up to 2 weeks). Irritability, abdominal discomfort and even suicidal thoughts may accompany the depressive symptoms. Serotonergic antidepressants (e.g. SSRIs) can be very helpful. Premenstrual exacerbation of current depressive symptoms may also occur.

Box 8.5
Normal phases of grief

- Initial shock
- Numbing, detachment
- Anger
- Denial
- Somatic and emotional discomfort and withdrawal
- Acceptance
- Return to pre-bereavement level of functioning.

and will be determined by personality, past life experience, current life context, cultural traditions and expectations, and the nature of the loss. The experience may include absence of emotion ('numbing' or 'detachment'), overwhelming distress, anger, denial of the loss and/or preoccupation with the lost object. Auditory, visual and even other modalities of hallucinations may occur, are mostly reassuring and positive, and are not pathological in nature. Sometimes the individual is unable to integrate the loss constructively into their experience of life (*pathological grief*) and transitions into a depressive disorder (see Box 8.5 and Box 16.2, page 266).

Box 8.6

General medical conditions sometimes associated with depressive disorders (an incomplete list)

- Cerebrovascular events (stroke)
- Hypothyroidism
- Hypomagnesaemia
- Cushing's syndrome
- Addison's disease
- Hypocalcaemia
- Viral infections including Epstein-Barr virus and Human Acquired Immunodeficiency Virus
- Delirium presenting in apathetic form
- Dementia of various pathologies
- Deficiencies of vitamin B group; possibly vitamin D and others
- Medications including corticosteroids, antineoplastic medications, etc
- Intracerebral neoplasia
- Autoimmune cerebral vasculitis
- Acquired brain injury; trauma.

Grief and other distressing reactions to unpleasant life circumstances which are persistent and interfere with function but do *not* meet criteria for a depressive disorder are diagnosed as *adjustment disorders*, further specified by the predominant symptoms (e.g. with depressed mood or anxious mood).

Schizophrenia is often accompanied by depressive disorder and negative symptoms of schizophrenia may be confused with depressive disorder (see Chapter 7). Depressive disorder comorbid with schizophrenia can be severe, with a high risk of suicide.

A number of *general medical disorders* can provoke depressed mood (see Box 8.6), but the depression may persist after these have been treated. The sufferer may present with emotionally focused depressive symptoms, such as persistently depressed mood or anhedonia, or less specific symptoms such as insomnia, anergia or weight loss. The contribution of depressive illness to these symptoms may be significant and treatment of the depressive illness may bring about significant improvement. However, usually the symptoms are mixed in origin and the outcome will be optimal when both the medical condition and depressive disorder are treated. Indeed, each will usually affect the other and treating both will give the best outcome.

The separation of physical symptoms of a general medical disorder and major depressive disorders can be challenging, particularly in the elderly. Anhedonia is a useful symptom for helping to distinguish, as the loss of the capacity for pleasure is unusual in all but the most severe of medical disorders. The history will often give very useful information to differentiate, with depression carrying a background of developing dysphoria and other typical depressive symptoms. Diurnal mood variation is unusual in most general medical disorders, although it can be seen with non-specific stress. Psychotic depression may arise in association with medical disorders, but is usually part of a

Case examples: Depressive disorders

- An 18-year-old student presented with difficulty studying and complained of being unable to concentrate, suffering a loss of interest in her subjects and exhibiting a decline in personal hygiene for months. Cognitive and behaviour therapy was employed, and while she made some progress her core symptoms of impaired concentration and poor motivation for self-care persisted. The addition of fluoxetine was very helpful and she was able to resume her studies the following year.

- A 28-year-old casual factory hand presented with financial problems because he had not been able to work and was only paid when he attended work. He complained that he had great difficulty getting going in the mornings and by the time he did get up, felt it was too late to go to work. Treatment with cognitive and behaviour therapy, combined with desvenlafaxine, was very rewarding, and he was able to resume full time work after several months. The focus of management moved to a better understanding of the development of his illness and the strategies he could use to prevent further relapse.

- A woman of 26 presented 6 months after the birth of her first child with lack of interest in her baby and intense guilt about not wanting the child. She stated: 'I feel like throwing her at the wall when she cries and then feel overwhelmed with guilt. I just can't go on like this'. She responded well to an antidepressant and cognitive-behaviour therapy, and gained benefit from admission to a psychiatric facility that specialised in perinatal disorders. However, she suffered a relapse of her depressive disorder 2 years later and has struggled with recurrent episodes since that time.

- A man of 68 presented at the insistence of his children because he was increasingly forgetful and disinterested in his personal hygiene. He said he had never been the same since his wife died. He was diagnosed with melancholic depression and responded to a course of ECT and supportive psychotherapy, including grief therapy. There was no evidence of underlying dementia following completion of treatment and he has remained well.

- A 45-year-old medical practitioner presented saying she felt stupid coming for such a silly reason but she had been finding that she was struggling to take an interest in her patients, was sleeping poorly and lacked energy. She thought she might be depressed but had always thought that her knowledge of medicine should enable her to cope with depression by herself. She responded to a combination of an antidepressant and cognitive behaviour therapy, and addressed the challenges of managing a busy general practice while raising two teenage children.

- A man of 50 presented saying that he had been drinking much more alcohol than ever before and was recently charged with driving while intoxicated. He could not sleep without drinking and was worried he might lose his job because of his drinking. His wife was very worried and said he had 'not been himself for almost a year' and was unusually aggressive and unpleasant. He responded to detoxification from alcohol in hospital, with the addition of an antidepressant and subsequent cognitive behaviour therapy, but was later found to suffer from an early frontotemporal dementia.

comorbid depressive illness. As mentioned in Chapter 6, 'when in doubt, think organic', and when depressive disorder is suspected comorbid with medical disorder, treat for both.

Aetiology of depressive disorders

Genetic factors

Pedigree studies in depressive disorders show a significant increase in the risk that first degree relatives of sufferers will also develop similar disorders. The odds ratio for the development of depressive disorders in these relatives is about 2.8, suggesting a significant role for heritability in depressive disorders generally.

Twin studies show a heritability for depressive disorders in general of between 30% and 40%, with evidence that individual environmental factors contribute about 60% to 70% of the variance in incidence of these disorders. Shared environmental factors do not seem to contribute beyond individual experience. *Adoption studies* confirm a similar pattern.

A number of *gene polymorphisms*, including those for the serotonin transporter (5-HTTLPR-short form) and brain-derived neurotrophic factor (Val66Met), appear significant in depressive disorders. The presence of either or both specific polymorphisms is associated with a significantly higher risk of developing a major depressive disorder (it is highest when both are present), when combined with early life stress. Modulation of epigenetic processes that involve protein-modification of DNA/histones also appear significant, and other genetic differences probably also contribute to increased vulnerability.

Neuroimaging

Reduced metabolic activity and blood flow within the prefrontal cortex and anterior cingulate gyrus have been shown in depressive disorders. Limbic regions such as the amygdala may show increased activity.

In chronic depression the hippocampus is often reduced in size (perhaps because of reduced neurotrophic factor release) and other regions may show similar changes. MRI scanning has shown that in later age small areas of brain injury associated with hyperintensity correlated with the severity of depressive disorder.

Figure 8.1 shows computer-generated images of a Single Photon Emission Computerised Tomography (SPECT) scan of a patient with a depressive disorder.

Neurochemistry

Amines

Among the hundreds of neurotransmitters in the human brain the amines serotonin, noradrenaline and dopamine (see Box 8.7) appear particularly important in depressive disorders. This conclusion has followed a series of observations, including the propensity of certain drugs to provoke depression, altered physiological responses to certain drugs, measurements of metabolites of these amines in depressed people, and the observation that substances that relieve depressive symptoms enhance the release of these amines. Defective response of the *serotonin*-releasing nerve pathways impedes the capacity of the brain to cope with stress, including high circulating cortisol levels, excessive activity in glutamate-releasing nerve pathways and changes in immune function. Defective activity in the *noradrenaline*-releasing nerve pathways impedes the activation of important brain

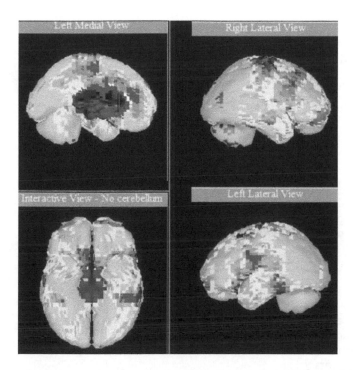

Figure 8.1 Scan shows moderately reduced blood flow to prefrontal cortex, temporal cortex, cingulate gyrus and medial frontal cortex which are features sometimes associated with severe depressive disorders (Courtesy of Dr Joe Cardaci)

Legend:
medium grey = two standard deviations above or below the mean blood flow in healthy people
white = between two and three standard deviations below the mean
dark grey = between three and four standard deviations below the mean
very dark grey/black = five or more standard deviations below the mean

Box 8.7
Summary of action of serotonin, noradrenaline and dopamine

- *Serotonin* has a significant role in modulating mood, aggression, sleep and appetite
- *Noradrenaline* has a role in modulating drive, focusing of thought, mood and appetite
- *Dopamine* has important roles in pleasure, sex, thinking and psychomotor function

mechanisms that are regulated by these pathways. The absence of activity in the *dopamine*-releasing nerves pathways reduces the experience of pleasure (dopamine is the key transmitter in reward pathways) and ease-of-thought processing.

Intracellular signal transduction

Alterations in signal transduction, such as altered activity of phosphokinases A and C (including from the action of 'radical oxygen species'), have been detected in various forms of depressive illness and appear relevant through their effect upon the translation of cell receptor activation to DNA transcription.

Peptides and acetylcholine

While the focus has been heavily upon amines in depression, gamma aminobutyric acid (GABA), corticotropin releasing factor (CRF), thyrotropin releasing factor (TRF), glutamate, somatostatin, a range of neurotrophic factors, tachykinins and other peptides have been implicated in depressive disorders. CRF is critical to the response to stress and activation of the hypothalamic-pituitary-adrenal axis (HPA axis), discussed under Endocrinology.

Endocrinology

Excessive activity of the HPA axis appears associated with many depressive disorders. Individuals with depressive illness show increased production of CRF, with disruption of the feedback loop between cortisol production and the hypothalamus, because of altered function of glucocorticoid receptors.

Thyroid hormone release is altered in many people with depressive disorders because of reduced output of thyrotropin releasing factor (TRH). At the same time, adding liothryronine in depressives disorders can be therapeutic, perhaps because of increased sensitivity to amines.

Immunology

Cytokines are heavily involved in the inter-cellular signalling processes that accompany immune functions. They also have effects upon glucocorticoid receptors and synaptic activity through modifications in transmitter activity. Interleukins 1 & 6, plus tumour necrosis factor-α are recognised as particularly relevant, and probably others are also involved. As numerous hormones (CRF, cortisol, TRH, growth hormone, growth hormone releasing factor, etc) significantly modulate cytokines and other immunological processes, the complexity of the neurobiology of depressive disorders is evident.

Sleep

Sleep process is usually disturbed in depressive illness, with increased duration of rapid eye movement (REM) sleep, earlier onset of REM sleep episodes, increased eye movement during REM periods (REM density), reduced deep sleep (stages 3 and 4) and significant changes in total sleep duration (mostly reduced and sometimes increased). Further, it is known that disruption of circadian rhythms may significantly aggravate depressive disorders.

Psychosocial contributions

Thoughts, relationships, life events and personality development all contribute significantly to the onset of depressive disorders and to relapse. Certain *personality traits* have been found to be relevant. These include a heightened tendency to become anxious (neuroticism or high trait anxiety), poor self-esteem, prominent sensitivity to interpersonal interactions, a perception of relative helplessness, prominent dependence upon others (particularly someone who is highly admired), prominent need to be highly independent and perfectionistic, or a combination of these traits.

Psychoanalytic theorists have suggested that significant disruption of the early mother/infant relationship distorts a person's capacity to cope with loss (particularly of significant people or relationships) or may severely disrupt a person's capacity to relate to others intimately, leaving them vulnerable in close relationships.

Cognitive therapists have emphasised the power of a person's thoughts about themself, their past and their future. Persistently negative or destructive beliefs promote persistent self-destructive thoughts and feelings, particularly at times of life stress. These beliefs are called 'schemas' and emerge during the developmental years. With time they become entrenched and are easily activated by life stresses. Learning to challenge these entrenched beliefs, assumptions and attitudes can be very relieving. When a depressive disorder has become chronic in nature, learning to tolerate and accept the negative aspects of this illness while striving to find new ways of approaching life positively, can again be very relieving.

Some psychological therapists have emphasised the impact of distorted learning from repeated negative experiences, thus producing a state of '*learned helplessness*'.

Finally, there are those therapists who emphasise the nature of close relationships or *systemic distortions* in the development of mood-related symptoms. The person may experience symptoms that reflect these distorted relationships or the 'system' in which they are living.

Management of depressive disorders

The management of the depressed patient requires a comprehensive assessment, engagement, and a treatment plan that addresses biological and psychosocial domains. The elements are summarised in Box 8.8.

Basic clinical strategies and challenges

The management of a person with a depressive illness begins with the process of assessment, which becomes potentially therapeutic (supportive psychotherapy) because the person has an opportunity to experience hope, to experience feeling understood and supported, and to release painful emotions and thought content.

During initial contact, the therapist must try to establish a working relationship by showing genuine interest in the person and their experience of depression. Crying is a common event and the patient may find this relieving and therapeutic. Often, crying and emotional expression generally, become less common with increasing severity of depressive disorder. A clinician should be concerned about the depressed patient who exhibits no emotion at all, but is functionally impaired. The therapist must strive to clarify the details of thoughts, feelings and perceptions, while maintaining flexibility to suit the needs of the person.

Suicidality

See Chapter 17 on emergency psychiatry.

Box 8.8
Depression: management summary

- Hope is fundamental; provide and maintain
- Safety is paramount; *consider suicide risk*
- Features of illness give direction to treatment
- Establish first depressive symptoms in lifetime
- Personality factors are highly relevant
- Review family history
- Consider sleep management
- Review substance use
- Consider general medical health
- Give information about depressive illness
- Offer immediate coping strategies
- Introduce medications if appropriate
- Introduce further psychological interventions when appropriate
- Always arrange follow-up
- Consider speaking with significant others
- Obtain past experience from previous therapists
- Monitor mental state, core symptoms and function

Psychological therapies

(see Chapter 16)

Supportive psychotherapy is the foundation of managing depressive disorders. Talking and empathic listening are relieving for most and open the opportunity for further treatment.

Cognitive therapy identifies and strives to correct those thoughts and thought patterns which are distorted and therefore provoke negativity and self-defeat.

Behaviour therapy addresses the behaviours that contribute to the depressed state, including lack of exercise, lack of pleasurable activities, avoidance of contact with significant others, and absence of self-care. In practice this is often linked with cognitive therapy, so-called *cognitive-behaviour therapy (CBT)*.

Interpersonal psychotherapy (IPT) explores a person's relationships and the impact of these upon that person's experience of themselves and others.

Psychodynamic therapies explore inner psychological experience and examine the impact of less obvious or 'unconscious' thoughts and feelings.

Family therapies focus upon the 'system' in which a person lives, their 'family,' and work to modify distortions in that system.

Biological therapies

(see Chapter 15)
While some people suffering from depressive disorders respond to psychological therapies alone, others do not. Biological therapies are most effective when used for depressive disorders of at least moderate severity and when somatic or melancholic features are evident. Some form of psychotherapy remains essential as antidepressants will not change styles of thinking, relationships or the management of life problems. However, antidepressant medications will facilitate cognitive and emotional functioning, restoration of energy, drive and motivation, and the recovery of basic biological functions such as appetite, sex drive, mobility, cognitive functions and self-care.

Antidepressant medications

These medications facilitate recovery of the biological elements of depressive disorders by modifying levels of amines in the brain and subsequently enhancing release of nerve growth factors. They are effective in about 60% to 70% of people who suffer more than mildly severe depression. Treatment with these medications should be for at least 6 months and often longer, including indefinitely in some patients (see Chapter 15).

Adjunctive medications and treatments

(see Chapter 15)
Omega-3 fatty acids: There is increasing evidence that supplements containing these fatty acids (e.g. fish oil capsules) are beneficial in major mood disorders. Doses of at least 3,000 mg per day are required.

Exercise: Regular cardio-pulmonary and strength exercise is highly advantageous to patients with psychological disorders of all kinds and particularly major mood disorders and schizophrenia.

Folic acid: Deficiency is destructive to mental state and supplements may be essential if deficiency is evident.

Magnesium and zinc: Deficiency is destructive to mental state and supplements may be appropriate.

Other physical therapies

(see Chapter 15)
Electroconvulsive therapy (ECT) is a highly effective, well tolerated and safe treatment for depressive disorders in which melancholic or somatic features are prominent, and/or psychosis is present. This is particularly relevant when depressive stupor or catatonia is present, and the illness is seriously life-threatening. It is effective in more than 90% of patients suffering from severe melancholic depression or psychotic depression.

Light therapy may be helpful for some patients whose illness shows a strong association with seasonal changes or who have severe disruption of their circadian rhythm.

Transcranial Magnetic Stimulation (TMS), *Vagal Nerve Stimulation (VNS)* and *Deep Brain Stimulation* are options for treatment of severely treatment resistant depression.

Prognosis

Many people who suffer an episode of depressive disorder will not suffer further episodes. Relapse increases the risk of further episodes of depressive illness, with the probability of relapse increasing with the number of episodes. The prognosis is worse when substance abuse, other major psychiatric disorder or physical disorder, family history of mood disorder or social isolation are present.

REFERENCES AND FURTHER READING

Castle, D., Kulkarni, J., Abel, K. (Eds.), 2006. Mood and anxiety disorders in women. Cambridge University Press, Cambridge.

Iosifescu, D., Nierenberg, A. (Eds.), 2007. New developments in depression research. Psychiatric Clinics of North America. Saunders, Philadelphia.

Joyce, P., Mitchell, P. (Eds.), 2004. Mood disorders: recognition and treatment. University of New South Wales Press, Sydney.

Krishnan, V., Nestler, E.J., 2008. The molecular neurobiology of depression. Nature 455, 894–902.

Parker, G., 1996. Melancholia: a disorder of movement and mood. Cambridge University Press, New York.

Parker, G., Manicavasagar, V., 2005. Modelling and managing the depressive disorders. A clinical guide. Cambridge University Press, Cambridge.

Tanner, S., Ball, J., 1991. Beating the blues. Southwood Press, Sydney.

CHAPTER 8

AN ELDERLY MAN NAMED FRED
CASE-BASED LEARNING

JOEL KING & ANDREW GLEASON

The following role-play requires two students: one to play the nights intern (candidate) and another to play two roles, that of a patient named Fred Jones and the examiner (actor).

OSCE Station Instructions

(Reading time: 2 minutes)

You are the nights intern in a small country hospital in the town of Harrisville. There is no psychiatry ward. You receive a page from Mary, a nurse on the surgical ward. She asks you to see Mr Fred Jones, an 80-year-old man from Itchy Bark, an even smaller town 100 km from Harrisville. He lives alone and fell yesterday, resulting in an open Colles' fracture, which required open reduction and internal fixation earlier today. He is due for discharge tomorrow morning. Mary is concerned that he looks very sad and wonders how he will cope at home.

Task (10 minutes)

- Take a history from Mr Jones that is relevant to Mary's concerns (8 minutes).
- After 8 minutes, you must terminate the interview and present a brief management plan for Mr Jones to the examiner (2 minutes).
- You do not need to physically examine the patient.

Actor role: Fred Jones

You are an 80-year-old man who lives alone in the small town of Itchy Bark. You lost your wife, Beth, to cancer six months ago and have not recovered from her death. Beth became unwell last year. You were married for over fifty years and have two children who live far away in the city. You met Beth at school and married in your twenties. You were very happy together. You worked teaching maths at secondary school until you retired at 65. Prior to Beth becoming unwell, the two of you enjoyed going to the bowls club and socialising with friends.

Your children have families of their own and you rarely see them. You would like to see them more and appreciate it when they call, but you understand that they are busy and live far away. Roger is 55 and works as a corporate manager. Nicky is 50 and in charge of the physiotherapy department at St Christopher's Hospital.

DEPRESSIVE SYMPTOMS

You have tried to get on with your life as much as possible since Beth's death. You spend most of your time watching TV and doing the gardening, but you have found it more and more difficult to tend to the house and garden. You have no motivation to go to the bowls club or play bingo any more. It is also hard to go out to buy groceries and cook. You make very simple meals and only eat twice a day. You're not very hungry and don't really enjoy food any more. You have lost a lot of weight, although you're not sure how much. Most of your clothes now fit very loosely. You find little pleasure in anything. You feel constantly tired and your body feels heavy. Your sleep is poor – you lie awake for a long time, wake earlier than usual, and the little sleep you do get is broken.

SUICIDAL IDEATION

For the last month or so, you've wondered why you bother living. You think it might be easier not being here. You have never thought about actively ending your own life because that would disappoint Beth too much, because she enjoyed life immensely, and you're afraid of pain. You have never attempted suicide. There is no family history of suicide.

OTHER PSYCHIATRIC HISTORY

You have never had any symptoms of anxiety, psychosis or mania. You have never used drugs and rarely drink alcohol. You find it difficult to concentrate and your attention is poor, but you have never been diagnosed with cognitive impairment.

COLLES' FRACTURE

This was a simple mechanical fall in the dark and you tripped on the porch step. There was no loss of consciousness, head trauma, or neurological symptoms. You have no gait problems.

MEDICAL HISTORY

You have no significant medical history and take no medications regularly. Before Beth became unwell, you were actively playing bowls without difficulty.

SOCIAL SUPPORTS

You have no immediate family nearby. You receive no assistance from community services. You have stopped seeing your friends from the bowls and bingo clubs over the last few months. You have not seen the town GP since Beth died. He did telephone once, but you told him that you were fine.

HOW TO PLAY THE ROLE

You should appear melancholically depressed. Your eyes should be downcast. Your voice is monotonous. You appear immensely tired and slowed down. You should try to cooperate with the doctor's questions as best you can. You are okay with going home tomorrow if the doctor suggests this.

Model Answer

The good candidate will recognise that there are two key tasks to this station. The first is to establish a diagnosis. Students should recognise that this man has a depressed mood and establish whether he has other symptoms of a depressive disorder (see Table 8.1, page 113). Students should establish the temporal course of Mr Jones's depression and the change in his baseline function. The death of Mr Jones's wife appears to be the precipitant to his current depression. Some students might wonder whether Mr Jones's current presentation is normal bereavement. Grief and mourning are common and natural after a significant loss (see pages 116–118). There is a grey zone between normal bereavement and something pathological. In this case, Mr Jones has symptoms that are clearly consistent with a major depressive disorder. These are more severe than one would typically expect with normal bereavement, of longer duration, and have a significant impact on his functioning.

The good student will recognise that there are multiple medical conditions that can masquerade as depression, especially in the elderly (see Box 8.6, page 118). Chronic illness, such as hypothyroidism, anaemia, heart failure and chronic obstructive pulmonary disease, cause many of the physical features of depression, such as poor energy, impaired concentration, and sleep and appetite disturbance.

The second key task in this station is to address the nurse's concern about Mr Jones's ability to cope at home. Mr Jones will be in a cast and a sling and this will impair his ability to do basic activities of daily living (ADLs), such as toileting, showering and cooking. This is compounded by the fact that he lives alone, has no family or community supports, and is depressed. Other risks, such as suicidality, should be considered.

As such, the prudent step is to delay the discharge until a safe plan can be established. This may involve calling family, setting up community supports, and obtaining psychiatric input in the treatment of Mr Jones's depression.

FOR THE MORE ADVANCED LEARNER

Delirium and dementia are common in the elderly and may masquerade as depression. Certain medications, such as beta blockers and interferon, can also cause depression. As such, the good student would factor exclusion of these differential diagnoses into the management plan.

Some students may mention starting various treatments for depression in their management plan, but they should show an understanding of the real world applicability of these treatments to this clinical scenario. Students should recognise that starting an antidepressant will not be effective immediately and will require ongoing monitoring for effectiveness and side effects. Psychological therapy, particularly supportive, interpersonal or cognitive-behavioural, may be useful, but this is unlikely to be feasible and immediately beneficial prior to discharge from a surgical ward. These therapies also require trained practitioners. ECT may have a role (see pages 125 and 249–251), but this would require transfer to a psychiatric unit, preferably one specialising in old age psychiatry.

Chapter 9

BIPOLAR AND RELATED DISORDERS

DARRYL BASSETT & DAVID J CASTLE

Bipolar mood disorders (BD) are characterised by the occurrence of elevated mood and (usually) depressed mood, either at different times or simultaneously (see Table 9.1, Box 9.1). The precise delineation between 'normal' mood swings, mood instability as part of a personality disorder, and mood swings that are an indicator of bipolar disorder, is complex. As in all mood disorders, the disruption of normal mood is not the only or even necessarily the most prominent element of the disorder. The core elements of bipolar disorders are summarised in Box 9.1.

Prevalence of bipolar disorders

The lifetime prevalence for bipolar affective disorder type I, with severe manic and depressed episodes, is about 0.8–1% of the population. The prevalence for those with type II bipolar disorder (with less severe 'hypomanic' mood swings) is about 2–3%. The prevalence of the whole bipolar spectrum of disorders (see below) is about 4–5%. Bipolar disorder I has an equal gender distribution, while bipolar disorder II and cyclothymia are more common in females.

Table 9.1

Features of bipolar affective disorder according to DSM–IV–TR and ICD–10 (synopsis)

DSM–IV–TR	ICD–10
Manic episode A distinct period of abnormally and persistently elevated, expansive, or irritable mood, lasting at least 1 week (or any duration if hospitalisation is necessary). **Hypomanic episode** A distinct period of persistently elevated, expansive, or irritable mood, lasting throughout at least 4 days, that is clearly different from the usual non-depressed mood.	**F31 bipolar affective disorder** A disorder characterised by two or more episodes in which the patient's mood and activity levels are significantly disturbed; this disturbance consisting on some occasions of an elevation of mood and increased energy and activity (hypomania or mania) and on others of a lowering of mood and decreased energy and activity (depression). Repeated episodes of hypomania or mania only are classified as bipolar.

Box 9.1

Core elements of bipolar disorder

- Mood swings with periods of elevated mood (manic phase) and periods of depressed mood (depressed phase).
- Manic phases of illness are accompanied by increased energy, expansive thinking, pressured speech, disinhibited behaviour and reduced need for sleep.
- Depressed phases are accompanied by reduced energy, negative thinking, poor self-esteem, psychomotor changes and impaired sleep.
- Depressed phases of illness are more common than manic phases.
- 'Mixed' states with more irritability and aggression than euphoric mood may occur.
- Pathological mood swings tend to be independent of life events, persistent for more than 2 days, and often incongruous for the circumstances.
- Manic and depressive episodes may include psychotic features.

Clinical features of bipolar disorder

Mania

Mania is a mental state in which motivation, energy, mood and/or thinking are elevated. The need for sleep is reduced, thought content is more grandiose, speed of thinking is increased, but thoughts remain connected ('flight of ideas'), distractibility is high, libido is increased, behaviour is more socially disinhibited (including excessive spending of

Box 9.2
Summary of management strategies

Mania

- Establish therapeutic rapport as much as possible.
- Employ compulsory treatment if personal welfare is seriously at risk or others are at risk because of this illness.
- Administer an atypical antipsychotic (see Chapter 15).
- Introduce a mood stabiliser (see Chapter 15).
- Provide individual psychotherapy and psychoeducation.
- Engage 'significant others' in psychoeducation and further management as appropriate.
- Group therapy may be appropriate.

Depression

- Establish therapeutic rapport as much as possible.
- Introduce a mood stabiliser (see Chapter 15).
- Introduce quetiapine or other atypical antipsychotic if severe or response to a mood stabiliser after 2 weeks is poor.
- Consider adding an antidepressant if response after at least 1 month of maximally tolerated doses is poor.
- Consider using ECT if progress is poor or illness is very severe.
- Provide individual psychotherapy and psychoeducation.
- Engage 'significant others' in psychoeducation and further management as appropriate.
- Group therapy may be appropriate.

money), judgement is impaired and often the person is more physically active than usual. The person is often intolerant of challenge and may become aggressive if frustrated. This can pose a major problem for 'significant others' when faced with very inappropriate behaviour. In a state of mania an individual may not only be a risk to others through inappropriate or aggressive behaviour, but may also place themselves at risk through dangerous behaviours (such as driving recklessly or trying to fly like Superman) or through damage to their reputation or finances.

The separation of mania and hypomania is the subject of some variation. Some authorities maintain that manic symptoms which do not significantly impair function or require hospitalisation constitute hypomania. Others insist that mania is defined by the presence of psychosis, and that absence of psychotic symptoms and signs in a patient with manic symptoms, constitutes hypomania. The latter definition is more objective and coherent than relying upon decisions regarding admission to hospital and the severity of disruption in life function, but the former is more commonly used in the literature.

Upon mental state examination the person may appear obviously euphoric, but if the thought content is more anxiety provoking or hostile, the facial expression may change

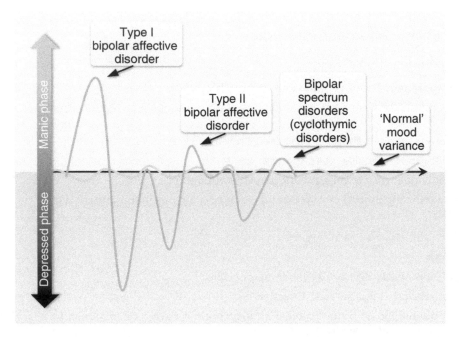

Figure 9.1 Different phases of bipolar disorder mood profile

accordingly. They may present with dramatic choice of clothing or none at all. Physical and intellectual capacity during a state of mania can be exceptionally high for that individual, sometimes with remarkable feats of ability. Assessment is usually facilitated by the person's lack of inhibition but insight may be poor and the diagnosis of mania may evoke rage and denial. The decision to seek help usually comes from a relative or other interested person rather than the patient.

Depressed phase of bipolar disorder

The clinical presentation is essentially the same as in depressive disorders (see Chapter 8) but is more likely to be severe, and associated somatic (melancholic) features are more likely. Abrupt onset of a severe melancholic depression in a young person (particularly an adolescent) may be a harbinger of bipolar disorder, and careful monitoring of antidepressant response (to check for manic switch) is required. 'Atypical' depressive clinical features are more common in bipolar disorders than other mood disorders. The different phases of illness are shown in Figure 9.1.

Course of bipolar disorders

In *bipolar I disorder*, episodes of both mania and severe depression occur. *Bipolar II disorder* is characterised by episodes of hypomania, interspersed by separate and often severe episodes of depression. *Rapid cycling*-type bipolar disorder refers to a subset of patients with either bipolar I or bipolar II disorder, whose illness includes more than four episodes of both mania/hypomania and depression per year. This form of the illness is particularly

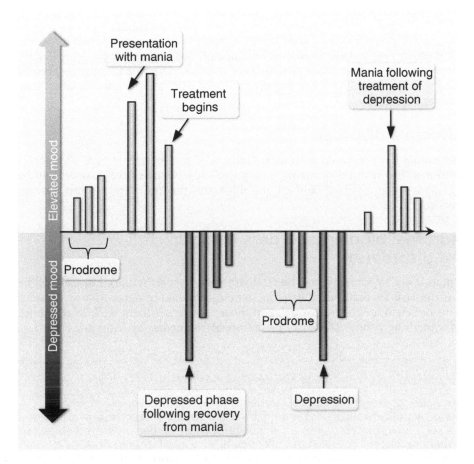

Figure 9.2 Example of longitudinal course of bipolar disorder in patient with bipolar I disorder

disruptive and may be provoked by substances such as antidepressant medications and stimulants.

Mania and hypomania often arise quickly, over a period of days, but may also show early signs for several weeks with reduced need for sleep and increased resilience to life stresses. Monitoring changes in sleep patterns can be helpful in identifying a manic or depressive change in a euthymic individual with known bipolar disorder.

Depressive episodes are the most common state in bipolar disorders, but a very small group of persons will suffer only manic symptoms. The most common sequence is for mania and/or hypomania to be followed by depression, but the reverse also occurs. Depression followed by mania or hypomania is often more resistant to mood stabilisers than the opposite sequence. Manic symptoms become less common with age in bipolar individuals and mixed manic and depressive symptoms more common. Figure 9.2 is a diagrammatic representation of a patient with bipolar I.

Mixed bipolar states

Manic or hypomanic symptoms may arise simultaneously with depressive symptoms in a mixture that is easily overlooked. Sometimes manic and depressive symptoms will arise in close succession and at other times symptoms of mania or hypomania may be present and combined with depressed mood or negative thought content. The affect is often irritable rather than euphoric.

Schizoaffective disorder

When an individual has presented with clear features of schizophrenia (see Chapter 7) and at other times clear features of mania, a diagnosis of schizoaffective disorder can be considered. This is a controversial concept and illustrates the limitations of our current diagnostic system.

Sub-syndromal bipolar disorders (bipolar spectrum disorders)

Some presentations of hypomania may be relatively mild (hyperthymia), but can still be recognised as unusual for that individual. The same can be said of depressive symptoms, which may be sufficient for the individual, and those who know them well, to recognise that there is something wrong. These can be reasonably named as cyclothymic disorder.

Case examples: Bipolar disorders

- A woman aged 22 presented to an emergency department because she had been found by police walking down a major street naked and waving at passing cars. She seemed intoxicated with a substance because of her pressured speech, flippant manner, blatant sexual seductiveness, high level of energy and impressive fitness (police had to run several blocks to apprehend her). However, tests revealed no evidence of substance use and her husband later reported that she had hardly slept for the 2 weeks after she started a new job. She had a history of depressive symptoms which began soon after menarche aged 12. *Management*: She required considerable persuasion to accept treatment, and had to be admitted to hospital. She responded to an atypical antipsychotic medication and began treatment with a mood stabiliser. Psychotherapeutic treatment was increasingly employed as she recovered.

- A 26-year-old man presented with an 8-year history of recurrent periods of hyperarousal, irritability, rapid speech, intolerance of others for being 'too slow', minimal need for sleep and high sex drive, alternating with periods of intense depressed mood, despair, lack of energy, excessive sleep and suicidal thoughts. He could not recall the last time he had not struggled with complaints about his behaviour from other people and said his job was at serious risk because he was regarded as 'unpredictable and difficult to work with' by his employer. *Management*: His treatment consisted of psychoeducation about his bipolar disorder, introduction of a mood stabiliser and further psychotherapy over time to help him cope with the impact of his illness. He did not lose his job and life became much more comfortable for him and his workmates.

Continued

Case examples continued

- A 40-year-old man with a 20-year history of bipolar affective disorder (type I) telephoned his psychiatrist to say he was about to board an aircraft to fly to Canberra to advise the prime minister that the world was at serious risk. He mentioned that he wanted his psychiatrist to know this so that he would not worry about failing to keep his appointment later that day. He said there was no need to send further prescriptions of his medications as he had found a new machine which used magnetic fields to improve his thinking and he had been managing much better off all medication. He was subsequently arrested in parliament.
Management: He required compulsory treatment in a psychiatric hospital. Treatment consisted of a sedative antipsychotic and reintroduction of his mood stabiliser. Regrettably, although this was effective at reversing his manic episode, he became psychotically depressed, and required a course of ECT. He subsequently required a complex combination of medications to keep him well and underwent extensive psychological treatment.

Differential diagnoses

Substance use disorders: Intoxication and withdrawal relating to a variety of substances can mimic or provoke bipolar disorders. These include corticosteroids, dexamphetamine, methamphetamine, methylene-dioxy-methamphetamine (ecstasy), cocaine, alcohol (notably binge pattern of intoxication), cannabis and lysergic acid diethylamide (LSD). The bipolar features may resolve when the substance use ceases, but may also persist independent of substance use.

General medical disorders: Multiple sclerosis, Parkinson's disease, various forms of dementia, epilepsy (notably temporal lobe epilepsy), cerebrovascular diseases (notably cerebrovascular accidents), acquired brain injury, neoplasia of the brain, neurosyphilis, acquired immunodeficiency syndrome and other disorders can all mimic or provoke bipolar disorders. The bipolar features may resolve when the medical condition improves but may also persist independent of the medical disorder.

Personality disorders: In some circumstances severe personality disruption can be accompanied by unpredictable fluctuations in mood, self-evaluation and behaviour. These 'highs' and 'lows' can be confused with bipolar disorder but are usually distinguished by the links to life events, their brevity, and strong response to changes in life circumstance (see Chapter 14).

Aetiology of bipolar disorders

Genetic factors

Genetic processes contribute significantly to bipolar disorders, with first degree relatives (adjacent generations to the patient: i.e. parents, siblings, children) having approximately seven times the risk of developing a bipolar disorder and twice the risk of developing unipolar depression compared to the general population. Twin studies have revealed 67% concordance in monozygotic twins and 19% in dizygotic twins. Unipolar depression is also over-represented in these monozygotic twins. In adoption studies, bipolar and unipolar mood disorders both appear more common in the biological relatives of adopted children than the families of adopting parents.

The precise genes involved in bipolar disorders remain elusive, but a number of possible genes of relevance have been identified. These include genes related to such activities as monoamine function, neurogenesis, neuronal signal transduction, synthesis of neurotrophic factors and neurotransmitters, synaptic activity, myelin synthesis and circadian rhythms.

Neuroimaging

Cerebral blood flow studies suggest an increase in temporal and limbic structures in mania and the reverse in the depressed phase of bipolar illness. Glucose metabolism appears generally reduced, but neuronal activity appears increased in the frontal lobes and basal ganglia, compared with controls.

In physiological terms, bipolar disorders appear to be related to disruption of the integration of frontal lobe (particularly anterior cingulate gyrus), basal ganglia (particularly caudate), thalamus and limbic system (particularly amygdala and hippocampus) activities.

Figure 9.3 shows computer generated images of a Single Photon Emission Computerised Tomography (SPECT) scan of a patient with mania.

Signal transduction pathways

Alterations in the intracellular processing of receptor activation in patients with bipolar disorders appear significant and may involve the phosphoinositide system, protein kinase C (PKC) activity, intracellular calcium activity, glycogen synthase kinase (GSK-3) and guanine nucleotide binding proteins (G proteins).

Neurocognition

Executive cognitive functions and memory are subject to subtle disruption in bipolar disorders and may represent endophenotypes of bipolar disorder. This probably relates to alterations in dendritic networks, glial cell function and myelin synthesis that disrupt brain function.

Endocrinology

These are similar to depressive disorders.

Neurotrophic factors

Neurotrophic factor production is impaired in bipolar disorders, as in depressive disorders. However, this impairment appears even more severe in manic than in depressed phases.

Psychosocial contributions

These appear similar to depressive disorders, but early life trauma (particularly emotional trauma) may be more important in bipolar disorders.

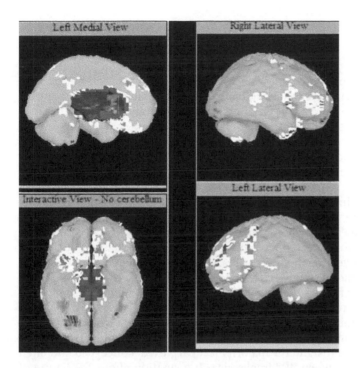

Figure 9.3 **The scan shows increased activity in the resting state in the prefrontal cortices, subgenual cortex, right anterior temporal and medial orbitofrontal cortices, which may be associated with mania** (Courtesy of Dr Joe Cardaci)

Legend:
medium grey = two standard deviations above or below mean blood flow in healthy people
white = two or more standard deviations above the mean
dark grey = between three and four standard deviations below the mean
very dark grey/black = five or more standard deviations below the mean.

Management of bipolar disorders

Clinical assessment

Direct observation of a person suffering from any disorder is essential and the opportunity to gather information from others is invaluable. The patient may present requesting help, or others may seek help for them. Mental state examination may reveal some or all of the clinical features noted above, but a history of symptoms and signs of altered behaviour reported by significant others will be worthwhile. It helps to routinely ask about manic symptoms (such as a reduced need for sleep without daytime fatigue) when assessing anyone who presents with depressive symptoms.

Management of mania

Mania is managed as an acute psychosis, but euphoria can rapidly change to rage and aggression when a person is confronted with proposed treatment and containment, however benevolent. An explanation of the need for treatment is essential, but is often not accepted by patients who are psychotic, and compulsory treatment may be required. Once the diagnosis has been made and the need for treatment established, the therapist must proceed as quickly as possible to administer effective treatment.

Medications should include an antipsychotic agent (see Chapter 15) and sometimes extra sedation in the form of a benzodiazepine. Some patients will accept oral medications and this is clearly preferable, but parenteral administration may be required.

Mood stabilisers should be introduced early in management to help contain the manic episode and also provide some prevention of a possible depressive swing.

Response to treatment with antipsychotic medications in mania is usually rapid, but relapse may occur if medications are reduced too quickly or adherence is poor. Many sufferers will subsequently move directly into a depressed phase of illness but it will often be sufficient to persist with a mood stabiliser as the mood instability settles. The management of hypomania essentially follows the same principles, but the patient is usually (not always) more accepting of treatment with medications.

With recovery, the opportunity for psychotherapy arises and patients will usually want to talk about their experience, including their embarrassment and even guilt. While some patients may not have significant insight, the majority feel perplexed, concerned and often depressed about their behaviour when ill. Simple, clear information about the nature of their illness and its treatment is required. Management of significant financial debts, disrupted relationships and the impact of illness in parents upon children must also be considered.

Sometimes mania may not respond well to medications and electroconvulsive therapy (ECT) can be invaluable (see Chapter 15).

Management of bipolar depression

The management of bipolar depression is best achieved using mood stabilisers, including second generation antipsychotic medications. There is evidence that quetiapine appears particularly effective; ziprasidone and other atypical antipsychotics may also be effective. Antidepressants which are SSRIs (particularly those with very little noradrenergic effect, such as citalopram and escitalopram) appear less likely to provoke manic switching than NASAs, SNRIs, tricyclic antidepressants, NRIs and irreversible MAO inhibitors (see Chapter 15).

A 'rapid cycling' pattern of mood swings or mixed affective states may develop in response to antidepressant treatment and they should be used with care. Increased irritability may also develop when antidepressants are employed in bipolar depression. There is controversy regarding how long to treat before removing antidepressants. They are best withdrawn once recovery has become established and a mood stabiliser is in use, whenever possible.

Electroconvulsive therapy (ECT) is invaluable in the management of bipolar depression when the severity is high and particularly when psychotic symptoms are evident.

Box 9.3
Summary of biological interventions

- *Mood stabilisers*: fundamental to the acute and chronic management of bipolar disorders.
- *Mood stabilisers and quetiapine*: first-line treatments for bipolar depression.
- *Antidepressants*: can be useful for bipolar depression, but can precipitate rapid cycling, as well as irritability and sometimes mood switching. Antidepressants should always be used with care in conjunction with a mood stabiliser.
- *Antipsychotic medications*: valuable in mania and its variants, as mood stabilisers and in the treatment of depression.
- *Benzodiazepines*: useful as adjunctive treatment in managing acute mania with marked hyperarousal.
- *Electroconvulsive therapy*: invaluable in severe and/or intractable mania and depression.

Management of bipolar spectrum disorders

The decision to treat with medications requires negotiation with the patient and perhaps their partner or families, as some may prefer to cope with psychological assistance alone or tolerate the mood swings without further intervention (see Box 9.3). Citalopram, escitalopram or lamotrigine appear particularly helpful.

Psychosocial interventions in the management of bipolar disorders

Individual and group psychotherapy that may use a variety of treatment models are very helpful with psychological adaptation to bipolar disorders and in the reduction of vulnerability to the precipitants of illness episodes. Identification of specific stresses and their meaning to patients is invaluable. See Chapter 16 for further detail about specific therapeutic techniques.

People with bipolar disorders are highly sensitive to the disruption of circadian rhythms and sleep cycle. Return to a regular daily life rhythm enhances mood stability. Regular exercise is very helpful, particularly during periods of depression. Regular time for relaxation and recreation each day will also be of assistance. This is known as interpersonal and social rhythms therapy (see Chapter 16).

Family-focused therapy and marital or relationship therapy are very helpful in the comprehensive management of bipolar disorders and their impact upon 'significant others'. The children of patients must be considered in such interventions.

The biological interventions used in the management of bipolar disorders are summarised in Box 9.4.

Box 9.4
Summary of psychosocial interventions

- Stress management strategies.
- Management of circadian rhythms and sleep.
- Individual and group psychotherapies.
- Family, marital and relationship therapies.

REFERENCES AND FURTHER READING

Brown, E.S. (Ed.), 2005. Bipolar disorder. Psychiatric Clinics of North America, Saunders, Philadelphia.

Goodwin, F., Jamison, K., 2007. Manic-depressive illness. Bipolar disorders and recurrent depression. Oxford University Press, Oxford.

Jamison, K., 1995. An unquiet mind. Knopf, New York.

Joyce, P., Mitchell, P. (Eds.), 2004. Mood disorders: recognition and treatment. UNSW Press, Sydney.

Parker, G. (Ed.), 2012. Bipolar II disorder. Modelling, measuring and managing. Cambridge University Press, Cambridge.

Yatham, L., Maj, M., 2010. Bipolar disorder. Clinical and neurobiological foundations. Wiley Blackwell, Oxford.

CHAPTER 9

A HUSBAND NAMED LAWRENCE
CASE-BASED LEARNING

JOEL KING & ANDREW GLEASON

The following role-play requires two participants: one to play the GP registrar (candidate) and another to play a man named Lawrence (actor).

OSCE Station Instructions

(Reading time: 2 minutes)

You are a GP registrar working in a busy metropolitan GP practice, under Dr Lee. Lawrence has come to see you today because he is very concerned about the behaviour of his wife, Vivian.

Task (10 minutes)

- Conduct the interview with Lawrence, determine the most likely diagnosis and discuss immediate management options.

Actor role: Lawrence

You are a 28-year-old accountant at a major city firm. You have been married to Vivian for one year. You live in an inner city townhouse. Vivian is a 26-year-old concert cellist with the city orchestra.

You are very flustered. You have come to the GP because you are concerned about Vivian. Her behaviour has been out of character for the last two weeks. Something has changed and she is not her usual self.

Vivian has been very irritable. You normally do not fight, but you have had a lot of arguments. She has been talking a lot and it's difficult to interrupt her. You estimate that she has slept about five hours this whole week, but she is still full of energy. She stays awake, composing sheets and sheets of music and she has just started a fashion blog. The other night, you found her awake at 3 am. She said, 'I've had the most brilliant insights about fashion trends of the future and I need to write them down now.' She believes that she can change the fashion industry and make it less dependent on cheap labour in developing countries and better for the environment. She went to the city last weekend and spent $5000 on clothes, fashion books and magazines. She thinks they are essential for her research.

You find that her sex drive has increased and she is much more lively. She seems to be a lot less introverted. She asks you all about your accounting department at work and comes up with numerous suggestions about managing your team. You went to a business dinner last week, but she was agitated and fidgety. She started flirting with one of your colleagues which was very out of character. You took her home soon after.

You can't get her to focus on anything. She gets distracted when making dinner, so you've been cooking all of the meals. At dinner she talks a million miles per minute about how she finally understands what Mozart and Beethoven must have gone through when they were composing their masterpieces and then runs off to the study to compose.

When you tell her that she's acting odd, she says that you're trying to oppress her and prevent her from reaching her full potential because she's a woman.

You asked her to come and see the GP, but she refused.

Usually Vivian is quiet, studious, and fairly introverted. She likes keeping to herself, often reading or posting on blogs. She dedicates several hours each day to practising the cello.

There have been episodes in the past when Vivian was full of energy and drive continuously for a few weeks. She does her best composing at these times, but you have never before seen her act the way she is now. Vivian told you that she had bipolar disorder in your first year of dating, which was diagnosed at age 20. She said that she was 'high' at the time. She was placed on medication (sodium valproate) and has been stable since, with no hospital admissions in her life. She saw a private psychiatrist 'for a while', but hasn't seen one for years. You did not know anything about bipolar disorder before and still do not know much about it. You do know that Vivian occasionally gets into 'sad funks' that last a few weeks. During these times she becomes quieter, more serious, not interested in going out, and sleeps in more. You usually leave her be, and she comes around after a few weeks without any intervention. She probably has three of these per year.

More recently, Vivian had three 'sad funks' over the last few months. You suggested that the two of you have a month-long holiday in Europe and Asia. Vivian was keen to go to the art galleries, museums and concert halls, as well as do some shopping. Neither of you had been to Europe before and wanted to make the most of it. The holiday went well, but you went to ten countries in four weeks and didn't get much sleep. There were also a lot of time zone changes. You got back a month ago.

Vivian has never talked about suicide or made an attempt, either recently or in the past. She takes an oral contraceptive. You do not know if she is still taking sodium valproate. She is usually pretty organised with that sort of thing.

Vivian doesn't have any past medical history that you are aware of.

You and Vivian share a bottle of wine over dinner on weekends, but do not drink more than this. Vivian does not use recreational drugs, but you occasionally have a joint of marijuana to help you relax, about once every month.

Vivian's aunt has bipolar disorder, but you have never met her. Her father smokes and has emphysema, but otherwise you think her family is healthy.

You married Vivian one year ago, after dating for two years. You met through friends. You were impressed by her intelligence and insightful, sharp sense of humour. For the most part, your marriage is very stable. You have similar interests. You spend your weekends going for walks and going to art exhibitions.

Statements you must make:
- 'Doctor, I've been really worried about Vivian and I really don't know what to do.'
- 'She's been acting very oddly over the last week.'
- 'She's been racing around and doing everything. It's like she's on a permanent caffeine high. I don't know what to do!'
- 'What do you think is wrong? What should I do?'

Model Answer

The good candidate will acknowledge that Lawrence is anxious and concerned. Ideally, this will involve empathic statements that assuage him, but in a manner that enables the candidate to continue taking a complete history before talking about diagnostic possibilities and suggesting management.

The candidate will identify confidentiality issues (e.g. does Vivian know he has come to see the GP?) and discuss ways of managing these with Lawrence.

A risk assessment is imperative and will dictate management. The candidate should explore the risks associated with mania. These include physical exhaustion, risky driving, costly or unwise financial decisions, inappropriate behaviour in the workplace or social circles, damage to relationships, drug and alcohol use, sexual promiscuity, physical assault or rape, sexually transmitted diseases, and unplanned pregnancy. Such risks can have an impact not only on Vivian and Lawrence, but also the wider community.

The likely diagnosis of a manic episode is clear, precipitated possibly by medication non-compliance or perhaps related to circadian rhythm disturbance from recent travels. The candidate should recognise that other possibilities exist, such as an organic condition or a psychotic episode (see page 137). The candidate will not only identify the likely diagnosis, but explain to Lawrence what a manic episode is and how it can be treated (i.e. that medication is required and that hospitalisation may be necessary). The candidate will also explain that other diagnoses are possible and need to be considered.

There is no ideal management strategy. The good candidate will recognise this and discuss the options with Lawrence. He could try again to take Vivian to the GP clinic, or to an appointment at a psychiatry clinic (although she has already refused to come, so this is unlikely). Lawrence can call the local psychiatry crisis service. The candidate should offer to tell Lawrence how to make contact. The crisis team may be able to assess Vivian at home. Lawrence may also be able to take Vivian to the local emergency department for assessment.

The candidate should make Lawrence aware of the local Mental Health Act and the situations in which it can be used. Lawrence may be worried about how he can get help if Vivian refuses to have treatment, but on the other hand he may also be worried that having her treated against her will would mean that she is going to be 'committed'. It is important to talk with Lawrence about crisis management. He should know that the police can be involved if things get out of hand, for example, if Vivian was to become aggressive. Lawrence may also worry about Vivian getting angry at him for seeking help. He will need reassurance that he is doing the right thing.

FOR THE MORE ADVANCED LEARNER

It is important that Vivian has a medical work-up with a view to assessing for complications of mania (such as dehydration, injury, or sexually transmitted infection if she is at risk), and organic causes of a manic syndrome. This includes a full history, physical exam, and basic blood tests (such as a full blood count, electrolytes, creatinine, liver functions tests, and thyroid function tests). She may need cerebral imaging if her episode is atypical or if she has neurological signs.

The candidate should also explain to Lawrence that the prognosis for Vivian is good. It is likely that she will settle and return to her usual self once treatment has been initiated.

Chapter 10

ANXIETY AND POST-TRAUMATIC DISORDERS

DAVID J CASTLE & DARRYL BASSETT

Anxiety is, of course, a perfectly normal phenomenon. Indeed, without any anxiety we would be comatose or dead! To perform optimally in any given situation we need a certain amount of anxiety/arousal. Sometimes it is appropriate for us to have a massive surge of anxiety, such as when we are confronted by a life-threatening situation: the so-called 'fight or flight' response. However, if one experiences too much anxiety most of the time and/or in excess to the level of 'threat', it can become incapacitating and un-useful. The Yerkes-Dodson curve (Figure 10.1) demonstrates this.

The neurobiology of anxiety and the underpinning brain pathways are increasingly being elucidated and this knowledge is informing effective treatments. Box 10.1 summarises these parameters.

The precise point at which anxiety becomes so severe as to constitute a 'disorder' is open to conjecture, and needs to be assessed on an individual basis. The general rubric – that the anxiety response is excessive/prolonged, causes the individual distress and impairs their psychosocial functioning – is a useful enough starting point. Note, though, that some anxious people are so good at avoiding their feared situation they might

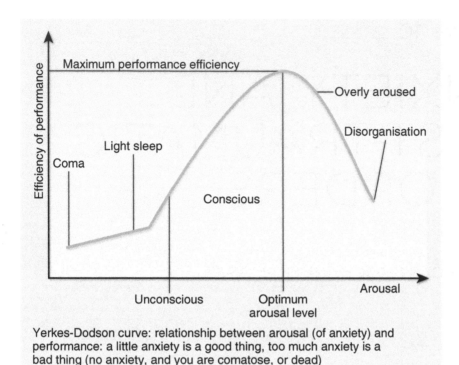

Yerkes-Dodson curve: relationship between arousal (of anxiety) and performance: a little anxiety is a good thing, too much anxiety is a bad thing (no anxiety, and you are comatose, or dead)

Figure 10.1 **Relationship between level of arousal and efficiency of performance**

effectively avoid ever becoming anxious, yet be objectively impaired in terms of the restriction this places on their life. For example, a woman in her 50s never left the house because of severe anxiety and panic attacks whenever she was in crowded situations. She never actually experienced anxiety because she completely avoided going out and relied on her family to do all her shopping and so forth. Indeed, she didn't see herself as 'disabled', raising the issue of so-called 'secondary gain', which is the benefit she accrued from being in the sick role ('primary gain' is the amelioration of the anxiety experience itself). The current DSM–IV–TR and ICD–10 classifications of the anxiety disorders are summarised in Table 10.1.

Anxiety symptoms can be seen as a manifestation of a number of physical and psychiatric disorders, and these need to be assessed and treated in their own right (see Box 10.2).

A *panic attack* is essentially a severe burst of anxiety, be it in response to a particular stimulus, or 'out of the blue'. There are somatic and psychic/cognitive features, as shown in Box 10.3. By definition, the attack should reach a peak within 10 minutes, but in many cases it is very abrupt. Panic attacks resolve with time, and can be attenuated with slow breathing or 're-breathing' (using a paper bag) techniques.

Box 10.1

The neurobiology of anxiety and anxiety disorders

Neuroanatomy

The amygdala forms the core brain structure in the derivation of emotional experiences and behaviours. There are links to:

- hypothalamus: notably HPA axis/cortisol release
- sympathetic nervous system: cardiovascular changes
- pons: vagal nerve activity, startle response, 'freezing' behaviours
- hippocampal complex: emotionally laden memories
- basal forebrain: arousal, vigilance, excitement
- prefrontal cortex: thought processing, modulation of arousal, fear content
- cingulate cortex: focusing of attention, execution of thoughts, integration of thoughts with emotions
- insular cortex: visceral experience of emotions; disgust
- septal nuclei
- parabrachial nucleus.

Common elements in anxiety disorders

- Limbic system
- Prefrontal cortex.

Neurochemistry

- Noradrenergic pathway activity
- GABA neuronal activity
- Serotonergic pathway activity
- Serotonin transporter activity
- Serotonin-1A receptor activity
- Serotonin-2 receptor activity.

Panic disorder

Of themselves, panic attacks carry no diagnostic specificity, and many people have them during their lives. Sometimes they are an indicator of an underlying physical problem, and these need to be investigated where appropriate (see Box 10.2).

If panic attacks occur habitually, with no clear organic cause and no particular predictable precipitant, a diagnosis of *panic disorder* should be considered. The panics themselves are often associated with interpanic anxiety, mostly relating to the thought of having another attack. Even if there is no clear precipitant, avoidance behaviour might ensue, particularly of situations in which the person considers their risk of another panic attack to be high. Classically, people find their home environment the most reassuring, and can become essentially housebound. The exception is those individuals who tend to wake from sleep in the throes of a panic attack.

Table 10.1

Classification of anxiety disorders according to DSM–IV–TR and ICD–10 (synopsis)

DSM–IV–TR	ICD–10
Panic disorder • with agoraphobia • without agoraphobia Agoraphobia without panic	Panic disorder Agoraphobia • with panic • without panic
Social anxiety disorder	Social phobia
Specific phobia	Specific phobia
Generalised anxiety disorder	Generalised anxiety disorder
Obsessive-compulsive disorder	Obsessive-compulsive disorder
Acute stress disorder	Acute stress reaction
Post-traumatic stress disorder	Post-traumatic stress disorder

Box 10.2

Causes of anxiety

Physical causes

Physical causes may be:

• exogenous (e.g. alcohol withdrawal, cannabis intoxication, amphetamines and caffeine), or

• endogenous:
  ○ inside the central nervous system (e.g. brain tumours, migraine, encephalitis and epilepsy), or
  ○ outside the central nervous system (e.g. cardiac arrhythmias, pulmonary insufficiency, anaemia, endocrine abnormalities, such as hyperthyroidism, hyperparathyroidism and phaeochromocytoma, hypoglycaemia and febrile illnesses).

Psychiatric causes

Psychiatric causes include:

• schizophrenia

• mania

• depression

• anxiety disorders

• post-traumatic syndromes

• obsessive-compulsive spectrum disorders.

Box 10.3
Features of a panic attack

Psychic/cognitive features
Psychic/cognitive features include:
- thoughts of imminent death (classically from a heart attack) or of 'going crazy'
- depersonalisation/derealisation.

Somatic features
Somatic features include:
- shortness of breath
- chest pain
- hyperventilation
- tachycardia/palpitations
- light-headedness
- tingling in the peripheries
- sweating
- nausea
- diarrhoea.

Treatment includes psychoeducation, breathing retraining, and, where indicated, formal cognitive therapy. Medications that are most effective include the selective serotonin reuptake inhibitors (SSRIs), although the initial energising effects can be bothersome and starting at a low dose is sensible. *Benzodiazepines* are sometimes resorted to in order to attenuate an acute attack. They can be very effective, although the message can be a disempowering one for the patient and benzodiazepines can become something of a 'crutch' for the individual, as well as being potentially habit-forming. Having said this, some people do find ongoing benefit from benzodiazepines without habituation or the requirement for dose increases.

Phobic disorders

Once anxiety becomes linked to a certain situation or thing and results in avoidance thereof to the extent that this impedes everyday life, the individual should be considered to have a *phobic disorder*. The important thing here is that, therapeutically, the psychological technique of exposure/response prevention (EX/RP) can be employed. Essentially, this involves mapping the behaviours, fears and avoidances, and helping the patient tackle their fears in a structured hierarchical way (i.e. starting with something relatively easy, conquering that, then moving on to the next step). An analogy is engaging in a step-wise exercise program, with the clinician as the coach.

Box 10.4

General guidance about when to prescribe antidepressants in people with anxiety disorders

- The patient simply does not engage in psychological treatment.
- The patient does not gain benefit from psychological treatment, or is left with significant continuing symptomatology and impairment.
- The symptoms are particularly severe, distressing and disabling.
- The patient has significant associated depressive symptoms.

Specific phobia

Specific phobia is common, but does not usually come to medical attention. There is fear and avoidance of particular or myriad objects or situations: spiders and snakes often feature, probably due to inherent evolutionary preconditioning. *Treatment* is EX/RP, usually in a step-wise hierarchical manner, but sometimes *flooding* is employed, where the individual is exposed to one of their worst fears and needs to 'stay with' the fear until the anxiety subsides.

Agoraphobia

Agoraphobia (literally 'fear of the market place') is characterised by a fear of situations where the individual feels trapped. These include busy supermarkets, heavy traffic and public transport; open spaces are also often feared and avoided, and home is seen as 'safe', resulting in the 'housebound housewife'. DSM–IV–TR specifically links agoraphobia among the phobic disorders with panic disorder, although panic can actually occur with any of the phobic disorders. More often than not, agoraphobia begins with a panic attack in an agoraphobic situation, resulting in withdrawal from the situation and subsequent avoidance. Technically, agoraphobia can occur without panic attacks, but this is usually seen in those patients who habitually avoid the situations in which they might panic. *Treatment* is psychoeducation, EX/RP, and, if required, SSRIs or serotonergic and noradrenergic reuptake inhibitors (SNRIs). In general, medications should be used in the anxiety disorders if those features in Box 10.4 are present.

Social anxiety disorder (SAD)

Social anxiety disorder (SAD), also known as social phobia, is now a well-established disorder, despite initial cynicism that it was merely a pathologising of normal shyness. People with SAD are significantly impaired by their disorder, which often begins in the teens and thus impacts on the normal social developmental trajectory.

There are two main forms:

- *Non-generalised SAD* is akin to performance anxiety and is restricted to performance situations. People with this problem do not usually seek professional help unless performance is key to their livelihood (e.g. musicians). *Treatment* involves psychoeducation, teaching breathing techniques, and possibly the use of a beta-blocker, such as low dose propranolol to assist with the performance situation itself.

- *Generalised SAD* is a more common clinical problem, although it is clear that many sufferers never seek treatment, perhaps through lack of knowledge about treatment potential and/or embarrassment. Severe generalised SAD can be very disabling, with restricted social networks, lowered performance educationally and vocationally, and excessive use of alcohol and benzodiazepines (often as 'self-treatment', which can become problematic in itself). There is significant depressive comorbidity. *Treatment* includes cognitive-behaviour therapy (CBT), especially dealing with the core negative cognition of making a fool of oneself in front of others, and a hierarchical approach to the behavioural avoidance: group treatment can be particularly useful. SSRIs and SNRIs are useful adjuncts, with the general guidance shown in Box 10.4.

Blood-injury phobia is unique among the phobic disorders in that the physiological response to the sight of blood is a vaso-vagal one, with profound hypotension and fainting. Of interest too is that it seems to be strongly genetic, with an autosomal dominant pattern having been shown in some families. *Treatment* is complex, but CBT techniques can be applied with modifications to encompass the vaso-vagal response to the 'exposure'.

Generalised anxiety disorder (GAD)

Generalised anxiety disorder (GAD) has become something of a residual diagnosis, being effectively 'trumped' by panic disorder. There is considerable comorbidity with depression, and some researchers consider it should be subsumed under the affective disorders. However, a clinical syndrome with predominant 'free floating' anxiety is certainly seen in practice. GAD usually begins insidiously and is predominant in females, seeming to grow out of an anxious personality structure. Symptoms include anxiety about just about everything, including what might or might not happen to the patient themselves, to their loved ones, or to the world in general. Many patients with GAD also focus on their physical health, with a strong tendency to somatise and present to doctors with physical symptoms (see Chapter 13). Muscle tension, headaches and abdominal discomfort are common. Sleep is often restless and unrefreshing.

Treatment includes psychoeducation and, in particular, teaching relaxation techniques. Problem-solving is useful: the patient is taught about prioritising important tasks and tackling them in a paced manner, rather than being so overwhelmed by everything that nothing is achieved. More formal CBT can be usefully employed, with a focus on challenging catastrophic thinking and modifying associated un-useful behaviours, such as doctor-shopping or benzodiazepine abuse. SSRIs and SNRIs are a useful adjunct, particularly in the face of mood disturbance. Pregabalin and buspirone can also be used for GAD, but they lack antidepressant properties. The atypical antipsychotic quetiapine has also been shown to be effective for GAD and has the benefit of hypnotic and antidepressant effects.

Case examples: Anxiety disorders

Panic disorder

An 18-year-old woman presented to the emergency department with an abrupt onset of chest pain, shortness of breath, nausea and intense fear; she was convinced she was going to die. Physical examination and electrocardiogram (ECG) were normal, and with reassurance and encouragement to slow-breathe, her anxiety

Continued

Case examples continued

settled to the extent that one could have a conversation with her about the nature of anxiety and the way panic attacks can evolve. On review 2 days later she revealed that in fact she had experienced a number of previous similar episodes and was constantly concerned about having another attack. *Treatment* was to exclude physical causes (such as thyroid dysfunction), psychoeducation and CBT.

Agoraphobia with panic

A 38-year-old woman presented for treatment with her husband, who reported that she had been suffering panic attacks and could not leave the house without him there to reassure her. The woman described her first panic attack during a Christmas shopping expedition at a crowded regional shopping centre. She said it 'just happened', and she felt intensely fearful, thought she was going to collapse, and had to sit in a quiet corner and call her husband to collect her. Ever since that event she had feared a repeat episode and had consequently avoided crowded shops and public transport. She was not pervasively depressed and was motivated to address her problem. *Treatment* entailed a step-wise EX/RP program, with her husband as 'co-therapist'.

Generalised anxiety disorder

A 41-year-old woman was referred to a psychiatrist by a physician colleague who had investigated her extensively to find a cause for her headaches, but could find no obvious physical pathology. The woman said she had always been a worrier and in particular had had ongoing concerns regarding various aspects of her physical health. She described being constantly tense, that she worried about 'everything and nothing' and had restless and unrefreshing sleep. Her mood was low, she lacked energy and concentration, and was concerned her husband was going to leave her because she considered herself 'such a pain to live with'. *Treatment* included a full exploration of symptoms, and an assessment of mood, including of suicide risk. She was offered extensive psychoeducation (with her husband) about the anxiety-depressive spiral. Simple psychological measures, such as problem-solving, and the introduction of a SNRI (started at low dose and built up slowly), helped both her mood and her anxiety.

Post-traumatic syndromes

Interindividual variation in response to trauma has been noted for centuries, and it is remarkable how some people can deal with what others regard as horrific trauma, with equanimity, while others can be severely incapacitated by exposure to what might objectively seem 'trivial'. Thus, trauma is in part in the eye of the beholder, and the subjective view of it is critical. Specifically, if the trauma is perceived as potentially life-threatening or likely to cause physical harm and injury, then it is more likely to cause *post-traumatic stress disorder* (PTSD). Apart from the trauma itself, the main risk factor for a pathological post-traumatic syndrome is the make-up of the individual, both in terms of past psychiatric problems and past experience of and response to trauma.

The course of symptoms can be perturbed to some extent by legal issues such as compensation, but the notion of a *compensation neurosis*, where symptoms resolve once compensation is settled, has largely been scotched.

Box 10.5

Stages of CBT treatment for PTSD

1 Stabilisation and engagement

2 Education and information

3 Anxiety management

4 Trauma exposure

5 Cognitive restructuring

6 Relapse prevention and maintenance.

Acute stress disorder (a DSM–IV–TR term not shared by ICD-10) shares many features with PTSD (see below), but by definition occurs from 2 days to 1 month following a traumatic event. *Dissociative symptoms* (e.g. depersonalisation, detachment, dissociative amnesia) are given particular prominence, although this might be reviewed in DSM-5.

A diagnosis of PTSD is made if symptoms persist (for at least a month in DSM–IV–TR). The classic triad is:

- *hyperarousal*, with symptoms akin to GAD, and including an exaggerated startle response

- *avoidance* of places or things associated with the event, and a triggering of symptoms in response to reminders of the event; and *emotional numbing*, or detachment from others and the world around one

- *reliving experiences*, including nightmares and flashbacks regarding the event.

Arguably, it is this last set of symptoms that sets PTSD apart from other psychiatric disorders.

Comorbidities are common and include depression and benzodiazepine, alcohol and illicit substance abuse. Chronic pain syndromes following injury sustained during the event can lead to (prescribed) opiate addiction. Loss of physical integrity, work capacity and role can compound matters.

Treatment of PTSD is complex, and needs to encompass all facets of the disorder, and also address, where indicated, comorbid substance use, depression and pain syndromes. Specific approaches include a variety of psychological treatments, including CBT (see Box 10.5) and EX/RP. Group therapy can be particularly useful in terms of mutual support from group members, and the other benefits of the group process, as outlined in Chapter 16. SSRIs and SNRIs are commonly prescribed for anxiety and depressive symptomatology. Hypnotics or low dose atypical antipsychotics (see Chapter 15) can assist sleep. Benzodiazepines are best avoided apart from initial short-term use.

A particularly contentious issue is that of *debriefing* following traumatic events, as a prophylactic measure. The weight of evidence is that this should not be done on a universal basis, but the offer of general support and the opportunity to ventilate feelings about the event are seen as helpful.

Case example: Post-traumatic stress disorder

A 50-year-old man was referred to a psychiatrist after having been involved in a motor vehicle accident and having subsequently experienced significant anxiety and disability. He described the accident in vivid detail, and how he had felt sure he was going to die, waiting for the rescue crew to cut him out of the wreckage. He cried as he related how his wife had been killed in the accident, and that he 'just can't keep the image of her dead body beside me, out of my mind'. He blamed himself for the accident, saying 'it should have been me, not her'. He described restless sleep with violent dreams, felt generally anxious and startled easily. He had not been able to get into a car again, and had been spending much of his time on his own; he had started drinking a bottle of whisky a day to 'settle my nerves and help me sleep: I just want to shut everything out'.

Treatment entailed a comprehensive psychological and medical strategy, with attention to suicide risk. A psychologist specialising in PTSD assisted with the generalised anxiety and avoidance symptoms. An SSRI was introduced to help his mood and dampen his anxious arousal. A short-term hypnotic was employed to aid sleep. His alcohol use was addressed as part of an integrated treatment plan.

REFERENCES AND FURTHER READING

Andreasen, N.C., 1995. Posttraumatic stress disorder: psychology, biology, and the Manichaean warfare between false dichotomies. American Journal of Psychiatry 152, 963–965.

Castle, D., Hood, S., Kyrios, M. (Eds.), 2007. Anxiety disorders: current controversies, future directions. Australian Postgraduate Medicine, Melbourne.

Castle, D., Hood, S., Starcevic, V., 2012. Anxiety disorders: current understandings, novel treatments. Australian Postgraduate Medicine, Melbourne.

Gelder, M., 1989. Panic disorder: fact or fiction? Psychological Medicine 19, 277–283.

Marshall, R.D., Spitzer, R., Liebowitz, M.R., 1999. Review and critique of the new DSM–IV diagnosis of acute stress disorder. American Journal of Psychiatry 156, 1677–1685.

Orr, K.G.D., Castle, D.J., 1998. Social phobia: shyness as a disorder. Medical Journal of Australia 168, 55–56.

Tyrer, P., 1984. Classification of anxiety. British Journal of Psychiatry 144, 78–83.

CHAPTER 10

AN ELECTRICIAN NAMED SCOTT
CASE-BASED LEARNING

JOEL KING & ANDREW GLEASON

The following role-play requires two participants: one to play a GP registrar (candidate) and another to play the role of a patient named Scott Mercer (actor).

OSCE Station Instructions

(Reading time: 2 minutes)

You are a first-year GP registrar working in a country practice. You are asked to see Mr Scott Mercer, a 25-year-old electrician. Scott has come to see you because he is having difficulty sleeping.

Task (10 minutes)

- Please interview Mr Mercer with the aim of establishing a diagnosis (8 minutes).
- After 8 minutes, you must terminate the interview and tell the examiner your provisional diagnosis (or diagnoses), together with a justification (2 minutes).
- You do not need to physically examine the patient.

Actor role: Scott Mercer

You are Scott Mercer, a 25-year-old man. You have lived most of your life in the country town of Nolansville, apart from your time in the army. You served in the army for five years. In your last year you were deployed overseas in a communications unit, responsible for laying down network cables. Towards the end of your tour of duty your unit came under enemy mortar fire. Your commanding officer, Lieutenant Reidy, was killed instantly and two other members of your unit died in the following barrage. You found cover, radioed for help, and waited for ten minutes until a helicopter destroyed the mortar team that was attacking you.

Two months later you received an honourable discharge and returned home to live with Chloe (24 years old), your girlfriend since high school. You found a job as an electrician working for Bill, a well-established electrician in the town. You settled back into civilian life quickly and enjoyed going out for drinks with friends on Friday nights, having three beers most nights, and playing tennis with Chloe on the weekend. You had a good circle of friends, were well-respected for your military service, and did not have symptoms of a depressive or anxiety disorder.

Three months ago, you and Chloe attended a town festival that featured the firing of long sequences of fireworks. During the fireworks you began to breathe quickly and shallowly. There was a sick feeling in your stomach. You began to sweat profusely. Your heart began to race and you felt dizzy and weak in your legs. You did not feel that you were in your own body anymore and felt out of control. Chloe noticed this sudden change and took you to the local base hospital.

At the local hospital you waited an hour until Dr Vikas came to see you. By this time your symptoms had abated. After a physical examination, Dr Vikas could not find anything wrong and attributed your symptoms to dehydration and heatstroke. He advised you to go home, drink plenty of water and rest.

Since the fireworks three months ago you have experienced difficulties falling asleep and staying asleep. Your sleep is often punctuated by fragmented nightmares of explosions and unidentified people screaming. You often wake up in the middle of the night, cannot go back to sleep, and walk around the house. You feel that you are constantly on edge and cannot relax. You have found it difficult to concentrate at work. When Bill commented that you had wired something incorrectly, you shouted at him and threatened to hit him. He fired you a week later.

DRUG AND ALCOHOL HISTORY

You started going to the pub on weeknights in addition to weekends, eventually going without friends when no one was available. After you were fired, you stayed home and drank beer and spirits throughout the day, rarely going outside, except to buy more alcohol. Initially, the alcohol helped you sleep, feel relaxed and forget your worries. You never intended to drink on a daily basis. Now, you find that you need more and more alcohol to get the same relaxed feeling and you drink roughly six to twelve beers a day. You often drink to the point that you pass out and cannot remember the events of yesterday. When you do not drink, you experience sweating, palpitations, insomnia, nausea, agitation and anxiety. These symptoms abate when you drink again.

You know that drinking this much alcohol is not good for you, but you find that you cannot stop. You do not think anything else can help you as much as the alcohol. You have tried to stop drinking twice, but this led to increased anxiety and discomfort, which led you to resume drinking. You have never vomited blood or had a seizure. You have never used an illicit drug.

COMORBID SYMPTOMS

Over the last three months you have noticed a drop in your mood, appetite, energy and libido. You feel plagued with feelings of hopelessness, helplessness and guilt. You feel that you are not a good person, the world is not a good place, and the future looks bleak and dark. You no longer get any enjoyment from playing tennis or other activities. Being hung over or drunk also contributes to you not doing things. You no longer feel that you have any loving feelings for Chloe and feel detached from her and other people in your life. You cannot project yourself into the future and do not expect to live a normal lifespan, although you have no active suicidal ideation, intention or plan. When Chloe asks what is wrong you find that you cannot tell her. When she suggested that it may be related to the fireworks, you went to the bedroom, curled into the foetal position and refused to talk to her. You have also stopped watching television and reading the newspaper, because you find the frequent articles about accidents, disasters and wars too distressing and anxiety-provoking, making you feel like you did during the festival fireworks.

RELEVANT NEGATIVES AND PAST HISTORY

You have never had manic symptoms. Apart from the incident around the fireworks three months ago, you have had no further acute panic attack symptoms. You do not have any obsessions or compulsions. You do not have social anxiety. You have no specific phobias. You have never seen a mental health professional and have no psychiatric history. You have no significant medical history and take no regular medications. You have no forensic history.

PERSONAL HISTORY

You were born and raised in Nolansville. You are an only child. Your developmental milestones were normal. Your father was a plumber who drank very heavily and beat your mother when he was drunk. Your father left the family when you were 8 and you were raised solely by your mother, who held down three jobs to send you to an independent Catholic school. Academically, you were an average student. You had a wide circle of friends, never got into serious trouble, played on a school football team, and met Chloe when you were 16. You graduated from secondary school at age 18 and spent two years backpacking around the world with Chloe. When you came back, you felt rather directionless and decided that you needed a vocation and a stable job. You joined the army and became a qualified electrician, attaining the rank of sergeant. When you had leave you returned to Nolansville to visit Chloe, who worked as an office clerk.

Your relationship with Chloe has deteriorated in the last three months. Last week, Chloe told you that she thought you had a serious problem and that she could no longer tolerate you sitting at home drinking all day. She told you that she would leave you if you did not seek help. This is why you have come to the GP clinic today.

Model Answer

This station is relatively straightforward with the single purpose of making a diagnosis. Patients often present with several comorbid conditions, as seen in this station. Scott is experiencing a cluster of symptoms that meet the established criteria for post-traumatic stress disorder (PTSD), major depressive disorder, and alcohol dependence. The latter two are common comorbidities of PTSD.

The good student will have a systematic approach to this station, initially focusing on demographics and the history of presenting complaint. The time course of symptoms is important, as it indicates that Scott's PTSD has had a delayed onset. Students should recognise that PTSD symptoms can be triggered at a later stage by events that re-enact the initial trauma. The student should ask about the various symptom groups of PTSD, which include persistent and intrusive re-experiencing of the traumatic event (sometimes called flashback phenomena, but this is a misnomer as patients do not experience straightforward flashbacks), avoidance of stimuli that remind the patient of the trauma, and symptoms and signs of autonomic hyperarousal (see pages 154–156).

Scott also had a panic attack during the fireworks. As anxiety disorders often co-exist, the good student will screen for other anxiety disorders. Asking about whether the patient had further panic attacks may lead to a diagnosis of panic disorder. If recurrent panic attacks exist, asking about whether this stops the patient from going to certain places for fear of being trapped or unable to get help may lead to a diagnosis of panic disorder with agoraphobia. It is best to either clearly elicit the symptoms of a panic attack or describe what this is to the patient in order to avoid confusion (see Box 10.3, page 151). For example, 'A panic attack is a discrete episode of intense anxiety that comes out of the blue and reaches its peak in ten minutes. During a panic attack you might feel like your heart is beating hard and fast, your breathing is fast and shallow, you are sweaty, you have a tremor in your hands, you feel nauseous, you feel dizzy, your legs get weak, you feel the world is coming to an end or you feel out of control. Have you ever had an episode like that?'.

Students may ask whether the patient is afraid of situations where they may be exposed to ridicule or embarrassment, such as public speaking, to screen for social phobia (see pages 152–153). Asking specifically, 'I wonder whether you get intrusive thoughts or images that come into your mind and cause you lots of anxiety, and you can't get them out of your head?' may indicate obsessions, providing they are recognised as products of one's own mind and seen as unpleasant, which will delineate them from delusions. If a patient does have an obsession, it is worthwhile trying to categorise the type of obsession, such as contamination-based, symmetry-based or security-based, and searching for a paired compulsion by asking, 'I wonder whether you feel you need to do things, say things, or think certain things in order to lessen the anxiety from those intrusive thoughts?'.

Moving through accepted criteria for depression and asking about negative cognitions is essential in a case of PTSD. This should lead to asking about alcohol use, as alcohol is initially anxiolytic and causes a short-term euphoria with disinhibition, but can lead to long-term physical and psychological consequences (see Chapter 22). Scott displays clear physiological tolerance and withdrawal, as well as the psychological features of alcohol dependence, which include narrowing of the coping repertoire, recognition that alcohol is detrimental but feeling unable to cut down, and increased salience of alcohol in his life. Asking about alcohol-related phyiscial sequelae, such as haematemesis and seizures, can also assist in establishing the severity of alcohol misuse.

FOR THE MORE ADVANCED LEARNER

The good student should establish the psychosocial impact of these symptoms on Scott's life. This includes the domains of finance, housing, recreational activities, vocation, education, relationships and sexual relationships. Asking about the various psychosocial domains is important not only in diagnosis, but management as well. Highlighting the past and potential losses and the different outcomes with treatment forms the cornerstone of motivational interviewing for people with substance use problems. Furthermore, key social contacts, such as Chloe and Bill, may be recruited as allies in Scott's ongoing treatment, which is likely to be a combination of psychosocial and pharmacological treatments.

Chapter 11

THE OBSESSIVE-COMPULSIVE DISORDERS

DAVID J CASTLE & DARRYL BASSETT

Obsessive-compulsive spectrum disorders are characterised by the presence of:

- *obsessional thoughts*, which are recognised by the individual as their own, are intrusive, anxiety-provoking and distressing, and are essentially ego-dystonic
- *compulsions*, which are ritualised acts or mental processes responsive to the obsession and which reduce (at least in the short term) the anxiety associated with the obsession.

These phenomena can also be seen in other psychiatric disorders and occur in psychiatrically healthy people. They thus lack specificity. Indeed, obsessions and some degree of compulsive behaviour are quite normal, and arguably a degree of 'carefulness' in terms of, for example, checking behaviours, is both adaptive and useful in everyday life.

Obsessive-compulsive disorder (OCD)

When obsessional thoughts become excessively intrusive, and the obsessions and compulsions become time-consuming (nominally over an hour a day) and interfere with daily functioning, the individual can be considered to have *obsessive-compulsive disorder (OCD)*, as long as other psychiatric and medical (organic) causes have been excluded.

Box 11.1

Subtypes of obsessive-compulsive disorder (OCD)

Subtypes include:

• cleanliness obsessions and washing rituals

• uncertainty and checking rituals

• angry/religious/sexual obsessions without overt rituals

• primary obsessional slowness

• hoarding.

OCD symptoms can co-occur with other psychiatric symptoms, and the determination of which is 'primary' has important potential therapeutic implications, as demonstrated in the case examples in this chapter.

OCD itself can manifest in a number of ways. The most robust subtypes of OCD are shown in Box 11.1. There is overlap between these subtypes, and some patients present with symptoms from a number of them at the same time or at different time-points on their illness trajectory.

Hoarding is a behaviour (or set of behaviours) that does not sit well within the obsessive-compulsive rubric. It clearly delineates from the other subtypes of OCD clinically, and does not respond well to the classic OCD treatments, such as exposure/response prevention (EX/RP) and serotonergic antidepressants. Furthermore, it can manifest in a number of other disorders, including senile squalor ('Diogenes') syndrome, schizophrenia and dementia. It is likely that in DSM-5 it will be removed from OCD.

There has been a lack of consensus about how common OCD really is. A number of early studies probably underestimated the rate, while more recent large population-based studies, such as the Epidemiological Catchment Area (ECA) study in the United States, which relied on lay-interviewer diagnoses (based on a structured interview, the Diagnostic Interview Schedule (DIS), but open to interpretation), almost certainly led to overestimates. Application of DSM–IV–TR criteria to an Australian general population sample resulted in a rate estimate of 0.6%, and this seems a reasonable take-home figure.

There is less debate about gender differences in OCD, with most studies suggesting an equal lifetime risk for males and females, but with males having an overall earlier onset of illness (late teens versus early 20s for females). The longitudinal course of illness is variable, and symptoms often wax and wane, usually worsening at times of personal stress. OCD can be an extremely disabling disorder associated with profound long-term disability.

Management

The management of OCD encompasses psychological and biological domains.

Psychological domain

Psychological treatments generally include elements of EX/RP, with the patient helped to 'face their fears' in a structured, supported and hierarchical way. For example, the patient with contamination fears is encouraged to become progressively 'contaminated' (the exposure) and not immediately wash (the response prevention). Family members can be usefully included in the treatment plan to ensure they support the patient, but do not give in to reassurance-seeking behaviours that would undermine the exposure exercise (e.g. the checker of electrical appliances asking a family member to check that the appliance has been switched off).

Psychological treatment in patients without overt rituals is rather more complex, but various strategies can be used. These include *distraction*, with the patient taught to bring pleasant or neutral thoughts into their mind to counter the obsession; *thought stop*, where a stop sign or some such image is used; *aversive conditioning*, such as snapping an elastic band on the wrist when obsessions arise; and exposure to a script or recording of their own thoughts. There is some debate as to how much a cognitive addition to EX/RP helps patients with OCD, as most patients readily admit that their fears are unreasonable. However, some patients do gain benefit from direct cognitive challenge. For example, a patient who believed every time she had sex that she had become pregnant, despite the use of a condom and being on a contraceptive pill, was tasked with establishing the objective risks of pregnancy in the setting of each of these precautionary measures, and shown how the risk of conception while using both was mathematically extraordinarily unlikely.

Biological domain

The most effective and well-established pharmacotherapy for OCD is *serotonergic antidepressants*, including the selective serotonin reuptake inhibitors (SSRIs) and clomipramine (see Chapter 15). Doses required are often higher than those usually needed for depression and it can take some months of treatment to see the full benefit. Many patients are left with residual symptoms, and some of these benefit from the adjunctive use of other agents such as *antipsychotics*. There is some evidence that patients with concomitant motor tics or schizotypal personality disorder particularly benefit from this latter approach. In very severe persistent OCD, *deep brain stimulation* (DBS) has been found to be effective in some cases, and this has supplanted the older irreversible neurosurgical techniques.

Obsessive-compulsive spectrum disorders

Obsessions and/or compulsions can also occur in a number of other disorders, as shown in Figure 11.1. These are sometimes grouped together into a so-called obsessive-compulsive spectrum of disorders (OCS). While the veracity of this approach is open to criticism, and some members of the spectrum fit much more snugly than do others, we use this overall structure here to address these groups of disorders in turn.

Disorders associated with bodily preoccupation

Body dysmorphic disorder (BDD)

Body dysmorphic disorder (BDD) is characterised by a preoccupation with a perceived imperfection or abnormality in physical appearance. It usually onsets in the teens and affects males and females roughly equally. Any aspect of appearance may be affected, but if the preoccupation is solely with weight and shape, then the diagnosis is of an eating disorder (actually there is a high rate of 'comorbid' BDD in people with eating disorders). The disorder has many similarities with OCD, but the intrusive thoughts are technically ego-syntonic, and are much more likely (about 50%) to be held with delusional conviction.

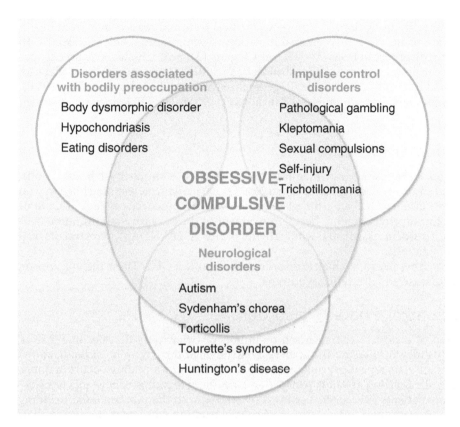

Figure 11.1 Obsessive-compulsive spectrum disorders

Rituals such as excessive and prolonged grooming can be very time-consuming; mirror checking can be either excessive or avoided as far as possible. There is also significant comorbidity with social anxiety disorder and depression.

Treatment includes various psychological techniques, notably cognitive-behaviour therapy (CBT) and EX/RP, and serotonergic antidepressants: as with OCD, high doses and prolonged treatment trials are required. Adjunctive antipsychotics can be helpful in some patients, but are not effective as solo agents, even if the patient has the delusional form of BDD.

Eating disorders

There is some debate about the inclusion of these disorders within the OCS, and they are covered separately in this book (see Chapter 12).

Hypochondriasis

This is a somewhat old-fashioned term which refers to a preoccupation with physical health, a belief one has a physical illness, and the seeking of help for this perceived problem from health professionals. Numerous medical tests and reassurance from health professionals are to no avail. It is one manifestation of somatisation, and is classed with the somatoform disorders in DSM–IV–TR (see Chapter 13). Hypochondriacal preoccupations can be seen in a number of other disorders, including depression (where they can reach delusional intensity; see Chapter 8), generalised anxiety disorder (see Chapter 10), and monosymptomatic hypochondriacal delusions (in DSM–IV–TR, delusional disorder, somatic subtype; see Chapter 7).

Neurological disorders

Obsessions and compulsions can manifest in response to a number of brain insults, including head injury and encephalitis lethargica. Of particular interest are children who have an abrupt onset of OCS after throat infection with streptococcus type A. This idiosyncratic autoimmune reaction has been grouped within the pervasive autoimmune neuropsychiatric disorders associated with streptococcus A (PANDAS). Treatments can include plasmapheresis.

A number of other neuropsychiatric disorders can manifest OCS. These include autism, Huntington's disease and Tourette's syndrome.

Impulse control ('habit') disorders

This is a group of disorders characterised by impulsive behaviours that become 'habits' which are very difficult to resist. The archetypal member of this group is *trichotillomania* (TTM), where sufferers repeatedly pull out their hair. Usually, hair pulling occurs in bouts, commencing with a feeling of being 'pent up', and 'needing' to pull to relieve this unpleasant affect. Some patients have a ritualised way of dealing with the plucked hair, including mouthing it and even ingestion: gastrointestinal obstruction can occur because of hair balls.

Treatment is difficult, with the most established mode being a behaviour modification technique called *habit reversal*, where a competing action (e.g. fist clenching) is encouraged to break the pulling cycle. Serotonergic antidepressants help some patients, but not very consistently.

Case examples: Obsessive-compulsive spectrum disorders

Depression with secondary hypochondriasis

A 45-year-old man presented with severe depression. He had become obsessed with his physical health, thinking he had bowel cancer (he was constipated) and kept seeking reassurance from medical doctors and requesting further investigations for his bowel problem. *Treatment* was primarily of the depressive process.

Obsessive-compulsive disorder

A 20-year-old nurse who had always been fastidious about personal cleanliness presented with intense anxiety revolving around the belief she had contracted hepatitis C following being inadvertently splashed by the urine of a patient with this condition. She was taking excessive precautions to avoid contact with any bodily fluids, including wearing safety goggles and three layers of gloves at all

Case examples continued

times at work. When she arrived home from work, she would strip off all her work clothes, place them in the washing machine, and don an 'uncontaminated' set of clothes for indoor use. She could no longer invite work colleagues to her home in case they contaminated it. *Treatment* was with a combination of EX/RP and a serotonergic antidepressant.

Obsessive-compulsive symptoms secondary to an atypical antipsychotic

After commencing the antipsychotic clozapine, a 40-year-old man with schizophrenia developed ritualised checking and cleaning behaviours, which for him became distressing and very time-consuming. The beliefs which drove the ritualised behaviours were quite independent of any psychotic beliefs, which had actually abated with the clozapine. *Treatment* was to continue the clozapine and treat the OCS with the established psychological and pharmacological techniques. (Note that the antidepressant fluvoxamine should be avoided as it interacts with clozapine.)

Body dysmorphic disorder

An 18-year-old was referred by a plastic surgeon. She had had two rhinoplasties by other surgeons, but was still unhappy with the outcome and was seeking a further procedure. She had been 'obsessed' by her 'hideous' nose since childhood, thought about it incessantly, constantly compared her nose with others and with models in magazines, and spent hours a day looking at her nose from different angles in the mirror. As soon as she was 16 she had persuaded her parents to pay for the initial cosmetic procedure. She was at first happy with the outcome, but soon began to think it was even worse than before, and resorted to covering it up with a plaster before she would even venture out of the house. She avoided social situations and had become significantly depressed. *Treatment* was with a combination of CBT and high-dose serotonergic antidepressants.

REFERENCES AND FURTHER READING

Castle, D., Groves, A., 2000. The internal and external boundaries of obsessive compulsive disorder. Australian and New Zealand Journal of Psychiatry 34, 249–255.

Castle, D., Phillips, K.A., 2006. The obsessive-compulsive spectrum of disorders: a defensible construct? Australian and New Zealand Journal of Psychiatry 40, 114–120.

Crino, R., Slade, T., Andrews, G., 2005. The changing prevalence of obsessive-compulsive disorder criteria from DSM–III to DSM–IV. American Journal of Psychiatry 162, 876–882.

Hollander, E., 2005. Obsessive-compulsive disorder and spectrum across the lifespan. International Review of Psychiatry in Clinical Practice 9, 79–86.

Stein, D.J. (Ed.), 2006. Obsessive-compulsive spectrum disorders. Psychiatric Clinics of North America 29, 343–613.

CHAPTER 11

A STUDENT NAMED STEPHEN
CASE-BASED LEARNING

JOEL KING & ANDREW GLEASON

The following role-play should be followed directly by the scenario in Chapter 16. This role-play requires two participants: one to play a GP registrar (candidate) and another to play the role of a patient, Stephen (actor).

OSCE Station Instructions

(Reading time: 2 minutes)

You are a GP registrar working in a suburban practice. You are asked to see Stephen, a 20-year-old university student. Stephen has upcoming exams and he is very concerned that he will not be able to cope.

Task (10 minutes)

- Take an appropriate history from Stephen to determine the most likely diagnosis.
- You do not need to conduct a physical examination or address management at this stage.

Actor role: Stephen

You are a 20-year-old man in your first year of your Commerce/Law degree at university. You live with your mother (Lauren) and father (Frank). Your mother is a tax accountant. Your father is a chemical engineer.

You have agreed to come to the doctor today because you have not been able to go to university for the last three weeks because of your thoughts. You are very worried about your first round of university exams in two months' time and believe that you will fail them.

Over the last three months, you have developed intrusive thoughts (obsessions) that door handles and other things that lots of people might grab with their hands are infected with germs and this might infect you. You are afraid that you'll get a golden staph infection and require hospitalisation, which would prevent you from sitting the exams.

You know that these thoughts are in your head and very out of proportion to reality. However, they cause you a great deal of anxiety and distress. You feel the need to wash your hands up to twenty times per day. You use one whole soap bar every three days. You only use antibacterial soap.

You also shower for an hour every time you come home, even if it is just to the milk bar. The hand-washing and showering temporarily relieves your anxiety.

You get very distressed when your parents come home and don't make a significant attempt to 'decontaminate' themselves, either by washing their hands thoroughly or showering. You scream at them, tell them that they're dirty, and plead with them to clean themselves.

PSYCHOSOCIAL IMPACT

These thoughts and behaviours have gradually become worse. They stop you from catching public transport and going to public places, like the movies, because lots of people might have touched the things in those places. They also prevent you from going out with your friends and to university. Your attendance has dropped off and you have not been to university in the last three weeks.

DEPRESSIVE FEATURES

As your thoughts and cleaning behaviours have become worse, you have developed numerous symptoms of depression over the last three months, including low mood, impaired concentration, poor energy, lethargy, and poor appetite. You have not had any changes in your weight or appetite and have not experienced feelings of worthlessness. You have never had suicidal ideation. You feel that your behaviours have led to you being excluded from your friends. You feel trapped and lonely.

OTHER OCD FEATURES

You do not have any other obsessive-compulsive symptoms, such as compulsions to touch, check, count, arrange things, or hoard. You do not have any underlying obsessions relating to sexuality or aggression.

OTHER ANXIETY SYMPTOMS

You do not have social anxiety (performance anxiety), panic attacks, PTSD, or specific phobias.

OTHER PSYCHIATRIC SYMPTOMS

You have no psychotic symptoms (such as delusions or hallucinations). You have no problems with body image or eating. You have never had any somatoform or conversion problems (unexplained medical symptoms).

PAST PSYCHIATRIC HISTORY

You have no past psychiatric history. You have never seen a psychiatrist, never received a psychiatric diagnosis, never been admitted to a psychiatric unit, or received a psychiatric medication. You have never seen a psychologist or counsellor.

You have never had these symptoms until three months ago.

You do not have a significant substance use history, medical history, forensic, or family psychiatric history.

DEVELOPMENTAL HISTORY

You were a planned pregnancy and born locally. Your gestation, delivery and developmental milestones were unremarkable. You have never been abused or neglected. Your parents are very loving and attentive, but also expect the best from you, having migrated so that you can have a good education and opportunities. They have organised private tuition and music lessons. You have never been good at sport.

You have always been brilliant academically and went to an elite single sex school on a full academic scholarship. You have never been teased or bullied, but have always been shy and have a small group of male friends who are similarly shy. You have never had a girlfriend, but you are interested in finding one. However, your shyness and unfamiliarity with the opposite gender make this difficult.

HOW TO PLAY THE ROLE

You should look shy, passive and intimidated. You do not provide information spontaneously, but answer any question put to you. You should say 'Doctor' a lot. You desperately want to get better but don't know what's wrong with you. You will agree to anything the doctor suggests.

Statements you must make:
- 'Thanks for seeing me, Doctor. I'm really worried about my exams.'
- 'I get really anxious because I'm worried I'm going to catch an infection and end up in hospital.'
- 'I'm so worried about getting germs that it's hard to go outside.'

Model Answer

This is a straightforward station, with a patient presenting with overt symptoms of obsessive-compulsive disorder, but also with a secondary depression. The candidate should employ a structured approach, starting initially with the demographics and moving to the presenting complaint.

Candidates should delineate obsessions – intrusive, distressing, recurrent thoughts and mental images – from compulsions – behaviours and mental acts that are employed to temporarily relieve the anxiety caused by the obsessions. Candidates should recognise that obsessions are often paired with certain compulsions, such as contamination-based obsessions with cleaning compulsions. Candidates should also be aware that there are numerous types of obsessions, such as those relating to order and symmetry (see Box 11.1, page 163). Obsessions relating to anxiety about being homosexual or aggressive are also possible, but patients are often very reluctant to disclose these for fear of embarrassment. Normalising the obsession can be useful in eliciting these features (e.g. 'Many people have this problem. I wonder whether it's the same for you?').

To establish the diagnosis of OCD, the candidate should clarify whether the thoughts are recognised as products of one's own mind and are excessive, in order to distinguish them as obsessions instead of delusions. The candidate should also quantify the amount of time spent on the obsessions and compulsions, as well as the psychosocial impact.

FOR THE MORE ADVANCED LEARNER

Individuals with OCD often have a secondary depression, as well as other anxiety disorders, such as social anxiety disorder (SAD) or panic disorder. Use of short-term anxiolytic substances, such as alcohol and benzodiazepines are common in anxiety disorders, so candidates should screen for this as well. Candidates are well-advised to screen for psychotic symptoms, because some cases of OCD are later re-diagnosed as psychotic disorders.

Chapter 12

EATING DISORDERS

PETER BOSANAC & DAVID J CASTLE

The eating disorders (apart from obesity, which is considered separately at the end of this chapter) are a group of conditions characterised by an overconcern with size and shape, leading to aberrant eating behaviours and other measures to try to obtain the thin ideal. Although DSM–IV–TR and ICD–10 classify eating disorders into distinct conditions, psychopathology may be shared and diagnostic crossover can occur over time. Some authorities classify these disorders within the putative obsessive-compulsive spectrum (see Chapter 11). A transdiagnostic approach to classification, which emphasises similarities rather than differences in eating disorders, has also emerged. The classifications according to DSM–IV–TR and ICD–10 are summarised in Table 12.1. The upcoming DSM-5 has not proposed any major changes to the classification of eating disorders beyond binge eating disorder becoming a free standing diagnosis, as well as the eating disorders category encompassing feeding disorders.

Table 12.1

Classification of eating disorders according to DSM-IV-TR and ICD-10 (synopsis)

DSM-IV-TR	ICD-10
The classifications are: • anorexia nervosa • bulimia nervosa, and • eating disorder not otherwise specified.	The classifications are: • anorexia nervosa • bulimia nervosa • atypical bulimia nervosa • overeating associated with other psychological disturbances • vomiting associated with other psychological disturbances • other eating disorders, and • eating disorder, unspecified.

Anorexia nervosa (AN)

Anorexia nervosa (AN) is a disorder characterised by a distortion of body image such that individuals 'see' themselves as fat when they are, in fact, thin. They have a 'morbid fear of fatness' and engage in activities to try to achieve a thin body ideal. By definition, AN is diagnosed when the individual 'refuses to maintain a weight over a minimal norm, leading to body weight less than 85% of that expected' (DSM–IV-TR) or is under a body mass index (BMI) of 17.5 kg/m² (ICD–10) (BMI = weight in kilograms/height in metres²). In growing children there is a failure to make expected weight gain during a period of growth. In post-pubertal girls there is the added criterion of amenorrhoea (some experts have challenged the amenorrhoea criterion as being redundant, and it may be dropped from the definition of AN in DSM-5). The current criteria are summarised in Table 12.2.

AN afflicts around 0.5% of young females (it is much less common in males) and onsets usually around puberty (mean age at onset 15–19 years). Patients engage in dieting behaviours, with either a purely *restrictive* pattern (i.e. restricting intake, especially of what are perceived as fattening foods), or encompassing *binge–purge* cycles, with episodic overeating followed by guilt, self-blame and purging. Dieting becomes an obsession, with avoidance of foods perceived as being fattening (some patients will avoid even smelling or touching such foods), calorie-counting, excessive weighing, and so forth. A variety of ritualised behaviours can occur, including around food preparation and meals, excessive exercise and weighing. Patients might also employ laxatives and diuretics. Box 12.1 lists some of the medical complications associated with AN.

Treatment of AN is rather complex, partly because sufferers often resent treatment and partly because the starvation cycle sets a very powerful train into motion. Education, nutritional rehabilitation and psychotherapy are the mainstays of management; psychotropic medications play an adjuvant role. This integrated approach is best coordinated among the general practitioner, psychiatrist, psychologist, dietician and other clinicians.

Although there is currently an overall lack of empirically established, evidence-based treatments for AN, this does not equate to ineffectiveness of treatment, and established key components of treatment include:

Table 12.2

Criteria for anorexia nervosa according to DSM–IV–TR and ICD–10 (synopsis)

DSM–IV–TR	ICD–10
Criteria are: • refusal to maintain body weight at or above minimally normal weight for age and height (less than 85% of that expected, or failure of expected weight gain during a period of growth) • intense fear of gaining weight or becoming fat, even though underweight • disturbance in the way body weight or shape is experienced, undue influence of body weight or shape on self-evaluation, or denial of the seriousness of low body weight • amenorrhoea in post-menarchal females • *specification* of restricting type or binge eating/purging type.	Criteria are: • weight loss (at least 15% below normal, or that expected for age and height) • weight loss is self-induced by avoidance of 'fattening foods' • self-perception of being too fat, with intrusive dread of fatness • widespread endocrine disorder involving hypothalamic-pituitary-gonadal axis.

Box 12.1

Selected potential medical complications of anorexia nervosa

Complications include:

• lanugo hair (fine excessive body hair)

• dry skin

• hypothermia

• atonic bowel from excessive laxative use

• constipation

• osteopaenia and fractures

• joint problems from excessive high-impact exercise such as running

• amenorrhoea

• reduced fertility

• ovarian atrophy

• death from starvation.

- restoration to healthy weight (menstruation and ovulation in females, normal sexual hormone levels in males and restoration of physical and sexual growth and development in children and adolescents)
- treatment of physical complications
- enhancement of motivation to restore healthy eating patterns and engagement in treatment
- education about healthy nutrition and eating patterns
- psychological intervention for related maladaptive thoughts, attitudes and feelings
- treatment of psychiatric comorbidity
- relapse prevention.

Treatment should, where feasible, always include the family, at the very least in terms of provision of education and support. More formal family therapy has proven to be of benefit for relapse prevention in younger girls. There are a number of family therapy approaches, including structural, strategic, behavioural and family-based treatment. *Family-based treatment* in adolescent AN, now regarded as first-line treatment in this group, was developed at the Maudsley Hospital in London, and is often called 'The Maudsley model'. In this treatment, which is applicable to teenagers, the parents of the patient are empowered to intervene actively with re-feeding; helped to renegotiate the relationship with the child to encompass issues other than just food; and aided in assisting their child to resume a normal developmental pathway without an eating disorder. The majority of patients who engage in this treatment (and not all are willing and/or have a family who is amenable) appear to have sustained benefit (5 years) in terms of remission.

If the patient is *significantly underweight*, such that they are medically compromised, re-feeding is required as a matter of urgency. Guidelines about hospitalisation are based on expert opinion, but differ between the American Psychiatric Association (APA) in North America and the National Institute of Clinical Excellence (NICE) in the United Kingdom. Thus, the APA recommends hospitalisation for markedly underweight patients, while NICE endorses that most patients be treated as outpatients, with inpatient care being reserved for when there is a poor response to outpatient treatment; a significant risk of suicide; and at least moderate physical risk.

Nutritional rehabilitation and medical monitoring during re-feeding are essential features of treatment for AN patients who are significantly underweight. Nutritional rehabilitation involves normalising three meals and snacks with 4000–6400 kilojoules per day initially, and up to 10,000–16,500 kilojoules per day. Weight gain of 0.25–0.5 kg per week as an outpatient, and 0.5–1 kg per week as an inpatient are appropriate trajectories. Patients have a better prognosis and are less likely to relapse if they are discharged from inpatient settings with a BMI ≥ 16 kg/m^2.

Vital signs, fluid and food intake, serum electrolytes (magnesium, phosphorus and potassium), thiamine and blood glucose require monitoring during re-feeding. *Magnesium* levels can drop over the first 5–10 days (causing weakness, cramps, impaired short-term memory and difficulty with visual accommodation) and intravenous replacement (20 millimoles per day over 5–10 days) may be required. *Phosphorus* levels also fall over the first few days of re-feeding and can be life-threatening once at or below 30–50% of the lower laboratory limit; symptoms might include delirium and/or cardiac failure. Intravenous *glucose* can worsen hypophosphataemia and should therefore be avoided at this time, particularly when hypoglycaemia is not present. *Phosphate* can be supplemented at 500 mg three times a day, or intravenously. If serum phosphorus is low and falling, then it may be necessary to cease the re-feeding in the interim, while phosphate replacement is occurring. Falls in *potassium* levels (weakness, palpitations and polyuria) during re-feeding are usually gradual; this occurs in hypovolaemic states with urinary potassium loss (> 10 mm/L) in exchange for sodium to maintain extracellular volume, and when volume status is normal while serum magnesium is low.

Thiamine deficiency, which can result in Wernicke's encephalopathy, can occur during re-feeding and may require thiamine and concurrent magnesium replacement. Hypoglycaemia can also occur during re-feeding and result in post-prandial hypoglycaemia; the response to 1 mg intravenous glucagon should increase blood glucose to around 7 millimoles/L; otherwise, there is a risk of post-prandial hypoglycaemia. The latter may require 10–20 days of re-feeding to restore hepatic glycogen. Dietician advice is crucial. Adjunctive medications, notably atypical antipsychotics such as olanzapine, can be helpful in reducing anxiety or distress associated with re-feeding or body image disturbance. However, it is not known whether these medications may confer benefit specific to the core symptoms of AN.

Case history: Anorexia nervosa

A secondary school student had taken up dancing 8 months earlier. According to her parents, she had always been a shy and stoic girl, but had become increasingly irritable and argumentative with her parents over the previous year. She had begun distance running 10 months earlier and became 'vegetarian'. Her parents had become increasingly worried about her looking gaunt and rarely eating a meal with them, but when they tried to talk to her about this she accused them of being domineering and 'upsetting' her, and also alluded to their marital difficulties and accused them of 'having nothing better to do with their time than criticise me'. Nonetheless, she reported that it was becoming more tiring when dancing, and she was worried that she would lose her place in the dance troupe because she was not 'fit enough'. She was also concerned that she lacked 'tone' around her thighs and abdomen, especially when wearing her dance attire. She had not menstruated for 4 months and her BMI was 17 kg/m^2.

Bulimia nervosa (BN)

Bulimia nervosa (BN) shares with AN an overvalued belief in a thin ideal, but by definition sufferers are not underweight (in many cases they are actually heavier than the normal range). Again, girls are more often affected than boys (see above). Mean onset is in the early 20s. Some bulimic activity is common in high school girls, but BN itself has a prevalence of around 1% in such groups. BN became much more common over the latter decades of the 20th century, and is more prevalent in so-called developed countries, and in higher socioeconomic groups.

BN usually begins with dieting behaviour, which becomes predominantly a binge–purge cycle. Thus, sufferers perennially starve themselves, but ultimately become overwhelmed by the desire to eat, whereupon they binge, usually on high-calorie foods such as chocolates, biscuits or bread. Patients describe how once they start they simply cannot stop eating, and can consume a vast amount of food over a short period. This is often done in secret, and the person is usually ashamed of the behaviour. Sometimes food is stolen. After the binge, there is inevitable shame and guilt, which may lead to self-induced vomiting, usually by putting a hand down the throat. They might also resort to misuse of laxatives, diuretics, enemas and appetite suppressants. Table 12.3 summarises the criteria for BN, and Box 12.2 lists some of the potential medical complications of the condition.

Treatment of BN is usually done on an outpatient basis, using cognitive-behaviour therapy (CBT) techniques. There is an emphasis on regular meals and snacks to break the starvation–binge–purge cycle, as well as monitoring of shape and weight concerns, and the challenging of related negative thoughts. Other core components of treatment include:

- addressing binge eating and related compensatory behaviours, such as purging or excessive exercise
- exploring and challenging underlying psychological issues, such as self-esteem, body image and other disturbances of thinking

Table 12.3

Criteria for bulimia nervosa according to DSM–IV–TR and ICD–10
(synopsis)

DSM–IV–TR	ICD–10
Criteria are: • recurrent episodes of binge eating • recurrent inappropriate compensatory behaviours to prevent weight gain • binge eating and inappropriate compensatory behaviours on average at least twice a week for 3 months • self-evaluation unduly influenced by body shape and weight • disturbance does not occur exclusively during episodes of AN • *specification* of purging type and non-purging type.	Criteria are: • recurrent episodes of overeating (at least twice a week over 3 months) • persistent preoccupation with eating and strong desire or sense of compulsion to eat • attempts to counteract the 'fattening' effects of food • self-perception of being too fat, with intrusive dread of fatness.

Box 12.2

Selected potential medical complications of bulimia nervosa

Complications include:

- oesophageal excoriations from acid in the oesophagus
- oesophageal rupture
- erosion of dental enamel from stomach acid
- parotid gland swelling in response to stomach acid in the mouth; this can lead to a paradoxical 'fat faced' look
- abrasion of the knuckles from putting the hand down the throat (Russell's sign)
- hypokalaemic alkalosis from vomiting up high-potassium stomach acid
- cardiac arrhythmias
- constipation.

- treating comorbid psychiatric conditions, such as mood disorders and substance misuse
- providing nutritional counselling
- treating physical complications (see Box 12.2), and planning relapse prevention strategies.

Although CBT is the predominant psychological intervention in BN, it has evolved beyond a focus on weight and shape concerns to encompass self-esteem, tolerability of mood and interpersonal experiences (in second-generation CBT); emphasis on exposure to the body (in enhanced cognitive-behaviour therapy, or CBT–E); and integrative approaches with greater emphasis on emotional and cultural factors.

Other psychological interventions that are effective for some patients with BN include: self-help, with some professional guidance; interpersonal psychotherapy, which addresses interpersonal roles, stressors and transition through them; and dialectical-behavioural therapy, focusing on behavioural change, interpersonal relationships, mindfulness and regulation of emotion with acceptance and tolerance of distress. Family-based treatment may also hold promise in adolescent patients with BN.

Antidepressants have an established place as adjunctive treatments, with a reduction of binge eating and purging behaviours. There is similar efficacy among serotonergic and other antidepressants. The effect of antidepressants in BN is not as great as with CBT, and the therapeutic effect is often not maintained on cessation. The combination of CBT and antidepressants appears to be superior to either treatment on its own. Of course, if the patient is also depressed, one is more likely to employ an antidepressant.

Case history: Bulimia nervosa

A 14-year-old girl had just entered puberty; she was developing breasts and had started her menstrual periods. At a school social she had overheard one of the boys talking about 'fat chicks', and immediately assumed he was talking about her. She had decided to diet, but found that it was difficult to be consistent about her food habits, and became increasingly frustrated at her 'lack of willpower'. She started to weigh herself daily and to restrict her dietary intake. Every 3 or 4 days, she would become overwhelmingly hungry, and feel an urge to eat sweet things. She would buy large volumes of chocolate and sweets and eat them all in a single episode, by herself and often in the middle of the night, so that no one else would know about it. She immediately felt 'bloated and disgusting' and would put her fingers down her throat to make herself vomit. She also bought many packets of laxatives, and used these in increasing quantities to help her 'feel empty'.

Other eating disorders

The terms *binge eating disorder* and *eating disorder not otherwise specified* (EDNOS) are applied when the eating disorder does not meet criteria for AN or BN. The fact that many people with eating disorders are placed in these categories is an indication of the imperfections of the current classification systems. DSM-5 criteria will address these problems to same degree.

> ## Case history: Binge eating disorder
>
> A 42-year-old obese woman had struggled with her weight since childhood. She had experienced several severe episodes of depression, which she attributed to ongoing difficulty 'coping with excess weight'. She reported 'comfort eating' chocolates or biscuits when feeling anxious or stressed about her social isolation and finances. She ate at least two plates for her main meal each day, and although she tried, could not stop eating even when full. Although she had tried dieting in the past, she had not engaged in other strategies to try to lose weight.

Box 12.3

Classification of obesity

The US National Heart, Lung and Blood Institute classifies obesity as:

- *overweight*: a BMI of 25–29.9 kg/m²
- *obesity*:
  - class I: a BMI of 30–34.9 kg/m²
  - class II: a BMI of 35–39.9 kg/m²
  - class III: a BMI > 40 kg/m².

(US National Heart, Lung and Blood Institute)

Obesity

Although obesity is not considered primarily a psychiatric disorder, there is an increased incidence of obesity in some psychiatric disorders (e.g. binge eating disorder and night eating syndrome, major depressive disorder and schizophrenia), as well as being a potential risk with psychotropic medication (such as antipsychotics). Obesity is compounded by increased mortality and morbidity, including cardiovascular disease, dyslipidaemias, diabetes mellitus, stroke, malignancy and sleep apnoea (which is also associated with depression and diurnal fatigue). The prevalence of obesity is increasing, particularly in Western countries, with a significant health economic burden. The interaction of multiple genes, neural and hormonal regulation of appetite and activity, and the interface with environmental factors (meal size and physical activity) are significant in the aetiology of obesity. Intervention in childhood obesity may be of more enduring benefit than later in life. Box 12.3 shows the US National Heart, Lung and Blood Institute classification of obesity.

Improved eating habits, lifestyle change and exercise are the treatments of choice for overweight and moderately obese people. Psychotherapy is not a primary treatment for obesity, but may improve self-esteem and motivation for a healthier lifestyle and treatment.

Weight loss medication, such as orlistat, a gastrointestinal lipase inhibitor, may be considered for a BMI > 30 kg/m² without comorbid medical conditions such as diabetes, or for a BMI > 27 kg/m² when such comorbidity is present. Such medications added to behavioural treatment of obesity may result in relatively modest weight loss of 2.5–8 kg, with weight regain highly likely on discontinuation. The safety and efficacy profile of these medications beyond 1 year is not known. Obesity surgery (commonly known as 'lap banding') appears to be the most effective treatment for people with a BMI > 40 kg/m^2 or a BMI of 35–39.9 kg/m^2 with associated medical conditions, but again long-term outcomes are not clear.

REFERENCES AND FURTHER READING

Attia, E., Walsh, B.T., 2009. Behavioral management of anorexia nervosa. New England Journal of Medicine 360, 500–506.

Berkman, K.A., Lohr, K.N., Bulik, C.M., 2007. Outcomes of eating disorders: a systematic review of the literature. International Journal of Eating Disorders 40, 293–309.

Birmingham, C.L., 2002. The art and science of refeeding. In: Burrows, G.D., Bosanac, P., Beumont, P.J.V. (Eds.), Selected papers from the first Asian Pacific eating disorders congress, 10–14 November. University of Melbourne and Mental Health Foundation of Australia, Melbourne.

Brownley, K.A., Berkman, N.D., Sedway, J.A., Lohr, K.N., Bulik, C.M., 2007. Binge eating disorder treatment: a systematic review of randomized controlled studies. International Journal of Eating Disorders 40, 321–336.

Bulik, C.M., Berkman, N.D., Brownley, K.A., Sedway, J.A., Lohr, K.N., 2007. Anorexia nervosa treatment: a systematic review of randomized controlled studies. International Journal of Eating Disorders 40, 310–320.

Fairburn, C.G., Cooper, Z., 2011. Eating disorders, DSM-V and clinical reality. British Journal of Psychiatry 198, 8–10.

Honigman, R., Castle, D.J., 2007. Living with your looks. University of Western Australia Press, Perth.

Lock, J., 2011. Evaluation of family treatment models for eating disorders. Current Opinion in Psychiatry 24, 274–279.

Shapiro, J.R., Berkman, N.D., Brownley, K.A., Sedway, J.A., Lohr, K.N., Bulik, C.M., 2007. Bulimia nervosa treatment: a systematic review of randomized controlled studies. International Journal of Eating Disorders 40, 321–336.

Treasure, J., Schmidt, U., 2008. Eating disorders. In: Murray, R.M., Kendler, K., McGuffin, P., Wessely, S., Castle, D.J. (Eds.), Essential psychiatry, fourth ed. Cambridge University Press, Cambridge.

Wadden, A.T., Stunkard, A.J. (Eds.), 2004. Handbook of obesity treatment. Guilford Press, New York.

CHAPTER 12

A MEDICAL STUDENT NAMED PAT

CASE-BASED LEARNING

JOEL KING & ANDREW GLEASON

The following role-play requires two participants: one to play a medical resident (candidate) and another to play the role of a junior medical student named Pat (actor).

OSCE Station Instructions

(Reading time: 2 minutes)

You are a resident on the general medical ward. You have a very keen junior medical student, Pat, who is eager to learn from you.

Your consultant has asked you to show Pat how to perform a physical examination on Zoe, a 25-year-old woman with established anorexia nervosa. Zoe has been admitted voluntarily to the medical ward with a BMI of 14 and is receiving monitored oral re-feeding. Zoe was very impressed with Pat's empathic approach when Pat was clerking her earlier. As such, Zoe has consented to this demonstration for Pat's education and is okay with you describing what you are doing.

Task (10 minutes)

- Conduct the physical examination and highlight possible physical signs seen in the patient with anorexia nervosa.
- You should vocalise what you are looking for as you go through the physical examination.
- You will not be provided with any physical examination results.
- The role of Zoe will be played by a mannequin.

Actor role: Pat

You are Pat, a junior medical student attached to the medical ward. This is your first clinical placement. You are very excited and eager to learn. You think that being on the medical ward is the greatest thing ever, after endless lectures.

You have learnt that there is a patient on the ward who has anorexia nervosa and have been told by the consultant, 'Yes, they're quite interesting patients. You should examine her because they can have quite a myriad of physical signs. I'll ask the resident to demonstrate how to do this.'

You suspect that the consultant was trying to get you out of his outpatients room because you kept asking questions, but you are keen to learn nonetheless and run off to explore this learning opportunity.

HOW TO PLAY THE ROLE

You watch the candidate perform the physical examination with great interest. They should perform a thorough physical examination starting with the vital signs, commenting on general inspection, then moving through the hands to the head and down the rest of the body. The candidate should explain what he or she is looking for at each point. Occasionally, write down notes. If the candidate becomes silent, ask what they are looking for.

If the candidate becomes angry, dismissive or annoyed, state, 'I'm sorry, Doctor. I'm just trying to learn.'

If the candidate asks you a question, just respond:
- 'I'm sorry, Doctor. I don't know the answer to that question. What's the answer?' or
- 'I'm sorry. I don't know the answer. I'll write it down, look it up in the textbook tonight and tell you before the round tomorrow.'

Statements you must make:
- 'Thanks for agreeing to demonstrate how to examine someone with anorexia nervosa, Doctor.'
- 'Do you mind just telling me what you're doing so I can write it down in my notebook?'
- 'I found this past exam question: Name TWO important investigations you would order for a patient with anorexia nervosa. What do you think the answer is?' (at 8 minutes).

Model Answer

This station highlights the physical sequelae that can occur in patients with anorexia nervosa. These are serious and should be recognised by all doctors (Box 12.1, page 174). It requires competency in performing a basic multi-system physical examination. Students should consult a physical examination textbook for reference.

The candidate should greet the medical student and the patient confidently and warmly. They should acknowledge that informed consent has been obtained and explain what will happen during the physical examination. Despite the patient being a mannequin, the candidate should act as if this was a real patient and show the appropriate respect, particularly around disrobing the patient.

The physical examination should start with a general inspection. The candidate may note an emaciated frame, psychomotor retardation, and possible altered consciousness. The candidate may ask for the observation chart and note hypotension (which can be postural), bradycardia, hypothermia, and an altered respiratory rate. The respiratory rate can be decreased in metabolic alkalosis with prolonged vomiting and the associated loss of hydrochloric acid from the stomach contents, or more rarely increased in metabolic acidosis due to the production of ketones from lipid metabolism. Laxative abuse can cause metabolic acidosis or alkalosis.

From here, a good approach is to start with the hands, move up to the head and down the rest of the body. Cold and blue hands may indicate peripheral shutdown. Russell's sign may be present, which is callus formation on the dorsum of the hand overlying the metacarpophalangeal and interphalangeal joints. Russell's sign is caused by repeated contact of the incisors to the skin of the hand that occurs during self-induced vomiting. The nails may be brittle. The skin may have an orange colour, suggesting carotinaemia, due to slowed breakdown of carotene or consumption of large quantities of low-energy carotene-containing vegetables such as pumpkin and carrots. Easy bruising may indicate deficiency of vitamin K dependent clotting factors or thrombocytopaenia. The candidate should look for lanugo, which is fine, downy, minimally pigmented hair, and may be found on the back, forearms and abdomen.

The head is a treasure trove of various signs. The eyes may be sunken. Parotidomegaly may be found. The mucosal membranes may be dry due to dehydration. The teeth may show corrosive changes secondary to continuous vomiting of the stomach's acidic products.

Moving to the chest, the candidate may discover breast atrophy and a lack of other secondary sexual characteristics. Cardiovascular examination may reveal signs of cardiac failure. Respiratory examination may reveal pneumonia, as infections are more common in the compromised immune system of the anorexic patient. Abdominal examination may reveal abdominal tenderness secondary to gastritis, constipation, or superior mesenteric artery syndrome.

Neurological examination of the peripheries may reveal proximal myopathy. This is most easily done by asking the patient to perform a squat test. Peripheral neuropathy may also be present. Calcium deficiency may manifest in fractures. The lower limbs may show evidence of oedema, which can result from low albumin and cardiac failure.

Upon completion of the physical examination, the candidate should ensure that the patient is dressed and thanked appropriately. To answer Pat's question about investigations, the candidate should state that an electrocardiogram (ECG) and electrolytes (particularly potassium, calcium, magnesium, and phosphate) should be performed. Hypokalaemia from vomiting may result in prominent U waves and a prolonged QTc interval on the ECG. Potassium and the other electrolytes are important to monitor over the next three to four days as re-feeding syndrome may occur, which can lead to acute cardiac and respiratory failure, renal failure, and encephalopathy.

Chapter 13

SOMATISATION AND THE SOMATOFORM DISORDERS

MICHAEL SALZBERG, DAVID J CASTLE &
DARRYL BASSETT

For most doctors in clinical practice, somatisation and somatoform presentations of psychiatric illness are the single biggest class of symptoms they will encounter. This is a big claim but easily substantiated by a large body of studies. Anxiety and depressive disorders frequently present with physical complaints, rather than by patients saying 'I'm anxious' or 'I'm depressed'. Complaints of fatigue, headache, insomnia, pain, palpitations and dizziness are everyday presentations to general practitioners and specialists, and often are the surface manifestation of depression or anxiety. Depressed patients often become hypochondriacal, in the sense of becoming more anxious about and more attentive to physical symptoms, and more ready to consult a doctor about them.

In addition to these high-prevalence presentations, there is a range of less common somatoform disorders, as shown in Table 13.1. Although all are collected together under

Table 13.1

Selected somatoform disorders (DSM–IV–TR)

Disorder (synopsis)	Comments
Somatisation disorder: multiple symptoms occur over several years without demonstrable physical cause. Symptoms include: • four pain symptoms (e.g. head, back, joints, chest or rectum; or during intercourse, menstruation or urination) • two gastrointestinal symptoms other than pain (e.g. nausea, bloating or intolerance of certain foods) • one sexual problem other than pain (e.g. sexual indifference, irregular menses, excessive menstrual bleeding, or erectile or ejaculatory problem), and • one pseudo-neurological problem other than pain (e.g. conversion symptoms or dissociative symptoms)	This is a rare and extreme disorder involving the experience of multiple symptoms in multiple body systems. Given its onset in adolescence or young adulthood, the way life revolves so completely around symptoms and help-seeking, its pervasive effects on relationships, and the fact that it often emerges from adverse early life experiences of emotional neglect, abuse or loss, some have argued it is a form of personality disorder.
Conversion disorder: motor or sensory deficits (or seizures) suggesting a neurological or medical cause, but for which no physical explanation can be found.	For largely historical reasons, when somatisation takes the form of 'neurological' symptoms, it has been allocated a category of its own: conversion disorder. In general hospitals, the most common presentations are psychogenic non-epileptic seizures (PNES), functional gait disorders, paralysis (including aphonia) or sensory loss (including blindness). Dizziness presents to cardiologists and ear, nose and throat specialists, as well as neurologists. For 'fainting attacks' patients present to cardiologists as well as neurologists.
Hypochondriasis: preoccupation with having a serious physical disease, leading to seeking medical help, but failing to be reassured by 'negative' medical examinations and tests.	Typically, these patients are preoccupied with one symptom (or a set of related symptoms) at a time, in contrast to somatisation disorder. Some experts have argued this has a lot in common with anxiety disorders and, in recent years, cognitive-behaviour therapies have been developed and trialled with some success.

Continued

Table 13.1

Selected somatoform disorders (DSM–IV–TR)—cont'd

Disorder (synopsis)	Comments
Pain disorder: pain is the predominant symptom, and causes significant distress and disability; it is defined as acute if duration is less that 6 months, and chronic if greater than 6 months.	There are two types: • associated with psychological factors (i.e. psychological factors are considered the major factor associated with onset, severity, exacerbation or maintenance of the pain) • associated with both psychological factors and a general medical condition (i.e. both psychological factors and a general medical condition are considered to have important roles in the onset, severity, exacerbation or maintenance of the pain).

the heading of *somatoform disorders*, these are conditions with very different natural histories, causation and treatments. In addition, the group as a whole has contested uneasy borders with factitious disorder, malingering, the culture-bound syndromes and the concept of 'psychological factors affecting physical illness'. For completeness, it is worth mentioning that occasionally patients with psychoses, such as schizophrenia, can present with odd physical symptoms stemming from delusions about their bodies, or from somatic or tactile hallucinations.

Many doctors and medical students dislike and avoid this area of medicine. They find the ideas intellectually muddy and the terminology confusing. They may be sceptical that these are disorders, rather than malingering or 'attention seeking'. Even when sympathetic to the patient's plight, they feel ill-equipped to help. Doctors can quickly feel drained, angry and helpless when faced with the more severe forms of chronic somatisation; even if they retain their professional courtesy, their body language may betray their true feelings. Their reactions to patients may be constructive or destructive. It is common for patients to be told 'there's nothing wrong with you', with the implication that 'it's all in your head'.

Medical services overall still do not deal well with these disorders. They are often missed clinically, so that it remains common for patients to undergo extensive, unnecessary referrals and investigations, which can reinforce or amplify the patient's problem. In addition, doctors fear that in making a somatoform diagnosis they may miss a serious physical diagnosis. It is common for doctors to engage in 'either/or' thinking: it is either a 'real' illness (e.g. brain tumour), or it is 'psychological'. In reality, physical illness and somatisation frequently coexist. A good example is psychogenic non-epileptic seizures (PNES) (unfortunately, still often termed 'pseudoseizures', a term which patients experience as pejorative and which should be abandoned). PNES coexist with epileptic seizures in a substantial minority of epilepsy patients (i.e. some patients have both kinds of event).

Box 13.1

Psychiatric disorders in which somatisation occurs

Disorders include:

- somatic symptoms in the course of high-prevalence disorders, such as depression and anxiety disorders
- somatic symptoms in the course of low-prevalence disorders, such as schizophrenia
- somatoform disorders
- somatisation disorder
- conversion disorder
- hypochondriasis
- body dysmorphic disorder
- pain disorder
- factitious disorder
- psychological factors affecting medical conditions
- culture-bound syndromes.

For most somatisation symptoms and somatoform disorders, the evidence for psychological causation is compelling. For example, there are clear data from cohort studies that people subjected to childhood abuse and neglect are at higher risk of a range of disorders in later life, including somatising disorders. This fits with clinical experience and with the kind of evidence that emerges from detailed case studies, notably from psychotherapies of such patients. However, some argue that many of these disorders are better termed 'medically unexplained syndromes' (MUS) or 'functional somatic syndromes' (FSS). MUS and FSS are theoretically neutral terms: they simply say that a constellation of symptoms are observed (e.g. chronic fatigue syndrome and Gulf War syndrome) and remain agnostic about their causation. Causation may be psychological (e.g. trauma, attachment problems and anxiety), or physical (an unknown virus, environmental chemicals or cytokines), or some combination of these.

Despite the gloomy tone of the preceding paragraphs, many patients can be helped and, at the very least, protected from iatrogenic harm of over-investigation and unnecessary referrals. There is a toolbox of basic, readily acquired skills that most medical students and doctors can master.

Somatisation

Somatisation is a general, loosely defined term to describe the manifestation of psychological distress in somatic (physical) symptoms, and for help-seeking from doctors or other healers for these symptoms. Somatisation exists on a spectrum from transient and mild to chronic and severe. It also varies on a spectrum from normal to abnormal: transient somatisation is fairly common and normal in otherwise psychologically healthy children in situations of stress, and to some extent in adults as well. Box 13.1 lists those psychiatric disorders in which somatisation may be prominent.

Box 13.2

Sick role, illness behaviour and abnormal illness behaviour

- *Sick role* (Parsons 1964) is a sociological construct that says that people who are sick have certain rights (e.g. to stay home from work to be looked after), but also certain responsibilities (specifically, to follow the doctor's instructions about how to get better).

- *Illness behaviour* (Mechanic & Volkhart 1960) refers to the behaviours people engage in while sick (e.g. going to see a doctor and taking medication).

- *Abnormal illness behaviour* (Pilowsky 1978) is when illness behaviour is inappropriate. This may be driven consciously (e.g. malingering) or unconsciously (e.g. factitious disorder), and may be either illness-affirming (e.g. pseudoseizures) or illness-denying (e.g. 'flight into health', 'denial of illness').

Somatisation also has a complicated relationship with physical illness. In some cases, there may be little or no evidence of a physical substrate (physical examination and investigations may be normal); in other cases, the patient has an objective, proven physical disorder (e.g. coronary heart disease), but the symptoms and help-seeking are out of proportion to its severity.

Patterns of somatisation differ markedly across societies and cultures. In fact, it is probably impossible to have a culturally universal definition of somatisation, as norms vary greatly regarding what kinds of symptoms are considered trivial or serious, or how appropriate it is to talk about symptoms to others or to seek medical help. So it is equally impossible to say someone's somatisation is abnormal unless we have an idea of the person's sociocultural settings.

Two sets of ideas have been useful in thinking about the patterns of norms. The first is the *sick role*, which simply summarises core aspects of the social norms in 'advanced', industrialised societies about how people behave during occasions of illness (see Box 13.2). The second is the idea of *illness behaviour* and the derived idea of *abnormal illness behaviour*.

Case examples: Somatisation and somatoform disorders

Conversion disorder with major depression

A female patient aged 26 was working as an officer in a military force. She presented soon after being commissioned as an officer. She had originally enlisted and had been promoted to non-commissioned rank, but her service recognised her ability in her field and subsidised her attendance at university to complete a degree in civil engineering.

While at work she suffered fractures to several metatarsals in the left foot, which were satisfactorily managed. However, she developed persistent pain and loss of power in her left leg over several months, without any relevant pathology being defined. Extensive investigations followed, but no cause for her persistent symptoms could be found and she returned to restricted duties using a full leg splint.   *Continued*

Case examples continued

Despite her obvious symptoms of pain and restricted function in that leg, her affect remained euthymic and reactive. She was very concerned about her leg problem, but did not allow this to interfere with her capacity to function and to carry out her duties. Over a period of 6 months, a diagnosis of reflex sympathetic dystrophy was considered and established by several specialists. However, a number of other specialists maintained that her signs were inconsistent with this diagnosis and that there was no definable pathology.

On careful exploration it was found that this young officer was feeling very awkward in her new status and uncomfortable about being regarded as an officer by fellow servicemen and women, many of whom she had known when she had non-commissioned rank. She spoke of leaving the service because she felt that her future was now damaged by her persistent illness, but she felt guilty about leaving the service that had subsidised her further education and given her substantial new career prospects.

Over the next 6 months the patient became increasingly depressed and presented for psychiatric assistance. A diagnosis of conversion disorder, compounded by major depressive disorder was made and treatment introduced consisting of antidepressant medication and individual and group psychotherapy. Over a period of weeks her depressive illness improved and she came to recognise the dilemma that she now faced between the guilt of leaving the military service and the challenges of trying to persist in a situation she found very difficult to tolerate. Power returned to her leg over several weeks but her pain persisted. Her depressive symptoms responded well to treatment. She was given a medical discharge from military service and treatment continues.

Hypochondriasis

A female patient aged 55 years was divorced with two children. The divorce followed her husband's revelation that he was homosexual in orientation, but had never felt able to accept this or reveal this to her. They had been married for 24 years and the patient felt that her life was totally shattered. She and her husband remained friends, but they had proceeded with divorce. Within weeks of her husband's revelations, the patient developed abdominal pains which were fully investigated but no abnormality was found. However, her symptoms persisted and she underwent even more extensive and elaborate investigations. In the process, the patient became intensely concerned by the possible nature of her problem and insisted upon receiving copies of all investigations and reports. She read about physical symptoms extensively and began to attend a number of doctors to obtain further opinions. She was admitted to hospital in considerable pain and discomfort, but her symptoms resolved soon after admission, only to recur at a later time.

Over subsequent months she also suffered chest pains and some unusual difficulties with swallowing. Again, thorough investigations failed to reveal relevant pathology, but her presentations with significant symptoms and in crisis resulted in further admissions and further assessment. Syncopal episodes also developed, again without major pathology being identified. Her longstanding asthma deteriorated, but was managed successfully with appropriate medications.

Throughout this time her mental state had been assessed by her treating doctors to be depressed, but she insisted that her primary problem was her severe and extensive symptoms, loss of function, and frustration at not being able to resume her normal life. She considered her depressive symptoms to be 'understandable' given her multiple problems.

Continued

Case examples continued

As time passed, her depressive symptoms became more evident with typical features of depressed mood, sleep disturbance and anhedonia. However, the attempts to treat her depression with antidepressant medications were thwarted by particularly poor tolerance of those antidepressants introduced. With persistence she was able to tolerate mirtazapine and there seemed to be some improvement in her mental state. However, when she began to gain weight on this medication, she refused to continue and became concerned about the causes of her weight gain. The pattern of requesting copies of all reports and investigations continued.

Diagnoses of hypochondriacal disorder compounding a major depressive disorder were made and efforts were made to explore the unresolved grief surrounding the break-up of her marriage. She had previously resisted any attempt to explore these emotional issues, but with the persistence of multiple physical symptoms and her deteriorating quality of life, the patient became increasingly willing to consider other aspects of her life and health.

An antidepressant was slowly introduced and psychotherapy established on a regular basis. She was admitted to a private psychiatric hospital. Once in hospital, she was gently confronted with the extent of her illness preoccupation, high level of disease conviction and high level of disease phobia. These problems were approached as a reflection in her body of her emotional distress, rather than accusations of 'inventing symptoms'. Gradually, she was able to experience her despair in this supportive environment and felt able to reduce her preoccupation with her physical symptoms and investigations. Her treatment continues, but her presentations with physical symptoms have simplified and she remains under the care of one general practitioner and one psychiatrist.

Management: general issues

The first and most crucial principle is to establish and maintain a *positive therapeutic alliance* while setting a reasonable limit to medical investigations and treatment. Somatising patients can evoke very negative reactions in treating staff. Doctors, nurses and others may feel frustrated, hostile, angry or helpless. This may lead to subtle or gross forms of rejection, including referral elsewhere or over-investigation. Some doctors, in an effort to be sympathetic and helpful, resort to 'heroic' but not necessarily effective measures. Psychiatrically trained staff cope with the negative emotions of working with somatising and other challenging patients by mutual support (e.g. peer supervision groups) and/or one-on-one supervision. In this way, they are able to maintain a more objective, empathic and helpful perspective, with less risk of burning out.

Second, it is important not to invalidate the patient's experience. The language we use can make or break the therapeutic alliance. The message that 'there's nothing wrong with you' can be very damaging, rupturing trust and leading to the patient seeking help elsewhere. The antidote here is in part patient-centred interviewing. This means attempting to understand the patient's experience in his or her own terms, such as: 'When the dizziness started, what did *you* think was causing it?' or 'Were there any particular illnesses you were most concerned it might be?'.

It is useful to get to know the patient's own vocabulary to do with emotions and stress before offering your explanations using these terms. For example, some doctors try to explain a somatoform symptom using the term 'stress', only to have the patient say, 'But I don't have any stress in my life; everything's OK'. This kind of response can be expected; having limited emotional self-awareness or a limited emotional vocabulary are risk factors for somatisation and somatoform disorders.

Where possible, as in hospitals, it is often very useful for the diagnosis to be communicated to the patient by both physician and psychiatrist at the same time. This is something that can often be done when a psychiatrist is working in a so-called *liaison* relationship with a medical or surgical team, rather than just providing consultations.

Third, a useful strategy is to convey the 'good news' that thorough medical assessment has shown no evidence for any serious disease underlying the symptoms, and at the same time admitting the 'bad news' that we do not have a full understanding of the symptoms, but reassuring the patient we will continue to see them, periodically review their health, and thoroughly assess any new symptoms that might occur. The doctor suggests that in the meantime he or she helps the patient make the best of their situation by learning to cope more effectively with the symptoms and with life in general. This includes paying attention to the emotional aspects of day-to-day life and any stresses or predicaments the patient may be dealing with. Often, after several consultations, a transition does occur: patients talk less about their somatic complaints and more about very significant aspects of their lives that are likely to be linked to the psychological substrate from which the somatisation arose. This often occurs without any formal recommendation of or referral for psychotherapy.

Fourth, for chronically somatising patients it is useful to schedule *regular appointments*, even if infrequent (i.e. to be proactive rather than reactive). There is good evidence from randomised controlled trials in primary care that this leads to less overall health service use and better functioning.

Finally, for the more severe and chronic forms of somatisation, it is essential to have *excellent communication* between health services and practitioners. This takes time and effort, but pays useful dividends. In part, it is because it is easy for overt or covert disagreement to emerge about the patient's diagnosis. For those patients whose somatisation is accompanied by some form of personality disorder (especially borderline), this can lead to 'splitting', misunderstanding and hostility between services and practitioners, and iatrogenic prolongation of the patient's illness.

Specific treatments

Specific treatment depends on specific diagnosis. For much of the burden of somatisation in the high-prevalence disorders (i.e. depression and anxiety disorders), much of the management evolves around the underlying disorder. Usually, GPs and non-psychiatric medical specialists are able to do this effectively using medication and psychotherapy; in a minority of cases, referral to a psychiatrist is needed. Table 13.2 outlines techniques appropriate to the specific somatoform disorders.

Conclusions

The various forms of somatisation have been a relatively neglected topic within general medicine and surgery, despite their high prevalence, the associated suffering and dysfunction, their emotional impact on doctors and other health workers, and their huge

Table 13.2

Specific treatments for selected somatoform and related disorders

Disorder	Treatment
Somatisation disorder	Various forms of psychotherapy have been advocated, but the evidence base of randomised controlled trials is extremely small. Types of therapies have included psychoanalytic psychotherapy, cognitive-behaviour therapy (CBT), behaviour therapy, group therapy, supportive psychotherapy, psychoeducation and eclectic combinations of these. Involvement of partners and family can be very useful: they can benefit from psychoeducation, marital counselling and/or family therapy. There is no good evidence for pharmacological treatment of somatisation disorder itself (as opposed to treatment of, say, comorbid depression).
Conversion disorder	Many episodes of conversion resolve with non-specific general measures, as described in the text, including: reassurance that no evidence has been found of serious neurological disease; positive suggestion; physiotherapy and rehabilitation; and treatment of comorbid psychiatric problems. Many psychological therapies have been proposed and are used. Barbiturate or hypnosis-facilitated interview aims to reveal information about the psychological conflicts or trauma underlying the conversion and, with hypnosis, to help the patient achieve greater control over their symptoms. Trials have been reported of CBT, behaviour therapy, psychodynamic therapy, and biofeedback, among others.
Hypochondriasis	The evidence base is greater than for somatisation disorder. Uncontrolled and controlled trials (including randomised controlled trials or RCTs) suggest benefit from 'explanatory therapy', CBT, behaviour therapy (employing exposure and response prevention or EX/RP), and stress management, with little evidence of any one being superior to the others. In addition, there are case reports, open series and one placebo-controlled RCT suggesting selective serotonin reuptake inhibitors (SSRIs) are beneficial. The effect is small but useful and there is evidence of a high placebo response rate.

collective impact on health system costs. This has changed greatly, as shown by more extensive and better quality research, improvements in medical education and specialist training, and the development in many places of innovative medical services with closer, more effective forms of liaison between psychiatrists and physicians. However, there is a long way to go and, hopefully, these trends will continue.

REFERENCES AND FURTHER READING

Abbey, S.E., Wulsin, L., Levenson, J.L., 2011. Somatization and somatoform disorders. In: Levenson, J.L. (Ed.), American psychiatric publishing textbook of psychosomatic medicine. Psychiatric Publishing, Washington DC, pp. 261–290.

Asher, R., 1951. Munchausen's syndrome. Lancet 1, 339–341.

Drossman, D.A., 2011. Abuse, trauma, and GI illness: is there a link? American Journal of Gastroenterology 106, 14–25.

Guthrie, E., 2011. Psychotherapy. In: Levenson, J.L. (Ed.), American psychiatric publishing textbook of psychosomatic medicine. Psychiatric Publishing, Washington DC.

Hatcher, S., Arroll, B., 2008. Assessment and management of medically unexplained symptoms. British Medical Journal 336, 1124–1128.

Henningsen, P., Zipfel, S., Herzog, W., 2007. Management of functional somatic syndromes. Lancet 369, 946–955.

Kanaan, R., Armstrong, D., Barnes, P., Wessely, S., 2009. In the psychiatrist's chair: how neurologists understand conversion disorder. Brain 132, 2889–2896.

Lacey, C., Cook, M., Salzberg, M., 2007. The neurologist, psychogenic nonepileptic seizures, and borderline personality disorder. Epilepsy and Behaviour 11, 492–498.

Lipowsky, Z.J., 1988. Somatization: the concept and its clinical application. American Journal of Psychiatry 145, 1358–1368.

Lipsitt, D., Escobar, J., 2005. Psychotherapy of somatoform disorders. In: Gabbard, G., Beck, J., Holmes, J. (Eds.), Oxford textbook of psychotherapy. Oxford University Press, Oxford, pp. 247–258.

Mayou, R., Kirmayer, L.J., Simon, G., Kroenke, K., Sharpe, M., 2006. Somatoform disorders: time for a new approach in DSM-V. American Journal of Psychiatry 162, 847–855.

Mechanic, 1962. The concept of illness behaviour. Journal of Chronic Diseases 15, 189–194.

Mechanic, D., Volkart, E.H., 1960. Illness behaviour and medical diagnosis. Journal of Health and Human Behaviour 1, 86–94.

Parsons, T., 1951. Illness and the role of the physician: a socio-logical perspective. American Journal of Orthopsychiatry 21, 452–460.

Parsons, T., 1964. Social structure and personality. Free Press, New York.

Pilowsky, I., 1978. A general classification of abnormal illness behaviours. British Journal of Medical Psychology 51, 131–137.

Stone, J., Carson, A., Sharpe, M., 2005. Functional symptoms in neurology: management. Journal of Neurology, Neurosurgery and Psychiatry 76, 13–21.

Voigt, K., Nagel, A., et al., 2010. Towards positive diagnostic criteria: a systematic review of somatoform disorder diagnoses and suggestions for future classification. Journal of Psychosomatic Research 68, 403–414.

A WIFE NAMED MARGARET
CASE-BASED LEARNING

ANDREW GLEASON & JOEL KING

The following role-play requires two participants: one to play an intern (candidate) and another to play a patient's wife, Margaret Lombardi (actor).

OSCE Station Instructions

(Reading time: 2 minutes)

You are an intern on the first day of a neurology rotation. You briefly met Sam Lombardi this morning on the team ward round. He is a 52-year-old man who initially presented three weeks ago with a generalised seizure due to a benign left frontal meningioma. This meningioma was resected several days later. There were no postoperative neurological or cognitive deficits.

Mr Lombardi re-presented yesterday with a second seizure. During the ward round your consultant, Dr Gupta, said that a 24-hour video EEG recording captured a typical event but showed no signs of epilepsy. He said that Mr Lombardi had a non-epileptic seizure.

Dr Gupta asked you to get a psychiatry consult. You called the psychiatry registrar, who said that she will see the patient, but asked if you could first obtain a collateral history from a family member, looking for factors that might be contributing to Mr Lombardi's non-epileptic seizure. Mr Lombardi's wife is on the ward at present.

Task (10 minutes)

- Take a collateral history from Mrs Lombardi, focusing particularly on psychosocial stressors that may have contributed to Mr Lombardi's non-epileptic seizure (8 minutes).
- At 8 minutes, answer Mrs Lombardi's questions about the difference between non-epileptic seizures and epilepsy.

Actor role: Margaret Lombardi

You are 48 years old and live with Sam in your own home. You are a social worker at a charity that supports refugees. You have two children who both live with you, aged 18 and 21.

HISTORY OF PRESENTING ILLNESS

Your husband, Sam, is 52. About three weeks ago you and Sam were watching a movie at home. You went to get a drink and when you returned Sam was on the floor. His whole body was shaking and he didn't respond when you tried talking to him. After about 30 seconds Sam came to, but was quite confused. You immediately called an ambulance and Sam was taken to hospital. The doctors found a meningioma on a brain scan and said this had caused his seizure. They also did a recording with wires on his head and found that he had epilepsy. The tumour was removed and Sam returned home. The doctors told you they thought the tumour was cured. They also did some memory testing and said that his cognitive abilities had not been affected by the tumour.

Sam had another seizure yesterday. You were at work when it happened, but your daughter saw it. She said that Sam fell to the floor and began thrashing about. His eyes were closed and he was breathing heavily. The symptoms fluctuated but lasted for about 10 minutes in total.

There have been a number of stressors in Sam's life over the last three years. Sam has his own concrete business, which had been expanding and doing very well. This changed three years ago when a former customer took Sam to court claiming that Sam's business was responsible for some water damage in a building that his company had worked on. The case dragged on and had a profound effect on Sam. He began to have trouble managing the business. About two years ago it reached the point where his mood was low most days, he was having trouble sleeping, and he lost about 10 kg of weight over a six month period. Sam developed the belief that he was going to be sent to jail, but this seemed irrational as his barrister was certain the case would be resolved.

Things got even worse when Sam strained his back while lifting some equipment at work. He had a disc prolapse and had an operation, but continued to suffer from pain. He tried to go back to work, but wasn't able to manage. This led to another legal battle, this time over compensation from his insurance company. Sam eventually managed to get compensation about six months ago. His mood gradually improved after this and he began to return to being his usual self, although he still struggles with the fact that he hasn't been able to return to work because of the back pain. He has a strong belief that being the provider for the family is part of his role, and he hasn't been able to reconcile this with the fact that he is not working. The back pain was getting better, and it reached the point where he thought he would be able to return to work. Unfortunately, this was when Sam got the brain tumour.

After the brain tumour operation Sam was crying a lot when he returned home from hospital. You think he will pull through, but the tumour has been a lot to bear on top of all of the other recent difficulties.

PAST MEDICAL AND PSYCHIATRIC HISTORY

Sam has no past psychiatric history. He has no past medical history aside from the prolapsed disc.

DRUG AND ALCOHOL HISTORY

Sam drinks one to two beers each day after work. Sometimes when you have guests over he might have a whole bottle of wine to himself. He hasn't had anything to drink since he was diagnosed with the brain tumour. Sam doesn't smoke or use any drugs.

MEDICATIONS

Sam was put on an anticonvulsant after his first hospitalisation, but you can't remember what it is called. Sam also takes two paracetamol and codeine tablets four times a day for his back pain.

FAMILY HISTORY

Sam's father has arthritis. His mother has osteoporosis. They are in their late seventies and live independently nearby. Sam has one brother who had an episode of depression that was treated with sertraline by his GP.

   You and Sam have two children, who are well.

PERSONAL HISTORY

Sam's birth and milestones were normal. Academically he was an average student. Sam left school after finishing Year 10 and began to work at his uncle's concrete business. Sam's father is a very tough man who never showed emotions and never lets anything bother him. You think Sam takes after his father.

   You met Sam when he was 24 and got married shortly after. You have a good relationship. Sam has always been the cornerstone of the family. He used to laugh a lot, was very social, and took pride in your happy, stable family. Like his dad, he isn't someone who would let anyone know if he was sick or stressed, and he never missed a day of work until the last few years.

Statements you must make:
- Open with: 'Thanks for talking to me, Doctor. I have a few questions, but I know that you just began this job today and probably don't know a lot about Sam. Would you like me to begin by telling you what happened?'
- 'Dr Gupta, the neurologist, said that Sam had a non-epileptic seizure. What is this, and how is it different from epilepsy?'
- 'Does this mean that he is faking his symptoms?'
- 'How can you treat this sort of seizure?'

Model Answer

This is a difficult station, which is, in part, a reflection of the nature of somatoform disorders. This station requires the candidate to explain the difference between an epileptic seizure and a non-epileptic seizure in lay terms. Explaining this adequately is part of the treatment for non-epileptic seizures.

In lay terms, epileptic seizures are caused by abnormal electrical activity in the brain. While non-epileptic seizures can look similar to epileptic seizures, they are not associated with the type of abnormal electrical activity seen in epileptic seizures and are not the result of serious physical disease. Instead, non-epileptic seizures are physical manifestations of psychological distress. While non-epileptic seizures are related to 'stress', some people find that it is not easy for them to recognise or feel the stress.

It is essential to ensure that Sam and Margaret understand that his symptoms are involuntary and unconscious. When people are told that a physical symptom is due to psychological factors, many think that by implication the doctor believes the symptoms are made up. It should be very clearly reinforced that you believe the symptoms are real and not under Sam's volitional control. The event that Sam had was no less real than the epileptic seizure he had that led to the diagnosis of the meningioma.

Sam has clearly had numerous psychosocial stressors over the last few years, including the legal problems at work, further legal disputes over compensation, a back injury and chronic pain, followed more recently by the sudden diagnosis of a meningioma. Explaining his symptoms in the context of these stressors will make it easier for Sam and Margaret to understand what is going on, and will also help communicate that you are not saying there is nothing wrong.

Non-epileptic seizures may resolve with non-specific general measures. Formal psychological therapy is also an option if Sam has ongoing symptoms. He has also had significant depressive symptoms over the last few years and these could recur, in which case he may benefit from an antidepressant. Sam will need ongoing neurology follow-up.

Margaret and Sam will probably be confused by the fact that he has had an epileptic seizure and a non-epileptic seizure (many doctors often also find this confusing!). The advanced candidate will explain that it is not uncommon for people who have epileptic seizures to also have non-epileptic seizures. 'Physical' illness and 'psychological' symptoms commonly coexist.

A medical student doing this station should be able to elicit and identify the main psychosocial stressors the patient has experienced, and explain in a cogent and sensitive fashion that non-epileptic seizures are caused by psychological factors while epileptic seizures are due to abnormal brain activity. Interns are often asked questions that are beyond their expertise. Should this occur it is perfectly acceptable for the student acting the part of an intern to pass more difficult questions on to the psychiatry registrar or neurologist.

Chapter 14

PERSONALITY DISORDERS

DARRYL BASSETT & DAVID J CASTLE

Personality disorders represent 'a class of syndromes defined by the early onset of inflexible and maladaptive traits that are exhibited in a wide range of social and personal contexts and that are relatively stable over a period of years' (Pfol 1999). There are many theories and classifications surrounding personality and personality disorders. We have attempted to simplify this very complex field; refer to Further Reading at the end of this chapter for a more comprehensive understanding of the topic.

Personality

Personality is the persistent and integrated pattern with which a person perceives their internal experience and interacts with the world in general. This includes a person's beliefs and understanding of their subjective life experience and identity, as well as their behaviour in relationships with other people. Personality features or traits are to some extent enduring throughout adult life, but are still open to psychological modification and adaptation to a limited degree.

According to Robert Cloninger, personality can be considered to result from the combination of temperament ('emotional core') and character ('conceptual core').

Temperament

Temperament consists of developing personality traits manifested as emotional expression, level of activity and social interactiveness. Temperament is evident from birth and has strong biological roots, modified by environmental factors.

Temperament has four genetically determined dimensions:

- novelty seeking (tendency to explore)
- reward dependence (attachment seeking)
- harm avoidance (tendency to withdraw)
- persistence (tendency to persist).

Character

Character is the way individuals regard relationships with others and is derived from combinations of temperament, interactions with significant others and individual life experiences.

Character has three dimensions:

- cooperativeness (empathy with others)
- self-directedness (goal striving)
- self-transcendence (sense of 'spirituality' or notions such as beliefs, values, meaning in life, etc).

Personality disorders

The criteria for individual categories of personality disorders is lengthy and only a synopsis is presented in Table 14.1. We suggest that the respective manuals for DSM-IV-TR and ICD-10 be consulted for further detail about the specific criteria.

The concept of personality disorder requires judgements to be made about what is 'maladaptive' about persistent patterns of behaviour and self-perceptions. Determining what is maladaptive must take into account differences in cultural norms, social context and even moral values. However, loss of flexibility and adaptiveness in self-awareness and behaviour, which persistently and extensively impinge negatively upon relationships, can still be identified.

Recognising such difficulties clinically offers greater insights and opportunities for assistance for the persons involved. A diagnosis of personality disorder can be used pejoratively and can become destructive. It may also provoke challenges that the problems are 'normal variants' and do not justify treatment or special consideration as the consequences of illness. This ignores the destructiveness of personality dysfunction to both the patient and others, as well as the lack of choice experienced by such patients with their problems.

The current classifications first assign people with personality dysfunctions into clusters and then into specific disorders. Such categories have the value of identifying broad common features that illustrate the problems of rigidity and maladaptiveness mentioned above. They also illustrate the limitations of categories that do not reflect the many variations in human beings, both at any one time and over a period of time. However, the clusters can also be considered to reflect dimensions of personality dysfunction which have been grouped into broad categories for conceptual convenience (see Box 14.1).

Table 14.1

Classification of personality disorders according to DSM–IV–TR and ICD–10 (synopsis)

DSM-IV-TR	ICD-10
General diagnostic criteria for a personality disorder	**Disorders of adult personality and behaviour (F60-F69)**
A An enduring pattern of inner experience and behaviour that deviates markedly from the expectations of the individual's culture. This pattern is manifested in two (or more) of the following areas:	This block includes a variety of conditions and behaviour patterns of clinical significance that tend to be persistent and appear to be the expression of the individual's characteristic lifestyle and mode of relating to himself or herself and others. Some of these conditions and patterns of behaviour emerge early in the course of individual development, as a result of both constitutional factors and social experience, while others are acquired later in life.
1 cognition (i.e. ways of perceiving and interpreting self, other people, and events)	
2 affectivity (i.e. the range, intensity, lability, and appropriateness of emotional response)	
3 interpersonal functioning	
4 impulse control.	
B The enduring pattern is inflexible and pervasive across a broad range of personal and social situations.	Specific personality disorders, mixed and other personality disorders, and enduring personality changes are deeply ingrained and enduring behaviour patterns, manifesting as inflexible responses to a broad range of personal and social situations. They represent extreme or significant deviations from the way in which the average individual in a given culture perceives, thinks, feels and, particularly, relates to others. Such behaviour patterns tend to be stable and to encompass multiple domains of behaviour and psychological functioning. They are frequently, but not always, associated with various degrees of subjective distress and problems of social performance.
C The enduring pattern leads to clinically significant distress or impairment in social, occupational, or other important areas of functioning.	
D The pattern is stable and of long duration, and its onset can be traced back at least to adolescence or early adulthood.	
E The enduring pattern is not better accounted for as a manifestation or consequence of another mental disorder.	
F The enduring pattern is not due to the direct physiological effects of a substance (e.g. a drug of abuse, a medication) or a general medical condition (e.g. head trauma).	

Box 14.1

Personality disorders by cluster

Cluster A

These individuals tend to be persistently *cold, awkward* and *isolative* in their interactions with other people in their culture or social group.

Using Cloninger's model (1999) of personality structure, we suggest they exhibit 'low reward dependence, high harm avoidance, low novelty seeking, high persistence, low self transcendence, low cooperativeness and high self directedness'.

This cluster includes:

- *paranoid personality disorder:* characterised by pervasive distrust and suspiciousness of others, such that their motives are interpreted as malevolent.

- *schizoid personality disorder:* characterised by a pervasive pattern of detachment from social relationships and a restricted range of expression of emotions in interpersonal settings.

- *schizotypal personality disorder:* characterised by a pervasive pattern of social and interpersonal deficits marked by acute discomfort with, and reduced capacity for, close relationships, as well as by cognitive or perceptual distortions and eccentricities of beliefs and behaviour.

Cluster B

These individuals tend to be *emotionally highly dramatic*, *labile* and *distressed (particularly in relationships with other people)* in comparison with other people in their culture or social group.

Using Cloninger's model of personality structure, we suggest they exhibit 'high novelty seeking, high reward dependence, low harm avoidance, low persistence, low self transcendence, high cooperativeness and variable self directedness'.

This cluster includes:

- *antisocial personality disorder:* characterised by a pervasive pattern of disregard for and violation of the rights of others.

- *borderline personality disorder:* characterised by a pervasive pattern of instability of interpersonal relationships, self-image and affects, and marked impulsivity.

- *histrionic personality disorder:* characterised by a pervasive pattern of excessive emotionality and attention seeking, beginning by early adulthood.

- *narcissistic personality disorder:* characterised by a pervasive pattern of grandiosity (in fantasy, self-evaluation and behaviour), need for admiration, and lack of empathy for others.

Cluster C

These individuals tend to be persistently *anxious* and *inhibited* in relationships and behaviour, compared with other people in their culture or social group.

Using Cloninger's model of personality structure, we suggest they exhibit 'high harm avoidance, high reward dependence, low novelty seeking, variable persistence, high self directedness, high cooperativeness and high self transcendence'.

This cluster includes:

- *avoidant personality disorder:* characterised by a pervasive pattern of social inhibition, feelings of inadequacy and hypersensitivity to negative evaluation.

- *dependent personality disorder:* characterised by a pervasive and excessive need to be taken care of that leads to clinging and submissive behaviour, and fears of separation.

- *obsessive-compulsive personality disorder:* characterised by a pervasive pattern of preoccupation with orderliness, perfectionism, and mental and interpersonal control, at the expense of flexibility, openness and efficiency.

Frequently, patients present with the features of more than one personality disorder cluster. This emphasises the importance of avoiding rigid personality disorder categories and labels.

Case examples: Personality disorders

Cluster A – Schizoid personality disorder

A 32-year-old single lawyer working in legislative drafting has no friends and is regarded as a loner by his colleagues. However, he is extremely competent at his job and is very well regarded in this respect. He is courteous with people he meets, but does not converse beyond pleasantries. He presented for psychiatric assistance with persistent depressive symptoms of moderately severe intensity. Consultations are brief and very distant. When once offered brief psychotherapy for treatment of his depressive symptoms, he commented (without eye contact): 'What could you *possibly* say that would be of *any* use to me?' Management has been confined to antidepressant medications.

Cluster B – Borderline personality disorder

A 23-year-old woman presents in crisis after recently ending a highly traumatic relationship with an older man who physically and emotionally abused her. This was not the first abusive relationship she had been involved in and she recognised that her choice of partners had been poor. She recalled first suffering depressive symptoms aged 11 and had struggled with occasional episodes of severe depression ever since. In addition, she suffered distressing mood swings that might last only several hours, varying from deep despair to feeling almost elated. There did not seem to be any pattern to these mood fluctuations, and she was desperate for relief from this 'roller-coaster' existence. From early adolescence she found that cutting herself relieved her emotional distress, but she also attempted suicide by hanging on one occasion. The self-mutilation improved with the introduction of an antipsychotic medication in low dose and her persistence with individual psychotherapy over the past year. At times she could see a real future for herself and attended university intermittently. However, her despair and hopelessness would recur and disrupt her studies. Despite her major emotional upheavals, she is determined to go on and contacts her therapists frequently to obtain their help with a multitude of life problems.

Cluster C – Obsessive-compulsive/Anankastic personality disorder

A 27-year-old divorcee presents for help after her marriage of 4 years ended because her husband could no long tolerate her need for fastidious regulation of everything that happened in their lives. She demanded that their home was spotless and highly organised at all times but did not exhibit any cleaning or other rituals. All activities were recorded and planned in intricate detail, with her insistence that nothing could be undertaken spontaneously and without careful consideration. Items at home, including clothing and foodstuffs, had a designated place and there was a place for everything.

However, she did not see that there was a significant problem with her behaviour and said:

'I am very organised and I like things to be "just so". My husband said I was "too obsessional and controlling", and I suppose I found him chaotic and disorganised. His decision to leave me was very distressing for me and I wrote him lots of letters trying to understand his reasons for going. Surely he could see I just needed to be very organised?'

Treatment designed for obsessive-compulsive disorder was administered, but was ineffective despite her assiduous participation.

Comorbidity

Personality disorders are often associated with major psychological disorders and a variety of general medical disorders, more than expected by chance (see Box 14.2). Sometimes these comorbid conditions are present during the developmental period (including in prodromal form) and probably contribute to the distortions of development that promote the formation of personality dysfunction. Genetic factors may also have relevance here, as inheritance may be shared with other disorders. The presence of personality disorder comorbidly with other disorders often aggravates, distorts or prolongs those disorders. Treatment resistance may be enhanced and the risk of self-injury or injury to others increased.

Differential diagnoses

The differential diagnoses of personality disorders are critically important, as often the suggestion of personality dysfunction means that other possible diagnoses are not considered. This is particularly important when the onset of personality dysfunction is relatively recent or is evident before the age of 18 years. A diagnosis of personality disorder cannot be made before the age of 18 and should be considered putative until observed and confirmed by collateral evidence (such as the observations of others), over a period of several years. The separation from other differential diagnoses is usually established by further investigation and observation. The separation from autism spectrum disorders (ASD, see Chapter 18) can be particularly difficult with Cluster A personality disorders, but ASD is usually evident early in childhood and persist. In addition, most people with ASD do manage to maintain relationships, although they may encounter significant difficulties from time to time. A list of differential diagnoses for personality disorders is presented in Box 14.3.

All of the above disorders can present as personality disorders when in prodromal form as well as in overt diagnosed form, and may be responsible for persistent personality change.

Box 14.2

Specific disorders commonly comorbid with personality disorders or responsible for personality change

- Substance abuse: alcohol, illicit psychoactive substances (e.g. cannabis, stimulants of various kinds, hallucinogens), prescribed medications (e.g. benzodiazepines, opiates, ketamine), other varied substances with psychoactive effects (e.g. petrol, solvents)
- Bipolar disorder, including types I and II (particularly Cluster B)
- Depressive disorders, including major depressive disorders, dysthymic disorder
- Schizophrenia and related disorders (particularly Cluster A)
- Anxiety disorders of all kinds (particularly Cluster C).

Box 14.3

Common differential diagnoses for personality disorders

- Bipolar disorder (particularly for Cluster B personality disorders)
- Depressive disorders (all clusters)
- Schizophrenia (particularly Cluster A)
- Anxiety disorders (Cluster C)
- Acquired brain injury secondary to trauma
- Autism spectrum disorders
- Early dementia, including from multiple sclerosis, HIV/AIDS, Huntington's disease, neurosyphilis, frontotemporal dementias, vascular dementias such as secondary to vasculitis, and a variety of other infectious diseases
- Cerebrovascular disorders including cerebrovascular accidents (affecting frontal lobes)
- Cerebral malignancy (affecting the frontal lobes).

Aetiology of personality disorders

Neurobiological theories

Genetics

There is increasingly strong evidence that some personality disorders (e.g. borderline personality disorder) contain a significant genetic contribution, which appears to provide vulnerability to traumatic and meaningful life experiences during the developmental period. The relative contributions of inheritance and environment remain the subject of intense curiosity.

Developmental factors

Childhood and adolescent experiences interact with the genetic profile and promote change in the developing brain. Neurones create 'neural networks' forming the foundation for learning, both implicit (not available to conscious awareness) and explicit (available to conscious awareness). Deprivation of normal experiences and/or an overwhelming load of unpleasant experiences create neural networks that promote unhelpful patterns of physiological responses to a range of future life experiences.

Some patterns relate to excessive arousal (linked to excessive activity in the amygdala, hippocampus and sympathetic nervous system) and others to altered awareness which clinically is reflected as dissociative phenomena (linked to altered activity in the cingulate cortices and parasympathetic nervous system). In adult life these altered patterns of self-experience and behaviour result in a variety of problems coping with stress, relationships and occupation. The combination of intense arousal and dissociation can result in distressing behaviour, such as self-injury and mutilation. Sometimes experience of self-inflicted pain at these times is emotionally relieving and can become quite established as a maladaptive pattern of coping.

Early life trauma of various kinds (emotional, physical and sexual) appears to be a significant factor in the development of personality disorders. Sexual trauma is particularly significant in the development of borderline personality disorders. The perception (mostly based upon actual circumstances) that the child and/or adolescent cannot escape from this trauma or even talk about it, provides an even more noxious experience. This sense of entrapment in a context of serious abuse has been conceptualised as a 'complex post-traumatic stress disorder', although the accuracy of this concept in relationship to the development of personality disorders is not clear.

Psychosocial theories

Psychoanalytic theories

Sigmund Freud postulated that psychosexual development proceeds through the experience of basic instinctual drives and functions (e.g. survival through feeding, control of excretion, sexual drive and aggression) and the attempted mastery of these instincts in the context of frustrations and inhibitions drawn from the experience of key relationships during development. Consequently, conflictual emotions and thoughts are provoked, which are contained, out of conscious awareness, by a mechanism he called 'repression'. This is only partly effective and 'defence mechanisms' (see Chapter 16, Box 16.4) are employed to assist, but are experienced as symptoms.

Later psychoanalysts, including John Bowlby, Heinz Kohut, Donald Winnicott and others extended this thinking to focus more upon the relationships between children and their carers (usually parents), and considered the quality of these relationships is critically important. They considered that the integration of positive and negative experiences in those relationships offered an opportunity to develop positive self-esteem and resilience against unpleasant life events. Severe emotional deprivation and/or abuse disrupted development of self-esteem and impaired emotional resilience. There is increasing evidence that early life severe abuse (sexual, physical and emotional) are major contributing factors to the development of personality disorders (particularly Cluster B).

Social and cultural factors

Research has shown that only a part of personality development is related to genetics (about 50%) and suggests that a person's early experience of life (including intrauterine) is responsible for the remainder. Those experiences, which are not shared with other children, may be of particular importance. In addition, the impact of unpleasant experiences is strongly modified by significant positive relationships and social structures (including family and culture).

Cognitively-derived theories

Burrhus Skinner, Richard Lazarus, Albert Bandura and others began the process of examining personality in terms of learning and the modifications of learnt behaviours through experience. Their theories led to treatments that modified behaviour, both by repeated association and practice, the impact of consequences, modelling by significant others, and related changes in habitual learning. Aaron Beck and others followed with exploration of thought content and the patterns of thinking which become associated with personality development and disorders of feeling, thinking and behaviour. They suggested that these disorders could be changed by conscious effort to challenge maladaptive thought patterns or cognitions. The repeated challenge of such habitual patterns of thought and assumption change internal emotional experience and behaviour.

Jeffrey Young and others took this thinking further and expanded upon the complex plans of thinking or schemas that offer guidance for solving problems and interpreting information. Maladaptive schemas in Young's definition have the following features:

- A broad pervasive theme or pattern
- Comprised of memories, emotions, cognitions and bodily sensations
- Have regard to oneself and relationships with others
- Develop throughout childhood and adolescence
- Are elaborated upon throughout one's lifetime
- Dysfunctional to a significant degree.

Essentially, these maladaptive schemas result from fundamental emotional needs that are not met during childhood. They include disruptions of secure attachments to others, autonomy, competence and sense of identity, freedom to express needs and emotions, opportunity for spontaneity and play, and realistic limits and self-control.

Management of personality disorders

The management of patients with personality disorders can be difficult yet enormously rewarding. It is important to avoid pejorative labelling, and to work as effectively as possible with the individual to establish a good working therapeutic alliance.

Therapeutic alliance

A strong therapeutic alliance is critically important because of the difficulties patients with personality disorders have with important relationships, but this is also the site of frequent problems in treatment. These individuals frequently present with complaints of illness, but are often difficult to engage and maintain in treatment. They are sometimes very pleasant and clearly distressed, but can also often be hostile, demanding or clinging in behaviour. This provokes a mix of empathy, anger and sometimes distrust in health professionals, which then amplifies the patient's difficulties with self-identity and relationships.

Tolerating their intense mixed feelings is fundamental to further treatment of any kind. Negotiating a mix of behaviours that can be tolerated is also essential and will require both consistent boundaries (e.g. violence can never be tolerated), and reasonable tolerance of unpleasant emotions (e.g. some verbal abuse). Some form of simple contract is useful, establishing the expectations for frequency of contact, arrangements for crisis intervention, a policy regarding telephone contact between sessions and the expectations of further treatment.

Understanding that the negative emotion and behaviour is an established 'habit' and not a 'personal' issue with the therapist can help the therapist to cope more effectively. Further it helps to recognise that this is also a maladaptive but efficient strategy for conveying distress and eliciting assistance.

Crisis planning

Part of the management of patients with personality disorder, expressly Cluster B, must encompass the fact that they are likely to react to difficult life situations in maladaptive

Box 14.4

Crisis intervention

Presentations to emergency departments with self-mutilation, suicide attempts or intent, severe depression, severe anxiety and psychotic symptoms are very common.

Establish a therapeutic alliance by presenting a reasonably (but not intensely) caring attitude and focusing upon the immediate needs for intervention.

Obtain a history of the presenting complaint. Review of the complexities of past problems is usually best addressed after the crisis has resolved.

Perform a thorough mental state examination and all necessary physical examinations.

Safety is a major concern, but admission to hospital should be offered with care and planned (at least initially) to be brief and crisis focused. Avoid admission if safe and if a reasonable alternative management strategy can be offered. **Often individuals with personality disorders respond to admission with further psychological regression, returning to patterns of feeling, thinking and behaviour that are associated with much earlier times in their lives. The result can be loss of more mature coping strategies and unhelpful behaviour such as intense dependency, self-injury and/or aggressive behaviour. This is a risk with any psychological intervention in such patients, but intervention can be helpful in the management of a life crisis.**

Alternative strategies to admission to a psychiatric facility include offering rapid review by a therapist outside of hospital, accessing the support of significant others and – most importantly – a strong focus in treatment upon reinforcement of the patient's own psychological coping strategies (see below). Day hospital or 'partial hospitalisation' strategies have been usefully employed for borderline personality disorder.

Medications can be helpful to reduce anxiety, reduce intensity of depressed mood and thinking, reduce impulsivity, reduce psychotic symptoms and facilitate further intervention (see Chapter 15). These can include antipsychotic agents such as chlorpromazine, olanzapine, risperidone, etc (particularly for Clusters A and B, but sometimes also for Cluster C). Benzodiazepines can be useful to reduce anxiety, particularly for Cluster C, but the risk of dependence and abuse must be carefully considered in these patients.

ways, and self-harm might be one of these ways. Thus, the clinician and patient need to establish agreed ways of coping with and reacting to crises. Box 14.4 outlines the main issues relating to crisis plans.

Extended management and specialised treatment

Psychotherapy offers the greatest hope for patients with personality disorders to achieve worthwhile change in interpersonal function and relief of internal distress. Psychodynamic psychotherapies and related models have been utilised for many years, but in recent times cognitively orientated psychotherapies have given increasing benefits with less time and financial commitment (see Chapter 16).

Dialectical behaviour therapy (DBT) (aims to both accept maladaptive behaviours and emotions, and to challenge them over time) has shown particular promise with borderline personality disorder. Controlled studies of DBT have produced positive results, compared with less specific psychotherapies.

Mindfulness-based cognitive therapy and acceptance/commitment therapy (placing emphasis on 'self-soothing' and acceptance of self-worth) are of particular value in Cluster C disorders. Patients with Cluster A personality disorders are usually difficult to help with psychotherapy and often find the intensity of interpersonal involvement very disturbing.

Brief psychodynamic psychotherapy draws upon psychoanalytic theories, but is very brief (usually 10 to 30 sessions) and has some support from controlled trials. This form of psychotherapy is often useful when the patient is less amenable to 'cognitively orientated' psychotherapies.

Interpersonal therapy may be advantageous as this model of therapy focuses upon the nature and form of interpersonal interactions, without the need to explore the meaning of interactions, beyond the obvious. Thus this approach may be more acceptable and less emotionally confronting than some other models of therapy for some patients.

Generally speaking, patients with personality disorders become less intensely troubled with advancing age and become more amenable to psychotherapy of some kind. Change is slow and often spasmodic, with frequent disruptions in therapy and periods of emotional upheaval. The relationship with the therapist becomes very intense and provokes recall (often out of consciousness) of powerful and highly significant relationships from the past (particularly childhood and adolescence). This recall and association of the therapist with the past has been called 'transference' and can be very intense.

Because of the emotional intensity of the therapeutic relationship, the therapist will experience a similar process of recall and association, which has been called 'counter-transference'. Such processes, linking past to present, offer opportunities for substantial change that is otherwise not possible. They also make these therapeutic encounters very challenging for both patients and therapists. Thorough training and supervision is therefore essential for therapists entering this field, particularly when therapy of any kind (including even general medical treatment) continues for more than a few sessions. These links to the past are lowered by reduced frequency of contact, greater emphasis upon here-and-now experiences and problems, and a team approach to treatment.

Group therapy, using a variety of models, has also been employed and often has advantages, particularly for Cluster B individuals, because it offers the support of the group as well as a greater range of interpersonal interactions than individual therapy. Combining individual and group psychotherapies offers even greater efficacy than either on its own and can be particularly helpful with more challenging patients.

REFERENCES AND FURTHER READING

Bateman, A., Fonagy, P., 2001. Treatment of borderline personality disorder with psychodynamically orientated partial hospitalization: an 18 month follow-up. American Journal of Psychiatry 158 (1), 36–42.

Cloninger, C.R. (Ed.), 1999. Personality and psychopathology. American Psychopathological Association, Washington DC.

Gabbard, G., 2005. Psychodynamic psychiatry in clinical practice. American Psychiatric Publishing, Arlington.

Gabbard, G., Beck, J., Holmes, J. (Eds.), 2005. Oxford textbook of psychotherapy. Oxford University Press, Oxford.

Linehan, M., 1993. Cognitive behaviour treatment for borderline personality disorder. Guildford Press, New York.

Lugnegard, T., Hallerback, M.U., Gillberg, C., 2012. Personality disorders and autistic spectrum disorders. Comprehensive Psychiatry 53 (4), 333–340.

Millon, T., Davis, R., 1996. Disorders of personality: DSM-IV and beyond. Wiley, New York.

Pfol, B., 1999. Axis I and Axis II: Comorbidity or confusion. In: Cloninger, C.R. (Ed.), Personality and psychopathology. American Psychopathological Association, Washington DC, pp. 83–98.

Young, J., Klosko, J., 1994. Reinventing your life. Penguin Books Ltd, New York.

Young, J., Klosko, J., Weishaar, M., 2006. Schema therapy: A practitioners guide. Guildford Press, New York.

CHAPTER 14

A WOMAN NAMED STEPHANIE
CASE-BASED LEARNING

JOEL KING & ANDREW GLEASON

The following role-play requires two participants: one to play a GP registrar (candidate) and another to play the role of a patient named Stephanie Herman (actor) and the examiner.

OSCE Station Instructions

(Reading time: 2 minutes)

You are a GP registrar working in a suburban practice. Your next patient is Stephanie Herman, a 31-year-old woman. Stephanie works as a cashier clerk and lives alone. She has an established history of borderline personality disorder, diagnosed at age 25 by two eminent professors of psychiatry after multiple assessments with extensive longitudinal information. Stephanie sees an experienced psychotherapist weekly.

You have only seen Stephanie once. This was two months ago when she complained of a lump in her left breast. You performed a physical examination, palpated a small mass and sent her to a breast surgeon, Mr Black. Mr Black organised imaging and a biopsy. These came back as benign.

Stephanie is now returning for a routine follow-up. Your receptionist has told you that she seems quite angry about the breast surgeon. Stephanie is considering complaining about the surgeon to the Medical Board and wants to discuss this with you.

Task (10 minutes)

- Address Stephanie's concern about the surgeon (8 minutes).
- At 8 minutes, you must terminate the interview. The examiner will ask you TWO questions about the scenario (2 minutes).

Actor role: Stephanie Herman

You are a 31-year-old woman who lives alone.

PAST HISTORY

You were diagnosed with borderline personality disorder (BPD) by a consultant psychiatrist, Professor Tan, at age 23. This was confirmed by numerous other reputable psychiatrists.

You grew up in a lower-economic suburb and your parents divorced acrimoniously when you were 5. You witnessed significant domestic violence between them. You lived with your mother, who re-partnered with a man named John. You also watched a lot of fighting, both verbal and physical, between your mother and John. At age 13, John tried to molest you. You told your mother but she did not believe you. In the subsequent years you missed a lot of school and abused alcohol. You left home at age 16. At age 18 you were admitted to hospital in the context of a paracetamol overdose, after your relationship broke down with your first partner, Alfred, who had cannabis abuse problems. You were discharged after three days with community psychiatric follow-up that lasted a month.

You had an overdose of paracetamol at age 21, in the context of relationship rejection by another boyfriend, Fred. You had case management from the local mental health service and were prescribed fluoxetine 20 mg daily for what was described as a 'mild depression'. After four months your condition improved and you were discharged from the mental health service. You decided to stop taking the antidepressant two months later and did not experience any significant relapse of depressive or anxiety symptoms.

At age 25 you returned to psychiatric services as an outpatient feeling depressed, worthless and unloved in the context of a relationship breakdown with your third boyfriend, Bill. You improved with two months of case management. During this period you saw a psychiatrist, Professor Tan, several times. Professor Tan thought that you might have borderline personality disorder. He explained that this was a problem with the way you related to yourself and others and it stemmed from the lack of security, safety and trusting relationships you experienced as a child and teenager. You thought that this explanation made sense. He also explained that seeing a therapist on a regular basis might help you with your past traumatic experiences and the way that you see yourself and others today. He referred you to a private therapist, Molly, whom you have been seeing weekly since age 25.

You have not been in contact with public psychiatric services since this time and have been able to hold down a steady job as a cashier at a clothes store. Through your therapy with Molly, you have realised that you have significant issues around trust, going back to your early adolescence. You find that you trust people too readily and depend on them too much. Initial adoration and idealisation turns to denigration and disgust when you find that these people are not always there for you when you want them. This tends to lead to some very brief, intense relationships that end explosively. This has included rocky romantic relationships with men and short-lived friendships with women.

You are not taking any medication. Other than the benign breast lump, you have no medical history. There is no history of cutting, burning or disordered eating behaviour. There is no forensic history. Prior to age 25, you abused alcohol as a way of coping with stress and anxiety. However, since seeing Molly you have stopped drinking. You have never used recreational drugs.

RECENT EVENTS

Two months ago, you noticed a lump in your left breast while showering. You became very worried that you might have breast cancer. You went to see the GP (candidate) who performed a breast examination and was unsure whether it was benign or something more serious. The GP sent you to Mr Black, a breast surgeon, for further assessment. This was very anxiety-provoking for you and you had numerous sleepless nights. When you went to see Mr Black, you waited in the waiting room for an hour. You felt that he was a very rude man and did not talk to you much. You felt that he was very rough when he palpated your breast and you were reminded of the time when John tried to molest you. While you were still undressed, he told you that you needed a biopsy and some X-rays, and began filling out the forms. You felt that you did not have a choice in signing your name to tests that you did not understand.

You had the biopsy a month later at a local hospital and felt that the theatre staff were professional and respectful, but you felt neglected by Mr Black, whom you did not see during your stay. Instead, his resident saw you after the biopsy and sent you home. A week ago, Mr Black called you on the phone, curtly stating, 'Your pathology came back and it's benign. I don't need to see you again. Go back to your GP.' Although you were relieved by the pathology result, you felt dismissed and invalidated by Mr Black. You are very angry about Mr Black and are thinking about complaining to the Medical Board about his insensitive treatment. You think that he is the worst doctor ever and he should never be allowed to treat any more patients.

Your therapist has been away for the last three months on a sabbatical and is due to return next month. You miss not being able to discuss things with her and feel abandoned by her absence.

HOW TO PLAY THE ROLE

Although you have only met this GP once, you feel that this doctor's demeanour is far better than Mr Black's. In fact, you think that the GP is the best doctor in the world and your good pathology result can be attributed to the GP's excellent medical care. You bought a $2,000 watch to give to the GP for helping save your life.

You have no features of a mood, anxiety, psychotic, somatic or eating disorder. You do not have any suicidal ideation or ideation to harm yourself or others.

Statements you should make:

- 'First of all, that surgeon was the worst doctor in the whole world. He should never be allowed to treat any patients. I was thinking of complaining to the Medical Board about him. What do you think?'
- 'You are so different from Mr Black. He was arrogant and rude, but you're kind and patient with me. You must have been very smart at medical school.'
- 'I brought you a gift, Doctor, for helping save my life. If it wasn't for you, I wouldn't have found out that my lump was benign.'
- 'Do you like my gift, Doctor? I thought a doctor of your stature deserves nice things. Why don't you wear it now?'

EXAMINER'S QUESTIONS

1 Name ONE ego defence mechanism that Stephanie has displayed in this scenario.

2 Please describe ONE ethical issue in this scenario.

Model Answer

Personality disorders must be diagnosed upon comprehensive longitudinal assessment, including a clear developmental history. As such, they do not lend themselves easily to a brief cross-sectional situation such as an OSCE station. Instead, this station gives an already established diagnosis of borderline personality disorder (BPD). This is a rare station that does not focus on a psychiatric syndromal diagnosis or management planning. An approach that focuses too heavily on history-taking is likely to look dismissive and out of touch with the patient's concerns. Instead, the student must use their knowledge of this disorder in their interactions with the patient and to answer the examiner's questions.

Stephanie denigrates the surgeon, while idealising the GP registrar. While it is certainly possible that Mr Black was curt and dismissive and that the GP registrar has provided some good clinical care, it is highly unlikely that Mr Black and the GP registrar are the worst and best doctors in the world respectively. The astute student will acknowledge that this is likely **splitting**, which is an unconscious ego defence mechanism in which the individual does not reconcile both the positive and negative aspects of a particular object (or person). With splitting comes the related defence mechanism of **projection**, which has led to the GP registrar being perceived as all good and the surgeon as all bad. These defence mechanisms are common in individuals with borderline personality disorder, particularly when they are under stress or perceived attack, which may cause them to regress to these earlier, more primitive defence mechanisms. The candidate must be careful not to identify too strongly with Stephanie's projection and agree that they are a great doctor and Mr Black is terrible, which may reflect an unconscious process known as projective identification. Similarly, the candidate should not dismiss Stephanie's viewpoint completely as this is likely to lead to her feeling further invalidated and abandoned (see Box 14.1, page 201; Box 16.5, pages 274–275).

There are several ethical issues present in this scenario, but Stephanie's question of whether she could complain to the Medical Board and her giving a gift are the two most obvious. Both are tied to the aforementioned defence mechanisms of splitting and projection. The first raises issues of professional loyalties and impartiality, whereas the second raises significant boundary concerns. In both cases, the candidate can explore the reasons for Stephanie's statement or action and validate her experience: 'I'm trying to understand why you want to complain about Mr Black. Could you help me?', and 'It sounds like you're angry about your experience with Mr Black. Part of me wonders whether you felt a bit dismissed by what he said to you.'

From here, the candidate may be in a better position to politely state their role as a doctor and its boundaries. In terms of managing Stephanie's question about whether she should complain about Mr Black, the candidate may state, 'From what you've told me, you have felt angry and hurt by how Mr Black has treated you. I can't say whether you should complain to the Medical Board or not. That certainly remains an option for you, but I wonder whether you want to talk about this further and maybe explore some other options.'

Similarly, the candidate may approach Stephanie's gift by replying, 'I am glad that you had a good outcome with your test results. I'm very grateful for your gift and the appreciation that comes with it. Unfortunately, as your doctor, I am not allowed to receive gifts of such value, but thank you for the thought and effort that you put into choosing it.'

Chapter 15

BIOLOGICAL TREATMENTS

DARRYL BASSETT & DAVID J CASTLE

Psychopharmacology

Medications in psychiatry are used not only to reduce symptoms and modify maladaptive behaviour, but also to facilitate psychological therapies of various kinds. Many patients with mental disorders are significantly more vigilant and anxious about changes in bodily sensations than other people. Thus adverse effects tend to be identified and found to be poorly tolerable more often. However, tolerance usually improves with persistence and patients should be advised of this. It is essential that patients are made aware of common adverse effects, as well as the risk of less common ones (particularly when they are potentially serious or life-threatening). The majority of patients find it reassuring to be aware of potential problems and their management.

This chapter outlines medications that may be prescribed by the reader or encountered in clinical practice. It includes clinical tips and summarises common uses of medications. Less commonly used medications are included as a resource, should they be encountered in clinical practice.

Table 15.1

CYP isoenzyme inhibition by antidepressants

Antidepressant	1A2	2C9	2C19	2D6	3A4	2B6
Agomelatine	−	−	−	−	−	−
Citalopram	−	−	−	+	−	−
Escitalopram	−	−	−	+	−	−
Fluoxetine	+	++	++	+++	+	++
Sertraline	−	−	−	+	−	−
Paroxetine	−	−	−	+++	−	−
Fluvoxamine	+++	−	+++	+	++	−
Venlafaxine	−	−	−	+	−	−
Desmethylvenlafaxine	−	−	−	+	−	−
Duloxetine	−	−	−	+	−	−
Mirtazapine	−	−	−	−	−	−
Reboxetine	−	−	−	−	−	−
Bupropion	−	−	−	+	−	−

− = no clinically significant inhibition; + = potentially clinically significant inhibition, but only at high doses; ++ = moderately clinically significant inhibition; +++ = potent and highly clinically significant inhibition at all doses.

Drug interactions

Most medications are metabolised, at least to some extent, in the liver by the Cytochrome P450 enzyme group (CYP enzymes), and this includes most psychotropic medications. A number of psychotropic medications inhibit or induce isoenzymes of this enzyme group, creating potentially significant changes in the blood levels of other medications. Inhibition will promote increased levels, and induction, decreased levels. These effects need to be considered when prescribing medication combinations *and must be considered before prescribing*. CYP polymorphisms and levels vary from person to person, and also over different racial groups. Genetic testing is now available to determine the profile of these polymorphisms if there are specific clinical indications (see Tables 15.1, 15.10 and 15.11).

Some specific examples are noted below. Pharmacists can be very helpful with advice; computerised prescribing programs include warnings about potential interactions, and the internet site 'MedWatch' is useful. Tables 15.16 and 15.17 provide information regarding medications metabolised by CYP isoenzymes, and those which induce or inhibit those enzymes. This knowledge can greatly assist with clinical decision-making when combining medications.

Cigarette smoking induces CYP 1A2 and therefore blood levels of some medications (e.g. clozapine) may be lower in smokers than expected.

ABC membrane transport proteins (ATP-bound cassette membrane proteins) are heavily involved in the regulation of transport of multiple substances across cell membranes, including the gut, blood–brain barrier, placenta, kidneys and other organs. P-glycoprotein (Pgp) is one such membrane transport protein that has a significant role in the regulation of transport of medications and other substances and therefore pharmacokinetics (including drug interactions). Most psychotropic medications cross the blood–brain barrier by passive diffusion through their lipophilic characteristics, but Pgp can

Box 15.1

Serotonin syndrome

When medications that markedly increase the level of serotonin at nerve synapses are combined with other medications or substances with similar effects, the increase in serotonin levels can produce the symptoms of a *Serotonin syndrome*.

Common examples include an SSRI with a MAOI, an SSRI with lithium (often safe), an SSRI with clomipramine and an SSRI with a 'triptan' (e.g. sumatriptan) used to treat migraine. This is characterised by three potential groups of clinical phenomena:

- cardiovascular: flushing of the skin, increased sweating, tachycardia, increased or decreased blood pressure
- neurological: tremor, hyperreflexia, myoclonus, delirium, seizures
- gastrointestinal: nausea, vomiting, diarrhoea, abdominal pains.

The severity of the syndrome may vary from mild to life-threatening.

modify transfer against concentration gradients. A number of medications inhibit Pgp and therefore have interactive effects on the action of other medications. Examples of such inhibitors include most SSRIs and SNRIs (with the currently known exception of desmethylvenlafaxine), atypical antipsychotics, such as risperidone and olanzapine (less so paliperidone), and a variety of other medications. The tendency of Pgp to have common substrates with CYP 3A group of enzymes can also cause alterations in the bioavailability of several medications. Finally, various neurological diseases alter Pgp activity at the blood–brain barrier.

The combination of medications is a common and often necessary element of clinical practice in medicine. However, attention must always be paid to possible interactions, which can be complex and significant. At the same time, not all combinations are problematic and many interactions are trivial in effect.

The combination of antidepressants in the treatment of depressive disorders is an area of some controversy and any combinations should be approached cautiously and with attention to relative effects on CYP enzymes and Pgp. Most medications are carried in the blood bound to proteins. As many share the same carrier proteins, competition alters the level of 'free' drug and therefore effect. Alterations in the levels of warfarin, for example, are commonly important (see Box 15.1).

Absorption

Medication absorption and therefore bioavailability is affected by:

- the pharmaceutical preparation of the medication (e.g. wafer, enteric coated, controlled release)
- the timing in relation to food (which can also affect tolerance)
- the concurrent use of other substances (e.g. antacids)
- gastrointestinal function (e.g. diarrhoea).

Hepatic and renal dysfunction

Hepatic and/or renal diseases may interfere with medication metabolism and/or excretion.

Box 15.2
Practical notes

The use of:

* herbal remedies
* other 'over-the-counter' medicines and
* illicit substances

may promote significant interactions with prescribed medications.

Hypericum perforatum (St John's Wort) has weak antidepressant properties and contains a group of substances with antidepressant properties. Combination with serotonergic antidepressants can provoke a Serotonin syndrome (see Box 15.1). Several medicinal herbs either induce or inhibit CYP enzymes. Combination of these with psychotropic medications requires specific enquiry for each case.

Many 'recreational' substances can interact seriously with medications, and include alcohol, amphetamines (various forms), cocaine and opiates.

Adherence with medication regimens is improved with education about the medications, taking the medications when patients follow other habits (e.g. brushing teeth, after meals, upon retiring to bed), dosette boxes and bubble-packs filled by pharmacists.

Common adverse effects can be managed as suggested below:

* *Sedation:* take shortly before retiring to bed
* *Weight gain:* a planned, healthy diet with frequent small meals and regular exercise
* *Dry mouth:* frequent sips of water with lemon juice; chewing sugar-free gum; selected types of toothpaste (detergent-free); a variety of artificial saliva substitutes
* *Orthostatic hypotension:* stand up gradually in stages; add extra salt to the diet
* *Nausea:* take medications after food; use anti-emetic medications concurrently.

Age

The very young and the aged exhibit differences in fat/lean body ratios, medication absorption from the gut, hepatic and renal function, and tolerance of adverse effects from medications (see Chapters 18 and 19).

Specific medications

The categories used to classify medications are chosen by the manufacturer when first applying for registration with regulatory authorities. This means that medications may have multiple applications but are 'known' by their initial categorisation. Dose ranges given are *daily* and are suggested for 'routine' applications, but exceptions may arise. Adverse effects listed are those commonly encountered in clinical practice and those that are of particular seriousness. More detailed and comprehensive lists of adverse effects can be obtained in the section, References and further reading (page 257), and from various printed and electronic prescribing guides.

Most psychotropic medications reduce the seizure threshold but some have more potent effects than others and will be highlighted in the text. Box 15.2 provides further practical notes for the use of psychotropic medications.

Table 15.2

Doses, equivalents to diazepam and half-lives of anxiolytics

Drug Anxiolytics	Usual daily dose range (mg)	Approximate equivalent dose (mg) to diazepam 5 mg	Elimination half-lives of drug and active metabolites (hours)
Alprazolam	0.5–4	0.5	10–20
Buspirone	15–30	15	1–11
Clonazepam	2–8	0.25	20–60
Diazepam	5–30	5	12–72, 30–200
Flunitrazepam	0.5–2	1	20, 24, 30
Lorazepam	2–4	1	8–24
Oxazepam	45–90	15	3–25

Box 15.3

Clinical notes on anxiolytics

Diazepam is used frequently in presentations of acute anxiety and is useful for patients to keep for 'crisis' situations. Its rapid absorption by mouth and duration of action, lasting several hours, makes diazepam a flexible anxiolytic for all forms of anxiety disorder for short-term relief. Encourage patients to use this sparingly to minimise tolerance, dependence and adverse effects on the process of capacity to learn. Just knowing that the patient has ready access if in crisis can provide the confidence to manage without.

Alprazolam is preferred by many patients for short-term relief of panic attacks, but should not be seen as a substitute for cognitive and behavioural interventions. Clear education about the management of panic attacks is essential, in any event.

Anxiolytics

Indications

- Anxiety of any form.
- Best used for acute treatment of distressing anxiety and ceased as soon as possible.
- Useful in the first week when introducing antidepressant medications for anxiety or anxious depression.

Benzodiazepines

Alprazolam, clonazepam, diazepam, lorazepam, oxazepam (see Table 15.2 and Box 15.3).

General comments

- Anticonvulsant and muscle relaxing, in addition to anxiolytic properties, which can be useful at times.
- Has a high level of safety in case of oral overdose.
- Withdrawal of benzodiazepines after extended use (more than 2 weeks), must be slow and gradual because of physiological dependence.

Mode of action

- Activation of GABA receptors (the brain's 'braking system') reduces neuronal arousal generally.

Adverse effects

- Sedation is the most common adverse effect.
- Can interfere with cognition including memory, balance and reaction times, and may be addictive over time.
- Combination with alcohol or other sedative medications amplifies sedation and increases the adverse effect upon reaction times, reflexes and cognitive functions generally.
- Use should be intermittent if at all possible, as tolerance develops rapidly and there is significant dependence over time.
- They suppress respiration in very high concentrations (e.g. with bolus intravenous administration).
- Prolonged use may aggravate anxiety through alterations in the function of GABA receptors.

The major disadvantage of using benzodiazepines for anxiety is the reduced motivation to develop psychological coping strategies and, therefore, resilience. Memory and concentration are also easily adversely affected. Physiological and psychological dependence may develop, such that careful monitoring of their use is important. Brief and intermittent use for specific symptom control is optimal, although some patients with complicated problems may benefit from supervised use over extended periods. Long-term use of benzodiazepines may aggravate anxiety through changes in GABA receptors.

Clonazepam is sometimes used to assist with chronic severe generalised anxiety. While this may have short-term usefulness, the problems of aggravation of anxiety over time, impaired cognition, increased risk of ataxia and dependence, make this a less-than-optimal practice in all but the most exceptional circumstances.

Spirodecanediones

Buspirone

General comments

- Start at 5 mg and increase slowly because of dizziness, which usually resolves with time.
- Not addictive, well tolerated over time, does not affect cognition and easily withdrawn; not sedating.

Mode of action

- Buspirone is a serotonin receptor-1A partial agonist, providing optimal serotonergic activity.

Antidepressants

General comments

- All antidepressants relieve core symptoms and signs of depressive disorders with biological features (see Chapter 8).
- Also very effective in the treatment of all forms of anxiety disorders and particularly useful in treatment of resistant panic disorder, post-traumatic stress disorder and obsessive-compulsive disorder.
- Response in depressive disorders usually takes at least 1 week to be evident and 2 or more weeks to become significant. Optimal response will take several months.
- Response in anxiety disorders is slower than for depressive disorders (3 to 4 weeks) and usually requires relatively higher doses. Start with a low dose to minimise aggravation of anxiety early and increase gradually. Concurrent use of a benzodiazepine may be useful early in this treatment.
- Choice of antidepressant is usually initially based upon prominent symptoms (e.g. prominent anxiety might suggest a sedating antidepressant first), response, adverse effect profile and prescriber preference.
- Agomelatine, citalopram, escitalopram, sertraline, paroxetine, fluvoxamine, mirtazapine, duloxetine, tricyclic antidepressants and moclobemide all tend to be less activating than fluoxetine, reboxetine, venlafaxine, desvenlafaxine, bupropion and the irreversible monoamineoxidase inhibitors.
- Inappropriate secretion of anti-diuretic hormone (SIADH) may occur and result in hyponatraemia; most commonly with SSRIs and SNRIs; symptoms may include lethargy, muscle weakness, impaired concentration, and potentially hypotension and cardiac arrhythmias; the effect is usually temporary; most common in elderly patients; fluid restriction for a week or more may be required or the medication changed.
- The metabolism and, therefore, pharmacokinetics of most antidepressants are affected by polymorphisms of CYP enzymes, e.g. as found in racial variations. Desmethylvenlafaxine is not.
- Tricyclic antidepressants provoke mydriasis and may seriously aggravate closed-angle glaucoma. They may also aggravate sicca, again because of their muscarinic side effects.
- Many antidepressants (SSRIs, SNRIs, TCAs, MAOIs) can aggravate restless legs syndrome, particularly at night. If severe, pramipexole 125 to 250 mcg at night, can be very helpful.
- Changing from one antidepressant to another can lead to a period of intense discomfort (withdrawal can be very uncomfortable with dizziness, light headedness, impaired cognitive function, a sensation of 'electric shocks' and insomnia), a rapid return or deterioration in symptoms, and a delay in achieving the benefits of the new antidepressant. Suicide and other self-injury are a significant risk during the period of change (see Box 15.4). Slow withdrawal of one antidepressant, followed by a period of 'washout' without a new medication, followed by slow introduction of the new agent, is

Box 15.4
Antidepressants and the risk of suicide

- The risk of suicide increases around the time of presentation for treatment and in the early stages of treatment for depression or psychosis with **any** treatment.
- The highest risk occurs in the week *before* treatment.
- Some antidepressants may **increase** the risk of suicidal behaviour by enhancing impulsivity and aggression in the first 2 weeks of treatment, particularly in children and adolescents (notably males). However, care should be exercised with patients under the age of 25 as a sensible precaution.
- There is no evidence that antidepressants increase the risk of completed suicide in any age group and indeed there is evidence that after the first few weeks of consumption, antidepressants reduce the risk of suicide. The increased risk of self-injury and suicidal thinking may be reduced by concurrent use of anxiolytic and antipsychotic medications, and *may* be less with certain antidepressants (e.g. mirtazapine).

recommended by many authorities. However, the authors believe that from clinical experience, it is generally better to reduce the first medication to a low dose and simultaneously introduce the new medication in a low dose. There will be a risk of interaction (e.g. Serotonin syndrome) but this can be substantially minimised by careful consideration of the characteristics of each medication. We believe that it is usually safe to combine SSRIs, SNRIs, TCAs, NASAs, NRIs, RIMAs or agomelatine, with one other, in *minimal* doses for 1 to 2 weeks while a transition is achieved. The patient should be warned of possible symptoms of serotonin excess (heavy sweating, hot flushes, nausea/vomiting, diarrhoea, abdominal pains, tachycardia) and advised accordingly. The effects of these medications upon the metabolism of the new medication (e.g. through inhibition of CYP enzymes) and the half-life of the first medication, must be considered (e.g. fluoxetine and norfluoxetine have relatively long half-lives). *There must **always** be a washout period before and after the use of an irreversible monoamine oxidase inhibitor, as described later in this chapter.*

- Blood level monitoring of antidepressants is only occasionally useful, as the therapeutic ranges are very large indeed. However, adherence to treatment and unusual drug metabolic profiles can be checked with blood levels.
- Routine blood examinations can be useful as antidepressants can provoke abnormal function at times. Duloxetine and agomelatine can uncommonly adversely affect liver function and mirtazapine/mianserin can provoke blood dyscrasias.

Selective serotonin reuptake inhibitors (SSRIs)

Citalopram, escitalopram, fluoxetine, fluvoxamine, paroxetine, sertraline (see Table 15.4).

General comments

- Consumption after food reduces the intensity of nausea and reduces the risk of gastric erosion.

Table 15.3

Doses, half-lives and common adverse effects of TCAs

Drug	Usual daily oral dose range (mg)	Elimination half-lives of drug and active metabolites (hours)	Sedation	Postural hypotension	Anticholinergic	Weight gain
TCAs						
Amitriptyline	75–150	10–48	+++	++	+++	+++
Clomipramine	75–150	116–36	++	++	+++	++
Dothiepin	75–150	12–48	+++	++	+++	+++
Doxepin	75–150	8–36	+++	++	+++	+++
Imipramine	75–150	4–36	++	+++	+++	++
Nortriptyline	75–150	12–84	+	+	+++	+
Trimipramine	75–150	8–30	+++	++	++	++

Approximate frequencies of adverse effects: 0 (<2%) = negligible or absent; + (>2%) = infrequent; ++ (>10%) = moderately frequent; +++ (>30%) = frequent; +/− = variable intensity

Table 15.4

Dose ranges, half-lives and common adverse effects of SSRIs

Drug	Usual daily oral dose range (mg)	Elimination half-lives of drug and active metabolites (hours)	Insomnia	Sedation	Sexual dysfunction*	Agitation	Gastrointestinal#	Weight gain
SSRIs								
Citalopram	20–40	24–45	+	++	++	+/–	++	+
Fluoxetine	20–40	24–144 (parent) 200–330 (metabolite)	++	+	++	+	++	+
Fluvoxamine	100–200	10–30	+	++	++/–		+++	+
Paroxetine	20–40	5–65	++	++	+++	+	++	++
Sertraline	50–200	24–36 (parent) 60–96 (metabolite)	++	+	++	+	+++/–	+

Approximate frequencies of adverse effects: 0 (<2%) = negligible or absent; + (>2%) = infrequent; ++ (>10%) = moderately frequent; +++ (>30%) = frequent; +/– = variable intensity

*decreased libido, orgasmic delay or ejaculatory dysfunction

#nausea, vomiting or diarrhoea

- Some evidence of greater efficacy and greater efficiency with increased dose of escitalopram than with citalopram.
- Safe in overdose.

Indications

- Depressive and anxiety disorders with significant somatic/melancholic symptoms.

Mode of action

- By reducing the reuptake of serotonin and sometimes noradrenaline after release from pre-synaptic terminals, these medications improve the capacity of the brain to recover optimal function during depressive disorders or severe anxiety. Neurotrophic factor release is strongly enhanced.

Adverse effects

- Nausea commonly in the first few days, but usually improves with time.
- Disturbed sleep with initial and/or middle insomnia (unpleasant wakefulness after a period of sleep, followed by further sleep).
- Sexual dysfunction including orgasmic delay and suppression of libido; improves with time and sexual activity; particularly significant for females.
- Do not interfere with cognition.
- Movement disorders, such as restless legs syndrome, periodic limb movement disorder and bruxism, may be aggravated.
- Platelet adhesion and function is mildly impaired and may result in bruising, an increase in bleeding time and increased risk of gastric bleeding (clotting factors are not affected). This may be responsible for the small increase in the incidence of stroke in patients over the age of 65 taking SSRIs.
- Gastro-oesophageal reflux may be aggravated.
- Hyponatraemia; see 'general comments' on antidepressants.
- Withdrawal should be gradual as discontinuation can be very uncomfortable (e.g. dizziness, light headedness, insomnia, agitation, irritability); worst with paroxetine.
- Reduced male fertility.

Serotonergic and noradrenergic re-uptake inhibitors (SNRIs)

Desvenlafaxine, duloxetine, venlafaxine.

Indications

- Depressive and anxiety disorders with significant vegetative symptoms.
- SNRIs are popular in more severe disorders or when response to SSRIs is inadequate.
- Duloxetine can be very helpful in the management of chronic pain; other members of this group can also be of benefit in this regard.

Mode of action

- Similar to SSRIs, but with greater effect upon noradrenaline; duloxetine and desvenlafaxine have significant dual serotonergic/noradrenergic effect at usual doses; venlafaxine requires relatively high dose (more than 225 mg daily) to achieve significant noradrenergic effect.

Adverse effects

- Similar unwanted effects to SSRIs; adverse effects with venlafaxine appear clinically more severe than duloxetine and desmethylvenlafaxine.
- Withdrawal should be very gradual as discontinuation can be very uncomfortable (dizziness, light headedness, insomnia, agitation, irritability); appears most severe for venlafaxine and less severe for duloxetine and desvenlafaxine.
- Duloxetine may be mildly sedating at first or may be activating.
- Diastolic hypertension may rise; the increase is proportional to the dose; the effects of duloxetine and desmethylvenlafaxine appear less severe than for venlafaxine.
- Hyponatraemia: see 'General comments' on antidepressants.
- Duloxetine should be avoided when hepatic disease is present because of potential hepatotoxicity.

Selective noradrenergic re-uptake inhibitors (NRIs)

Reboxetine (see Table 15.5).

General comments

- Use of reboxetine is not accompanied by weight gain.
- The evidence for the efficacy of reboxetine as an antidepressant is increasingly less compelling.

Indications

- Depressive and anxiety disorders with significant somatic/melancholic symptoms.
- NRIs are activating and energising.

Mode of action

- By reducing the reuptake of noradrenaline after release from pre-synaptic terminals these medications improve the capacity of the brain to recover optimal function during depressive disorders or severe anxiety. Neurotrophic factor release is significantly enhanced.

Adverse effects

- Initial insomnia may occur.
- May provoke abnormal ejaculation and urinary retention in males; rarely, heightened genital arousal in females.
- Can amplify anxiety markedly, particularly early in treatment.

- Withdrawal is best achieved slowly, but is usually not uncomfortable.
- Movement disorders such as restless legs syndrome, periodic limb movement disorder and bruxism may be aggravated.
- Platelet adhesion and function is mildly impaired and may result in bruising and an increase in bleeding time and increased gastric bleeding.

Noradrenaline and specific serotonergic agents (NASAs)

Mianserin, Mirtazapine (see Table 15.5).

General comments

- Mirtazapine is used most commonly, as mianserin carries a higher risk of blood dyscrasia.
- Mianserin is usually more sedating than mirtazapine.
- Usually well tolerated in elderly patients and this can be an advantage (see Chapter 19).
- Mirtazapine appears useful in irritable bowel syndrome and less aggravating of restless legs syndrome than other antidepressants.

Indications

- Depressive disorders with significant somatic/melancholic symptoms and severe anxiety disorders.

Mode of action

- Inhibition of alpha-2 noradrenergic receptors, thus enhancing noradrenaline and serotonin release.
- Inhibition of serotonin 2a receptors enhancing noradrenaline, dopamine and glutamate release in the prefrontal region.

Adverse effects

- NASAs are very sedating and weight gain can be a significant problem; decreases with increasing dose (reverse of that usually expected).
- No or limited adverse effects on sexual function.
- Dry mouth, constipation and sometimes urinary retention can occur.
- Occasionally unusual and sometimes distressing dreaming may accompany NASAs; withdrawal is usually the optimal management, but they may resolve with persistence.
- Some evidence of an increased risk of seizures in vulnerable individuals.
- Blood dyscrasia occurs rarely.

Tricyclic antidepressants (TCAs)

Amitriptyline, dothiepin, doxepin, imipramine, nortriptyline, trimipramine (see Table 15.3).

General comments

- Tricyclics are very useful if tolerance of SSRIs and SNRIs is poor or those medications have failed to provide optimal response.
- Nortriptyline is a selectively noradrenergic tricyclic antidepressant, which can be useful when greater activation is required or when there is risk of serotonin syndrome.
- Tricyclics may have a 'therapeutic window' of blood level, with lower efficacy above and below certain blood levels. While these ranges have been suggested to be between 70–220 ng/mL for amitriptyline (amitriptyline + nortriptyline levels) and 60–150 ng/mL for nortriptyline alone, the variation between patients is considerable. It is clinically more helpful in the first instance to slowly achieve the highest tolerable dose and monitor the patient's clinical progress.

Indications

- Depressive and anxiety disorders with significant somatic/melancholic symptoms, as well as with chronic pain management.

Mode of action

- By reducing the reuptake of serotonin and noradrenaline after release from pre-synaptic terminals, and by enhancing noradrenaline, dopamine and glutamate release in the prefrontal region through inhibition of serotonin 2a receptors, these medications improve the capacity of the brain to recover optimal function during depressive disorders or severe anxiety. Neurotrophic factor release is significantly enhanced, but the mechanism remains uncertain.

Adverse effects

- Dry mouth and constipation are common (muscarinic) side effects. Optimal dosing is usually associated with these effects.
- Potentially lethal in overdose because of cardiac arrhythmia (impaired ventricular conduction).
- Blurred vision and urinary retention may occur, particularly at higher doses.

Noradrenaline and dopamine reuptake inhibitors

Bupropion (see Table 15.5).

Indications

- Depressive disorders and smoking cessation.
- Activating effects can be useful clinically.
- Sometimes used to counteract sexual dysfunction provoked by serotonergic medications.
- Some evidence of being less likely to promote manic switching in bipolar disorders than most antidepressants.
- Used in Australia mostly for treatment-resistant depression because of cost.

Table 15.5   Dose ranges, half-lives and common adverse effects of other antidepressants

Drug	Usual daily oral dose range (mg)	Elimination half-lives of drug and active metabolites (hours)	Insomnia	Sedation	Sexual dysfunction*	Agitation	Gastrointestinal#	Weight gain
other antidepressants								
Mianserin	60–90	20–60	0	+++/-	+/-	0	+	++
Mirtazapine	30–45	20–40	0	+++	+/-	0	+	+++
Duloxetine	30–60	12	+/-	++/-	+	0	+++/-	0
Reboxetine	8–12	12–14	+++	0	+	++	+	0
Venlafaxine	75–300	3–7 (parent) 9–13 (metabolite)	+	++	+++	++	+++	0
Desvenlafaxine	50–200	10–12	+	+	+	0	+	0
Bupropion	150–450	10–14	++	+/-	0	++	+	0
Agomelatine	25–50	1–2	0	+	0	0	+/-	0

Approximate frequencies of adverse effects: 0 (<2%) = negligible or absent; + (>2%) = infrequent; ++ (>10%) = moderately frequent; +++ (>30%) = frequent; +/- = variable intensity

*decreased libido, orgasmic delay or ejaculatory dysfunction

#nausea, vomiting or diarrhoea

Mode of action

- Uncertain mechanism but reuptake of noradrenaline and dopamine is reduced.

Adverse effects

- Dry mouth, nausea, sweating, insomnia and dizziness are relatively common.
- Rarely, seizures may occur.

Metabolism

- Bupropion is metabolised to hydroxyl-bupropion by CYP isoenzyme 2B6.

Monoamine oxidase inhibitors (MAOIs)

Moclobemide, phenelzine, tranylcypromine (see Tables 15.6, 15.11 and 15.12).

Indications

- Depressive disorders with significant somatic/melancholic symptoms and severe anxiety disorders.
- Reserved in clinical practice for treatment-resistant depressive and anxiety disorders.
- Moclobemide is best used for relatively mild depressive disorders.

Mode of action

- Inhibition of monoamine oxidase increases the quantities of serotonin, noradrenaline and dopamine available for release from pre-synaptic terminals.

Adverse effects

- Reversible inhibitors of monoamine oxidase type A (RIMAs) are very well tolerated, but are often not effective! Their relatively select inhibition of the A type of monoamine oxidase (MAO) is advantageous as this is found mostly in the brain and much less often in the gut. Consequently, the risk of excessive tyramine absorption from certain foods is very much lower (not absent) and use of the medications much safer and easier.
- MAOIs carry dietary restrictions because of increased tyramine absorption from foods (by reducing destruction by MAO in the bowel).
- Introduction of tyramine in foods or combination with serotonergic substances can result in rapid and severe hypertension, which can result in a cerebrovascular accident and even death (see Table 15.11).
- Typical early symptoms are:
  - severe headache (often of an 'exploding' quality)
  - severe neck stiffness
  - high temperature
  - sweating
  - tachycardia.
    Treatment can include sedation (e.g. with benzodiazepines), analgesia and vasodilating medications (e.g. phentolamine/diazoxide/nifedipine, etc). General medical

Table 15.6

Doses, half-lives and common adverse effects of MAOIs

Drug	Usual daily oral dose range (mg)	Elimination half-lives of drug and active metabolites (hours)	Sedation	Postural hypotension	Anticholinergic	Weight gain
MAOIs						
Phenelzine	45–60	1.5–4*	++/–	++	+++	++
Tranylcypromine	30–40	3*	+/–	+	++	+/–
Moclobemide	300–600	1–3	+/–	0	0	0

Approximate frequencies of adverse effects: 0 (<2%) = negligible or absent; + (>2%) = infrequent; ++ (>10%) = moderately frequent;

+++ (>30%) = frequent; +/– = variable intensity

*Phenelzine and Tranylcypromine inhibit all forms of MAO and their effects last 2 to 3 weeks

intervention with admission to hospital must be obtained urgently if any such symptoms or a rise in blood pressure occur.

- MAOIs also amplify the effects of monoamines (including noradrenaline, adrenaline and serotonin of any source) and serotonergic medications (including pethidine, lithium and most antidepressants) (see Table 15.7 and Box 15.5).

Serotonin receptor antagonists/melatonin receptor agonists

Agomelatine (see Table 15.5).

Table 15.7

MAOI dietary restrictions

High tyramine content – NOT PERMITTED	Moderate tyramine content – LIMITED AMOUNTS ARE SAFE	Low tyramine content – PERMISSIBLE AND SAFE
Aged, matured cheeses (unpasteurised) e.g. cheddar, camembert, stilton, blue, swiss Smoked or pickled meats, fish or poultry e.g. herring, sausage, corned beef Aged/putrefying meats, fish, poultry e.g. chicken or beef liver, pate, game Yeast or meat extracts e.g. 'Bovril', marmite, vegemite, brewers yeast, balsamic vinegar (beware of drinks, soups or stews made with these products). Note: 'Yeast breads' are safe Certain wines e.g. Chianti, sherry, vermouth Italian broad beans e.g. fava beans	Meat extracts e.g. Bouillon, consommé Pasteurised light and pale beers (tap beers preferred) Ripe avocado Soy sauce and soy milk	Distilled spirits (in moderation) e.g. vodka, gin, rye, scotch Red and white wines (in moderation – not Chianti) Cheese e.g. cottage cheese, cream cheese, mozzarella, ricotta Chocolate and caffeine containing beverages Fruits e.g. figs, raisins, grapes, pineapple, oranges Yoghurt, sour cream (commercial preparations)

Box 15.5

MAOI dangerous combinations

- Amphetamines
- Pethidine
- Opioids
- Lithium
- Serotonergic antidepressants
- *Hypericum perforatum*
- Tryptophan

Indications

- Depressive and anxiety disorders with significant somatic/melancholic symptoms.
- Frequently used for patients with a history of very poor tolerance of other antidepressants.
- Agomelatine is an attractive choice as a first-line antidepressant because of its relatively attractive side effect profile.

Mode of action

- Inhibition of serotonin 2c receptors with increased noradrenaline, dopamine and glutamate release in the prefrontal region.
- Enhancement of melatonin types 1 and 2 receptors.
- There appears to be synergism between the action upon serotonin 2c receptors and melatonin receptors.
- Agomelatine appears to enhance the maintenance of a regular circadian rhythm and may therefore enhance the quality of sleep in some patients.

Adverse effects

- Somnolence, dizziness, upper abdominal pain, migraine, nausea. The frequency of incidence is low.
- Mild increases in liver transaminase levels have been found in some patients but the clinical significance of this is not clear. Six-weekly tests of liver function are currently recommended.

Box 15.6 provides a framework for using the various groups of antidepressants in clinical practice. This is only a guide and clinical judgement must be exercised for clinical presentation.

Antipsychotics

General comments

The antipsychotic medications can be divided into 'generations': first, second and third. This reflects the history of their development and differences in some aspects of their actions and adverse effects.

Box 15.6

Clinical notes on antidepressants

Below are suggestions for the choice of antidepressants in common clinical situations, based upon research and personal experience/preference. The list is not exhaustive and clinical judgement must be used in each case, particularly when there is a history of antidepressant use. When treating depressive disorders, begin with the lowest manufactured dose (or less if the patient is anxious about adverse effects, in the treatment of panic disorder, or the elderly) and increase as quickly as tolerated to the recommended starting therapeutic dose. Increase the dose after 2 weeks if there is no evidence of any response, or persist for a further month if there are signs of some improvement, before increasing the dose further. In the treatment of panic disorder or highly anxious patients with depressive disorders, the addition of adjunctive anxiolytic medication (usually a benzodiazepine) during the first week of treatment can minimise the aggravation of the anxiety which often occurs with less sedating antidepressants (e.g. SSRIs, SNRIs, MAOIs). Anxiety disorders will sometimes require an increase in dose after 2 weeks to achieve an adequate response.

Depression – uncomplicated: consider an SSRI or agomelatine.

Depression – anxious: consider agomelatine or SSRIs (particularly citalopram, escitalopram, fluvoxamine, paroxetine). If severe, NASAs and TCAs can be useful.

Depression – retarded: consider fluoxetine, SNRIs, reboxetine, nortriptyline.

Depression – premenstrual: SSRIs.

Depression – severe: consider SNRIs, mirtazapine, TCAs.

Depression – failing to respond to or intolerant of SSRIs: consider agomelatine, SNRIs, NASAs, TCAs.

Depression – treatment-resistant: higher than usual doses of any antidepressants used; TCAs, MAOIs.

Depression – psychotic: consider SNRIs or TCAs; always combine with an antipsychotic medication.

Generalised anxiety disorder: SSRIs. Use SNRIs, NASAs, or TCAs if failing to respond to SSRIs.

Panic disorder: SSRIs combined with an anxiolytic for the first week to avoid provoking panic attacks. SNRIs, NASAs or TCAs if failing to respond to SSRIs.

Post-traumatic stress disorder: SSRIs. Use SNRIs, NASAs or TCAs if failing to respond to SSRIs; efficacy of antidepressants is limited.

Obsessive-compulsive disorder: SSRIs. Use TCAs (particularly clomipramine) if failing to respond to SSRIs. Relatively high doses may be required.

Social anxiety disorder, agoraphobia: SSRIs. Use SNRIs, NASAs or TCAs if failing to respond to SSRIs.

First generation antipsychotics (Neuroleptics)

Chlorpromazine, fluphenazine, flupenthixol, haloperidol, pericyazine, trifluoperazine, zuclopenthixol (see Table 15.8).

Second and third generation antipsychotics (Atypicals)

Amisulpride, aripiprazole, asenapine, clozapine (see Box 15.10), olanzapine, paliperidone, risperidone, quetiapine, sertindole, ziprasidone (see Tables 15.8 and 15.9).

- Rapidly disintegrating oral preparations of olanzapine (oral wafer), asenapine (sublingual wafer) and risperidone (tablet) are available.
- Slow-release preparations of risperidone (intramuscular depot), olanzapine (intramuscular depot), paliperidone (intramuscular depot and oral, slow-release capsule) and quetiapine (oral, slow release tablet) are available.
- Second and third generation antipsychotics have a lower tendency to provoke extrapyramidal side effects than first generation antipsychotics, but these may still occur with significant intensity. Akathisia is more common with ziprasidone, asenapine and aripiprazole than with other second generation antipsychotics. The profile of adverse effects of these medications generally is listed in Table 15.8.
- Quetiapine, ziprasidone and amisulpride tend to delay cardiac conduction significantly, with prolongation of the QT interval. Risperidone, paliperidone, olanzapine and clozapine may also have notable effect in some patients. This is not usually a clinically significant problem unless the patient is genetically very vulnerable or in combination with other medications which have a similar effect.
- The half-lives of atypical antipsychotics range from 6 hours (quetiapine) to 30 hours (olanzapine), with considerable individual variation and changes with different preparations.
- Most atypical antipsychotics are metabolised by CYP enzymes, with some glucuronidation (combination with glucuronic acid via uridine diphosphate glucuronyl transferase in the liver). Paliperidone is mostly excreted unchanged, largely in the urine. Asenapine is mostly glucuronated (and partly metabolised by CYP 1A2). Both are less sensitive to liver impairment than others (although metabolism of asenapine is significantly delayed in the presence of severe hepatic impairment), as a consequence.

Indications

- Antipsychotic medications all relieve psychotic symptoms of any cause to some degree. They reduce the intensity of sensory information drawn from the environment, improve the efficiency of reformulation of environmental stimuli and facilitate processing of information and perceptions. They can then gradually improve reality processing and facilitate more appropriate responses to their internal and external environment.
- The efficacy is high in schizophrenia, mania and psychotic depression but variable (sometimes ineffective) in psychosis secondary to general medical disorders or substance use (including prescribed medications), and in delusional disorders.

Table 15.8

Relative frequency of common adverse effects of antipsychotics at usual therapeutic doses

Drug	Usual daily oral dose range (mg)	Sedation	Postural hypotension	Anticholinergic	Extrapyramidal	Weight gain	Prolactin
Atypical drugs							
Amisulpride	400–1000 (acute psychosis) 100–300 (negative symptoms)	+	+	0	++*	+	+++
Aripiprazole	10–30	++/–	+	0	+	+	+/–
Clozapine	200–600	+++	+++	++	+	+++	+/–
Olanzapine	5–20	+++	+	++	+	+++	+
Quetiapine	300–750	+++/–	+++	+	+*	++	+
Risperidone	2–6	++	+++	0	++	++/–	+++
Paliperidone	3–12	+/–	+++	0	++/–	++/–	+++
Ziprasidone	80–160	++	+	+	+	0	+
Asenapine	0.5–20	++	+/–	+/–	+	0	0
Sertindole	12–20	+	++	++	+	0	+/–
Typical drugs							
Chlorpromazine	75–100	+++	+++	++	++	+++	++
Fluphenazine	5–20	+	+	+	+++/–	++	++
Haloperidol	1–7.5	+	+	+	+++	++	++
Pericyazine	15–75	+++	+++	++	++	++	++
Trifluoperazine	5–20	+	++	+	+++	++	++

Approximate frequencies of adverse effects: O (<2%) = negligible or absent; + (>2%) = infrequent; ++ (>10%) = moderately frequent;

+++ (>30%) = frequent; +/– = variable intensity

*rarely a problem at usual therapeutic doses.

Table 15.9

Relative frequency of common adverse effects of depot antipsychotics at usual therapeutic doses

Drug	Usual IM dose range*	Dosing interval (weeks)	Sedation	Postural hypotension	Anticholinergic	Extrapyramidal	Weight gain	Prolactin
Zuclopenthixol Acetate ^	50–150	2–3 days	+	++	+++/–	+++	++	+
Flupenthixol Decanoate	20–40	2–4	+	+	++	+++	++	+
Fluphenazine Decanoate	12.5–50	2–4	+	+	+	+++/–	+++	++
Haloperidol Decanoate	50–200	4	+	+	+	+++	++	+++
Risperidone Depot	25–50	2	++	+++	0	+	++	+++
Zuclopenthixol Decanoate#	200–400#	2–4	+	+	+++/–	+++	++	+
Paliperidone Palmitate	25–150	1–4	+/–	++	0	++/–	+	+++
Olanzapine Pamoate &	210–405	2–4	+	+	+/–	+/–	+++	+

Note: This is the frequency of occurrence of adverse effects, not the intensity with which they occur.

+++ (>30%) = frequent; +/– = variable intensity

*an initial test dose is recommended for all long-acting drugs especially if the patient has not been exposed to the class of antipsychotic drug previously

^single dose, not to be repeated for 2 to 3 days

#Patients switched from zuclopenthixol acetate do not require a test dose of zuclopenthixol decanoate and 'Post-injection syndrome' may arise within 1–2 hours of injection: sedation, confusion/delirium, agitation, hypotension, seizures, EPS

Mode of action

- All of the current antipsychotics have modulating effects upon dopamine activity in the brain. They all inhibit dopamine 2 receptors and this is directly related to their beneficial effects upon positive features of psychosis (see Chapter 7). The first generation antipsychotics all bind tightly to these (and some other) dopamine receptors throughout the brain. The second and third generation antipsychotics bind to the dopamine 2 receptors, as well as some others, but with differing affinity, activity and distribution in the brain.
- They all increase production of nerve growth factors in the brain (of considerable importance in schizophrenia particularly) and may have other useful effects upon neuronal and glial function.
- The second generation antipsychotics have the added effect of inhibiting serotonin 2a and 2c (post-synaptic) receptors, which reduces the likelihood of extrapyramidal side effects (through increased dopamine release in the substantia nigra and other regions of the basal ganglia) and positively affects negative features and cognitive functions (through increased release of noradrenaline, dopamine and glutamate in the prefrontal region).
- Aripiprazole and asenapine are different in that they act as partial agonists of dopamine 2 receptors.

Adverse effects

- The first generation antipsychotics do not appear to have significant benefit upon negative and cognitive features of psychosis (particularly schizophrenia), and can easily provoke a variety of extrapyramidal side effects (see Boxes 15.7 and 15.8).

Box 15.7

Practical notes regarding first generation antipsychotics

- Exposure to sunlight when taking chlorpromazine can provoke erythema, which can be uncomfortable and even painful (photosensitivity).
- Cholestatic liver dysfunction can occur, particularly with chlorpromazine.
- Intense heat should be avoided as temperature regulation may be impaired.
- Assistance with appetite and weight management is invaluable.
- Slow release intramuscular depot preparations of fluphenazine, flupenthixol, zuclopenthixol, and haloperidol are available.
- Zuclopenthixol acetate is available as a less prolonged-acting but relatively quickly absorbed (t-max = 4 hours) intramuscular injection, which has a duration of action of around 2 days. This can be very useful for the management of acute psychosis, but if severe adverse effects arise (e.g. laryngeal stridor), the prolonged action can be difficult to manage and potentially very dangerous.
- Extrapyramidal side effects are common (see Box 15.8).
- Chlorpromazine and other phenothiazines can provoke retinal pigmentation, particularly at high doses in genetically vulnerable patients. The other first generation antipsychotics can also cause damage but this is quite rare.
- Intramuscular chlorpromazine may produce sterile abscess formation.

Box 15.8

Extrapyramidal side effects (EPS)

General comments

- Inhibition of dopamine 2 receptors in the substantia nigra and basal ganglia provokes an imbalance of dopaminergic and cholinergic activity. This can produce clinical signs and symptoms usually associated with basal ganglia diseases such as Parkinson's disease.
- EPS are aggravated by anxiety.
- EPS are much less common with atypical antipsychotic medications, but occur more frequently with risperidone than others in this group, particularly at doses above 4 mg daily. Aripiprazole has a greater tendency to produce akathisia.
- Extrapyramidal side effects with depot preparations of medications can provide increased risks if severe, because of the long duration of action.

Acute forms

- *Tremor*: worst at rest.
- *Dystonias*: involuntary sustained muscle contractions, particularly of the head and neck; very unpleasant and can be painful; may include facial muscles, including the tongue.
- *Oculogyric crisis*: dystonia which affects the external ocular muscles.
- *Laryngeal stridor*: dystonia which affects the laryngeal muscles; potentially very serious.
- *Parkinsonism*: mask-like facial expression; muscle rigidity with tremor ('cog-wheel rigidity'); shuffling gait ('festinating gait'); retropulsion; reduced spontaneous arm swing.
- *Akathisia*: subjective sensation of very uncomfortable restlessness which is not relieved by movement (contrast 'restless legs syndrome'). Observation reveals frequent or constant movement and restlessness which is difficult to resist. The patient tends to walk as much as possible.

Management of acute extrapyramidal side effects

- Reduce dose of medication if possible.
- Anticholinergic medication such as benztropine 1 to 2 mg orally or intramuscularly, or benzhexol 2 to 5 mg orally.
- Beta blockers such as propranolol and benzodiazepines (notably diazepam) are most useful for akathisia.

Neuroleptic malignant syndrome (NMS)

- Serious but rare neurological reaction to antipsychotic medications characterised by severe hypertonia, high fever, autonomic instability and delirium.
- Idiosyncratic and unpredictable.
- Develops over hours to days with 'lead-pipe' rigidity as an early sign.
- Myolysis and myoglobinuria may occur, aggravated by dehydration.

Box 15.7 continued

- Creatinine phosphokinase levels rise sharply and can be very high; liver transaminases and neutrophil counts may also rise.

- Admission to a general medical Intensive Care Unit is essential given the life-threatening implications and complex management.

- Subsequent management requires specialist psychiatric care because of the risk of relapse.

Tardive forms

(delayed onset; sometimes many years)

These include: *Tardive dyskinesia:* mostly orobuccal-facio-lingual abnormal and involuntary movements; typically chewing movements and/or licking of the lips, and/or random tongue movements, and/or grimacing; may not be distressing to the patient; may be accompanied by more generalised choreoathetosis which can be severe; may be due to other causes (a range of neurological disorders and a number of other substances); can arise in schizophrenia without exposure to medications and are more common in this disorder than the general population.

- *Tardive dystonia:* late onset dystonias, as described above.

- *Tardive akathisia:* late onset akathisia, as described above.

- *Tardive Parkinsonism:* late onset Parkinsonism, as described above.

The prevalence of tardive extrapyramidal syndromes is not well documented, but arise in approximately 60% of chronic users of first generation antipsychotic (and related) medications. The prevalence in chronic users of second and third generation antipsychotic medications has not been adequately documented at this time, but is probably significantly less.

Management of tardive extrapyramidal side effects

- Benzodiazepines may give some relief and a change to atypical antipsychotic medications, particularly clozapine can be very helpful (see Box 15.9).

- Withdrawal or change to an atypical antipsychotic early in the appearance of tardive side effects can promote reversal of the movement disorder.

- May resolve spontaneously.

- Second generation antipsychotics are much less likely to produce these adverse effects (although they can occur); called 'atypical antipsychotics'.
- The second generation antipsychotics have beneficial effects upon negative features of psychosis and cognitive deficits.

Metabolic adverse effects

- Weight gain.
- Hyperlipidaemia: notably hypercholesterolaemia but sometimes triglyceridaemia.
- Diabetes mellitus (type 2).
- Metabolic syndrome: combinations of weight gain, diabetes mellitus (type 2), hypertension and hypercholesterolaemia.
- Metabolic complications are spontaneously more common in schizophrenia than with other disorders.

Box 15.9

Clinical notes on clozapine

- Clozapine is used in treatment-resistant schizophrenia, but is increasingly utilised early in treatment if the response to other antipsychotic medications is sub-optimal.
- It carries a significant risk of agranulocytosis and regular monitoring of haematological measures is mandatory.
- In addition, it carries risks of pericarditis/myocarditis (usually acute and extremely serious), cardiomyopathy (usually chronic and less serious) and epilepsy.
- However, the efficacy of clozapine in schizophrenia and (probably) in bipolar affective disorders is so exceptional that these risks can often be justified in patients with treatment-resistant illness.

Box 15.10

Clinical notes on antipsychotics

The starting dose will usually be the lowest manufactured dose, with increase determined by response over days to weeks.

Second generation antipsychotic medications are currently often used in preference to first generation antipsychotics because of the lower risk of extrapyramidal side effects and potential benefits upon negative and cognitive symptoms. Asenapine may have some advantages in the treatment of negative and cognitive symptoms. Weight gain, promotion of diabetes mellitus (type 2), hyperlipidaemia and metabolic syndrome from some of these medications are reasons for caution in practice.

First generation antipsychotics are cheaper than second generation medications and may be preferred for this reason.

Ziprasidone is best absorbed if taken with food.

Antipsychotics may prolong cardiac conduction (QTc interval) and examples include haloperidol, quetiapine, ziprasidone and sertindole. The risk is increased by concurrent use of some anti-arrhythmic medications, hypokalaemia, hypomagnesaemia and high dose. If there is any doubt, an electrocardiograph should be performed and serum electrolyte levels checked. If gastrointestinal disorders are present, including severe food restriction in anorexia nervosa, then a serum magnesium should also be obtained. A QTc interval of <500 msec is considered reasonable, but for safety <450 msec is preferable.

Atypical antipsychotics can also cause retinal damage, although this is very rare.

- Most prominent with the atypical antipsychotics clozapine, olanzapine and quetiapine. The risk is less prominent with asenapine, amisulpride, risperidone and paliperidone. Asenapine appears to have no significant effect upon the risk of diabetes mellitus (type 2) or hyperlipidaemia. Aripiprazole has very little risk and ziprasidone no adverse metabolic risks.

Cardiovascular adverse effects

- Postural hypotension (particularly with first generation antipsychotics such as chlorpromazine).
- Cardiac dysrhythmias (see Box 15.10).

Box 15.11

Clinical notes on lithium

Lithium is the 'gold standard' for mood stabilisers, but many patients are wary because of its side effect profile. Careful psychoeducation about its use and advantages is essential.

Mood stabilisers

Lithium

General comments

- Most effective mood stabiliser for bipolar affective disorder and neuroprotective in chronic mood disorder (see Box 15.11).
- Excretion half-life = 24–30 hours (once steady state has been established).
- Sampling of blood level: 10–12 hours after the last dose so that it is at the start of the excretion phase.
- Therapeutic index is low (low ratio of lethal dose to median effective dose and therefore a greater need for monitoring); aim for blood level between 0.5–1.2 mmol/L; *adjust for patient tolerance and efficacy.*
- 'Higher' blood levels are associated with subtle cognitive impairment (> 0.8 mmol/L)
- Interactions with other drugs: potential but rare serotonin syndrome when combined with serotonergic medications (*common when combined with MAOIs*); combination with anti-inflammatory medications, ACE inhibitors and thiazide diuretics increases the lithium level.
- Dehydration and hyponatraemia (with increased lithium resorption by the kidneys) can increase the lithium level significantly.
- Dose range: 250 to 1500 mg daily.

Indications

- Management of bipolar mood disorders both in acute care and in prophylaxis.
- Onset of action is over several weeks.
- Most effective in treating mania.
- Also effective as an augmenting treatment for depressive disorder.
- Exerts an 'anti-suicidal' effect.
- May reduce the intensity of aggressive behaviour.

Mode of action

- Complex range of effects upon signal transduction in neurons, alteration of some fundamental cell processes, an anti-apoptotic effect and increase in serotonin availability.

Adverse effects

- May damage the thyroid gland, impeding production and release of thyroid hormones; reversible early in the treatment, but may become permanent and require oral thyroid hormone supplements.

Box 15.12

Clinical notes on anticonvulsants

Sodium valproate is easily introduced at 500 mg daily in most patients and is preferred to carbamazepine in the first instance because of better tolerance and efficacy.

- May make skin/hair coarse and promote psoriasis.
- May cause increased urine production ('nephrogenic diabetes insipidus'); renal cortical damage can occur and, rarely, renal failure can follow.
- Toxicity can arise easily if poorly monitored; characterised by coarse tremor, dysarthria and ataxia; promoted by dehydration.
- Severe lithium toxicity can be fatal in some patients.

Anticonvulsants

Indications

- Management of bipolar mood disorders, both in acute management and in prophylaxis.
- Onset of action is over several weeks.
- Most effective in treating mania.
- Valproate and carbamazepine are effective in rapid cycling and mixed affective disorders (see Box 15.12).
- Lamotrigine is effective in bipolar affective disorder (type II) and bipolar spectrum disorders.

Mode of action

- Valproate and carbamazepine appear similar to lithium in some aspects of mode of action.
- Lamotrigine appears to modulate glutaminergic activity, possibly through its effects on sodium channel activity.

Hypnotics

Benzodiazepines

Flunitrazepam, nitrazepam, temazepam (see Table 15.11).

General comments

- Adverse effects are those of any benzodiazepines.
- Temazepam is most commonly used in practice.
- Disrupt sleep cycle with regular use and become addictive.
- Avoid flunitrazepam where possible because of the long duration of action, potent adverse effect on memory and frequency of abuse (dependency, 'date-rape drug').

Table 15.10

Usual daily doses and some adverse effects of anticonvulsants

Drug	Dose range	Adverse effects
Sodium valproate	500 to 1000 mg	Tremor, weight gain, alopecia (partial), blurred vision, thrombocytopaenia, hepatotoxicity
Carbamazepine	100 to 800 mg	Skin rash, dizziness, sedation, ataxia, dysarthria, thrombocytopaenia, agranulocytosis
Lamotrigine	200 to 400 mg	Serious rash (Stevens-Johnson syndrome; necrotising epidermolysis), headache, dizziness, diplopia, ataxia. Note that serious skin reactions are rare (about 1/1000) and management is usually very successful, providing lamotrigine is ceased immediately if any skin changes arise. The presence of fever, 'influenza-like symptoms' and mucosal blisters, enhance the probability of a serious hypersensitivity reaction. *Introduce 25 mg daily and increase slowly (25 mg daily for 2 weeks; then 50 mg daily for 2 weeks; then 100 mg daily for 2 weeks; then 200 mg daily) with care to check skin regularly for any unusual changes. Most skin changes are harmless and treatment can be resumed but ALWAYS withhold lamotrigine until the nature of the skin change has been clarified.*

Table 15.11

Doses, equivalents to diazepam and half-lives of hypnotics

Drug	Usual daily dose range (mg)	Approximate equivalent dose (mg) to diazepam 5 mg	Elimination half-lives of drug and active metabolites (hours)
Hypnotics			
Nitrazepam	5–10	2.5	15–48
Zolpidem	5–10	–	1.5–4.5
Zopiclone	3.75–7.5	–	3.8–6.5
Temazepam	5–20	10	3–25

Indications

- Distressing insomnia.
- Aim for intermittent and short-term use.

Mode of action

- As for other benzodiazepines.

Adverse effects

- As for other benzodiazepines.

Imidazopyridines

Zolpidem (see Table 15.11).

General comments

- Minimal effect on sleep cycle and appears to have relatively less addictiveness than benzodiazepines.
- Immediate release preparation has little effect on cognition after about 8 hours.
- Extended release preparation has little effect on cognition after about 10 hours.

Mode of action

- Activation of Ω-1 subset of GABA benzodiazepine receptors with more selective GABA-ergic effect; sedation.
- Significantly less activation of Ω-2 and Ω-3 subsets of receptor.

Adverse effects

- Odd but harmless effects (sleepwalking and hallucinations) if taken too early and in vulnerable individuals; try a low 'test dose' and avoid regular use.
- Unusual behaviours are strongly aggravated by concurrent alcohol.

Cyclopyrrolones

Zopiclone (see Table 15.11).

General comments

- Expensive but similar advantages to zolpidem.
- Longer acting than zolpidem.
- Some experience 'metallic taste'.
- Mode of action, as for zolpidem.

Indoleamines

N-acetyl-5-methoxytryptamine (melatonin).

General comments

- Produced endogenously by the pineal gland and a component of the normal sleep process, provoked by the reduction of ambient light.
- Given orally in a slow release formulation, augmenting endogenous melatonin.

Mode of action

- Activation of the suprachiasmatic nucleus of hypothalamus ('biological clock'); consequent inhibition of the ventrolateral preoptic nucleus; subsequent inhibition of a series of 'arousal' nuclei, promotes the induction of the sleep process.

Adverse effects

- Tolerance is usually excellent, but flushing of skin, diarrhoea, migraine and abdominal cramps have been reported. Box 15.13 provides a table of equivalent doses for guidance.

Other psychotropic medications

Oestrogen supplements

- Oestrogen deficiency in females is associated with an increased risk of depressive disorders; commonly observed in the perimenopause.
- Oestrogen supplements facilitate the management of depressive disorders at times of relative deficiency.
- Oestradiol is the only ocstrogen that crosses the blood–brain barrier and is therefore effective in the management of disorders that involve brain dysfunction.
- Mechanism of action appears to include modulation of serotonin, dopamine and neurotrophic factor activity in the brain.
- Adverse effects include nausea, increased risk of thromboembolism and enhancement of oestrogen-dependent neoplasia.
- The use of oestrogen in clinical psychiatric practice remains uncertain and routine use in psychiatry has not yet been achieved.

Vitamin D

- Vitamin D blood levels have been found to be significantly low in many patients with mood disorders.
- The use of vitamin D supplements may be helpful as this vitamin is essential for healthy neuronal and glial function.

Box 15.13

Clinical notes on medications for ADD

This is a controversial area because of public concerns about children being given medications (drugs) and the opportunity for abuse (a significant social reality). Their use should be restricted to specialists and carefully considered.

- However, there is currently insufficient evidence to confidently confirm the value of these supplements.

Omega-3 fatty acids

- Eicosapentaenoic acid (EPA) and docosahexaenoic acid (DHA), along with α-linolenic acid are essential unsaturated fatty acids in humans.
- These are vital for healthy cell membrane formation; EPA and DHA most notably.
- Deficiency of EPA and DHA is detrimental to cell membrane function and may be significant in a variety of psychological disorders, including schizophrenia and mood disorders.
- The value of supplements is uncertain, but there is increasing evidence to support their use in these disorders and in patients considered 'at risk' of these disorders.
- The most appropriate dose is probably about 3000 mg of omega-3 fatty acids daily.
- The risk of bleeding is enhanced by omega-3 fatty acid supplements.

Attention deficit disorders (ADD)

The following are used mostly for attention deficit disorders, but also for certain forms of brain injury and depressive disorders (see Table 15.12). They act to enhance dopamine, noradrenaline, serotonin and glutamate release in the prefrontal region, with benefits for regulation of attention and concentration.

Other stimulants

Modafinil is a stimulant which does not appear to operate through amine pathways, but the precise mechanism is unknown. Modulation of anterior hypothalamic nuclei may be relevant. Table 15.13 provides clinical information.

Table 15.12

Medications for ADD

Drug	Dose range	Comments
Dexamphetamine	5 to 30 mg	Improve attention and concentration in ADD Insomnia and reduced appetite common unwanted side effects Addictive but not usually a problem in ADD (correctly diagnosed) A slow release mix of amphetamine salts is available in other countries and from some formulating pharmacies in Australia.
Methylphenidate	10 to 30 mg	Similar to dexamphetamine Available in sustained release preparation.
Atomoxetine	10 to 120 mg	Not addictive and suitable for some patients.

Table 15.13
Modafanil

Drug	Dose range	Comments
Modafanil	100 to 400 mg	May have value in some patients with severe lethargy, apathy or abulia; non-addictive, expensive but well tolerated.

Box 15.14
Risks of pharmacological treatment during pregnancy and lactation

- Teratogenesis.
- Abortion.
- Growth retardation.
- Intra-uterine foetal death.
- Low birth weight.
- Baby developing rash after delivery.
- Baby developing delirium after delivery.
- Withdrawal symptoms including restlessness and poor feeding after birth.
- Pulmonary hypertension after birth.
- Hypotonia ('floppy-baby' syndrome).
- Baby suffering sedation or irritability after birth and with breast feeding.

Pregnancy and breast feeding

General comments

- Always seek specialist advice before prescribing a psychotropic medication to a pregnant or breast-feeding woman.
- Between 2 and 4% of all live births have some form of congenital deformity, across populations and cultures.
- *No psychotropic medication can be guaranteed safe in pregnancy or during lactation, but relative risks can be defined to some degree* (see Box 15.14). The fundamental principle is to carefully balance the risks of the patient's illness against the known risks of the treatment. However, excessive concern over adverse effects upon the foetus can sometimes leave mother and baby at significant risk and the decision about medication should be made carefully. Specialist assistance may be particularly useful.
- All psychotropic medications cross into breast milk, but the concentrations are less than 10% of those in the maternal blood. This means that the risks to the infant are very small. Lithium carries a greater risk because of the possibilities of lithium toxicity and damage to the infant's thyroid gland, but this is also very small.

- Sometimes mixed formula and breast-feeding, or expressing breast milk during 'troughs' in medication levels for use later can be helpful, particularly in premature infants.

Antidepressants during pregnancy and lactation

- Tricyclic antidepressants: the length of exposure to pregnant women without evidence of adverse effects *suggests* that these are relatively safe in pregnancy.
- Sertraline, fluvoxamine, citalopram/escitalopram appear to be largely safe in pregnancy, but neonatal hypoglycaemia may occur.
- Paroxetine *may* be associated with an increase in heart defects and is best avoided.
- SSRIs and particularly venlafaxine/desmethylvenlafaxine <u>can</u> be associated with pulmonary hypertension and discontinuation symptoms after birth. The dose should be progressively reduced before labour begins and can be increased again after delivery.
- Duloxetine: little is known about its safety in pregnancy, but there are no adverse reports at this time.
- Mirtazapine and mianserin *appear* relatively safe and there is no evidence to suggest that reboxetine has significant problems in pregnancy.
- Mirtazapine is also used for control of severe vomiting in early pregnancy, using doses of 7.5 mg to 30 mg daily.
- Bupropion *appears* relatively safe in pregnancy.
- There is some evidence that use of paroxetine and fluoxetine during pregnancy may be associated with a risk of cardiac malformations.

Anxiolytics during pregnancy and lactation

- There is some evidence that benzodiazepines may promote cleft palate deformity when used in the first trimester of pregnancy. The extent of this risk remains uncertain.

Antipsychotics during pregnancy and lactation

- Quetiapine has the advantage of significantly lower transmission across the placenta (greater binding to Pgp than other antipsychotics); risperidone and paliperidone appear next most advantageous, and olanzapine next.
- Most other current antipsychotic medications appear relatively safe in pregnancy.
- Metabolic complications, such as increased risk of gestational diabetes mellitus and weight gain, need to be considered.
- There is some limited evidence to suggest that aripiprazole and asenapine are better avoided in pregnancy.

Mood stabilisers during pregnancy and lactation

- Lithium can be uncommonly associated with major deformities of the heart and great vessels, and can also provoke hypotonia ('floppy-baby' syndrome) soon after delivery, from lithium toxicity in the infant. Damage to the thyroid gland of the foetus may occur, but is rare.

- Carbamazepine and valproate are both associated with serious neural tube defects, as well as other deformities in facial bone development. *They should be avoided in pregnancy if at all possible.* Folic acid supplements (5 mg daily) during pregnancy help to reduce these risks but are not fully effective.
- Lamotrigine may increase the risk of deformities if used during pregnancy but the risk appears small. Folic acid supplements (5 mg daily) during pregnancy help to reduce these risks.

Adjunctive medications and exercise

- Omega-3 fatty acids: there is increasing evidence that supplements containing these fatty acids (e.g. fish oil capsules) may be beneficial in major mood disorders. At least 3000 mg daily are required.
- Vitamin D: supplements of 5000 units per day may be helpful in patients with vitamin D deficiency, which appears common in major mood disorders.
- N-acetyl cysteine: this amino acid is converted to glutathione, an important antioxidant in the brain, and may enhance the long-term mental state of patients with bipolar disorders and schizophrenia. The recommended dose is 1000 mg twice daily.
- Exercise: regular cardio pulmonary and strength exercises are highly advantageous to patients with psychological disorders of all kinds and particularly valuable in depressive, bipolar and anxiety disorders.
- Folic acid: deficiency is destructive to mental state and supplements are essential if deficiency is evident.
- Magnesium and zinc: deficiency can be deleterious to mental state and supplements may be appropriate.

Physical treatments

Electroconvulsive therapy (ECT)

The nature of ECT

- Inducing a generalised seizure has a powerful therapeutic effect upon severe depressive disorders, but not all such seizures are therapeutic.
- A seizure is induced by passing an electric current through the frontal lobes, using a pulsed square wave form.
- A seizure is necessary but not sufficient to have a therapeutic effect. The extent to which the electrical charge exceeds the threshold for inducing a seizure, specific electrical features of seizure, and to some extent transient post-ictal blood pressure and heart rate increases (reflecting increased sympathetic activity), are useful guides to the likely efficacy of treatment.
- The treatment is given under a general anaesthetic to allow muscle relaxation and therefore reduced risk of musculoskeletal injury.
- The electrical stimulus is given either to both sides of the head (bilateral) or one side (unilateral). Unilateral placement reduces cognitive impairment significantly.
- A treatment course will usually require from 6 to 12 treatments to be effective.

Mechanisms of action of ECT (probably a combination)

- Anticonvulsant effect of ECT.
- Restoration of physiological frontolimbic interaction with reduced limbic activity and enhanced prefrontal activity.
- Increased and potent release of nerve growth factors (similar to antidepressants).
- Increased release of serotonin, noradrenaline, dopamine and prefrontal glutamate (similar to antidepressants).
- Hormonal changes including reduction in corticotrophin releasing hormone release.

Indications for use of ECT

- Severe melancholic depressive disorder; particularly with psychosis and/or catatonia. Improvement is almost always impressive, particularly with catatonia.
- Severe depression during pregnancy (relatively safer than medications) and puerperium (where a high risk of injury to mother and infant is present).
- Severe depression in the elderly (response is usually excellent).
- Mania.
- Schizophrenia with comorbid severe depression.
- Some neurological disorders.
- ECT remains the most potent and reliable treatment for severe melancholia and psychotic depression.

Contraindications

- Raised intracranial pressure is a total contraindication.
- Recent cerebrovascular accident (< 6 weeks).
- Anaesthetic risks as for any procedure.
- Severe cardiovascular disease; including within 10 days of a myocardial infarction.
- Other major medical disorders that might complicate treatment or recovery.

Adverse effects

- Cognitive impairment, notably memory dysfunction; mostly reversible except for events within days of the treatment.
- Cognitive impairment can be both retrograde and anterograde.
- Cognitive impairment is reduced by:
  - using unilateral electrode placement (over the non-dominant hemisphere)
  - using a pulsed square wave stimulus
  - using a pulse width of 0.3 to 0.5 msec
  - spacing treatments in time
  - giving good education to the patient about the nature and effects of the treatment.
- Cognitive impairment is aggravated by concurrent use of lithium or MAOIs.
- Persistent cognitive impairment has been reported as a rare phenomenon and appears related to multiple factors.

- Musculoskeletal injury from movement during the seizures.
- Transient cardiac dysrhythmias (mostly harmless unless accompanied by pre-existing cardiac pathology).
- Persistent seizures – relieved by intravenous anticonvulsants such as diazepam.
- Headache – common early in treatment and relieved by analgesics.
- Mania – easily relieved by further treatments or medications.
- Structural brain injury does *not* occur, despite many claims to the contrary.

Future developments

Magnetic stimulation therapy

This uses a pulsating magnetic field to provoke seizures and may offer equal efficacy with much less cognitive impairment than ECT.

Light therapy

Exposure to bright light each morning can relieve depression in disrupted circadian rhythms or seasonal affective disorder.

Transcranial magnetic stimulation

A treatment which uses pulses of magnetic field over the dorsolateral prefrontal cortex to relieve depressive disorders. There is no seizure and the patient remains conscious and comfortable, except for occasional local soreness early in treatment.

Table 15.14

Drugs metabolised by cytochrome P450 isoenzymes

CYP1A2	CYP2C9	CYP2C19	CYP2D6	CYP2E1
CNS	**CNS**	**CNS**	**CNS**	**CNS**
Agomelatine	Amitriptyline	Amitriptyline	Agomelatine	Clozapine
Amitriptyline	Imipramine	Barbiturates	Amitriptyline	Venlafaxine
Asenapine	Mirtazapine	Citalopram	Amphetamine	
Chlorpromazine	Phenytoin	Clomipramine	Chlorpromazine	**Other**
Clomipramine	Quetiapine	Diazepam	Clomipramine	Caffeine
Clozapine		Imipramine	Clozapine	Dapsone
Desipramine	**Cardiovascular**	Methyl-	Desipramine	Dextromethorphan
Diazepam	Fluvastatin	phenobarbitone	Donepezil	Enflurane
Fluvoxamine	Irbesartan	Moclobemide	Doxepin	Ethanol
Haloperidol	Losartan	Olanzapine	Duloxetine	Halothane
Imipramine		Phenytoin	Fluoxetine	Isoflurane
Mirtazapine	**Other**	Sodium valproate	Fluphenazine	Isoniazid
Nortriptyline	Celecoxib	Topiramate	Haloperidol	Methoxyflurane
Olanzapine	Dapsone		Imipramine	Ondansetron
Phenothiazine	Diclofenac	**Cardiovascular**	Mianserin	Paracetamol
Pimozide	Flubiprofen	Propanolol	Mirtazapine	Phenol
Tacrine	Glimepiride		Nortriptyline	Ritonavir
Thioridazine	Ibuprofen	**Other**	Olanzapine	Sevoflurane
Thiothixene	Indomethacin	Apomorphine	Paroxetine	Tamoxifen
Trifluoperazine	Mefenamic Acid	Lansoprazole	Quetiapine	Theophylline
Zopiclone	Metronidazole	Omeprazole	Risperidone	
	Montelukast	Pantoprazole	Selegiline	
Cardiovascular	Naproxen	Pentamidine	Sertraline	
Propanolol	Piroxicam	Proguanil	Thioridazine	
Verapamil	Ritonavir	Ritonavir	Tiagabine	
	Rosiglitazone	Tolbutamide	Trimipramine	
Other	Sildenafil Citrate	Warfarin	Venlafaxine	
Aminophylline	Tenoxicam			
Apomorphine	Tetrahydrocannabinol		**Cardiovascular**	
Betaxolol	Tolbutamide		Captopril	
Caffeine	Warfarin		Carvedilol	
Methadone	Zufirlukast		Flecainide	

Continued

Table 15.14

Drugs metabolised by cytochrome P450 isoenzymes—cont'd

CYP1A2	CYP2C9	CYP2C19	CYP2D6	CYP2E1
Metoclopramide			Labetatol	
Oestradiol			Metroprolol	
Ondansetron			Mexiletine	
Paracetamol			Perhexiline	
Ritonavir			Pindolol	
Ropivacaine			Propanolol	
Tamoxifen			Timolol	
Theophylline				
Warfarin			**Other**	
			Betaxolol	
			Chlorpheniramine	
			Codeine	
			Cyclophosphamide	
			Delavirdine	
			Dextromethorphan	
			Dihydrocodeine	
			Diphenhydramine	
			Dolasetron	
			Hydrocortisone	
			Loratadine	
			Methadone	
			Metoclopramide	
			Morphine	
			Ondansetron	
			Orphenadrine	
			Oxycodone	
			Papaverine	
			Pentazocine	
			Pethidine	
			Promethazine	
			Ritonavir	
			Ropivicaine	
			Tamoxifen	
			Tramadol	
			Tropisetron	
			Yohimbine	

Continued

Table 15.14

Drugs metabolised by cytochrome P450 isoenzymes—cont'd

CYP3A3/4	CYP3A3/4	CYP3A3/4	CYP3A3/4
CNS	Cerivastatin	Cyclosporin	Ondansetron
Alprazolam	Diltiazem	Dapsone	Oral contraceptives
Amitriptyline	Disopyramide	Delavirdine	Orphenadrine
Bromazepam	Enalapril	Dexamethasone	Paclitaxel
Bupropion	Felodipine	Dextromethorphan	Pantoprazole
Buspirone	Granisetron	Docetaxel	Paracetamol
Carbamazepine	Lignocaine	Dolasetron	Prednisone
Chlorpromazine	Losartan	Doxorubicin	Progesterone
Citalopram	Nifedipine	Doxycycline	Proguanil
Clomipramine	Nimodipine	Duloxetine	Quercetin
Clonazepam	Pravastatin	Erythromycin	Quinine
Clozapine	Quinidine	Etinyloestradiol	Repaglinide
Diazepam	Simvastatin	Etoposide	Rifampicin
Donepezil	Verapamil	Fentanyl	Ritonavir
Ethosuxamide		Fexofenadine	Salmeterol
Fluoxetine	**Other**	Finasteride	Saquinavir
Haloperidol	Alfentanil	Flutamide	Sildenafil citrate
Imipramine	Anastrazole	Glibenclamide	Tacrolimus
Midazolam	Apomorphine	Hydrocortisone	Tamoxifen
Mirtazapine	Astemizole	Ifosfamide	Teniposide
Nefazodone	Bromocriptine	Indinavir	Terfenadine
Pimozide	Budesonide	Itraconazole	Testosterone
Quetiapine	Busulfan	Ketoconazole	Tetrahydrocannabinol
Risperidone	Caffeine	Lansoprazole	Theophylline
Sertraline	Cannabinoids	Letrozole	Toremifene
Temazepam	Cimetidine	Loratadine	Tretinoin
Tiagabine	Cisapride	Methadone	Vinblastine
Triazolam	Clarithromycin	Miconazole	Vincristine
Venlafaxine	Clindamycin	Montelukast	Warfarin
	Cocaine	Navelbine	Yohimbine
Cardiovascular	Codeine	Nalfinavir	
Amiodarone	Cortisol	Nevirapine	
Amlodipine	Cortisone	Oestradiol	
Atorvastatin	Cyclophosphamide	Omeprazole	

Table 15.15

Inducers or inhibitors of the cytochrome P450 isoenzymes

CYP1A2	CYP2C9	CYP2C19	CYP2D6	CYP2E1	CYP3A3/4
Inducers	**Inducers**	**Inducers**	**Inhibitors**	**Inducers**	**Inducers**
Carbamazepine	Carbamazepine	Carbamazepine	Amiodarone	Ethanol	Carbamazepine
Charbroiled foods	Fluconazole	Phenobarbitone	Celecoxib	Isoniazid	Dexamethasone
Cigarette smoke	Phenobarbitone	Phenytoin	Chloroquine		Glutocorticoids
Cruciferous	Phenytoin	Rifampicin	Chlorpromazine	**Inhibitors**	Griseofulvin
vegetables (e.g.	Rifampicin		Cimetidine	Disulfiram	Nelfinavir
cabbage, brussels		**Inhibitors**	Clomipramine	Entacapone	Neviapine
sprouts, broccoli,	**Inhibitors**	Cimetidine	Codeine	(high dose)	Phenobarbitone
cauliflower)	Amiodarone	Entacapone (high	Delavirdine	Ritonavir	Phenytoin
Nicotine	Anastrozole	dose)	Desipramine		Primidone
Omeprazole	Chloramphenicol	Fluconazole	Dextropropoxyphene		Progesterone
Phenobarbitone	Cimetidine	Isoniazid	Diltiazem		Rifabutin
Phenytoin	Diclofenac	Ketoconazole	Doxorubicin		Rifampicin
Primidone	Disulfiram	(weak)	Entacapone (high		Rofecoxib (mild)
Rifampicin	Entacapone (high	Letrozole	dose)		St John's Wort
Ritonavir	dose)	Omeprazole	Fluphenazine		Sulfinpyrazone
	Flurbiprofen	Proguanil	Haloperidol		
Inhibitors	Fluvastatin	Ritonavir	Labetalol		**Inhibitors**
Anastrozole	Isoniazid	Teniposide	Lomustine		Amiodarone
Cimetidine	Ketocazole (weak)	Tolbutamide	Methadone		Anastrozole
Ciprofloxacin	Ketoprofen	Topiramade	Moclobemide		Azithromycin
Clarithromycin	Metronidazole	Tranylcypromine	Quinidine		Cannabinoids
Diltiazem	Omeprazole		Ranitidine		Cimetidine
Enoxacin	Ritonavir		Risperidone (weak)		Clarithromycin
Entacapone (high	Sodium valproate		Ritonavir		Clotrimazole
dose)	Sulfamethoxazole		Sodium valproate		Cyclosoprin
Erythromycin	Sulfinpyrazone		Thioridazine		Danazol
Ethynyl oestradiol	Sulfonamides		Venlafaxine (weak)		Delavirdine
Grapefruit juice	Trimethoprim		Vinblastine		Dexamethasone
Isoniazid	Warfarin		Vincristine		Diltiazem
	Zafirlukast		Yohimbine		Disulfiram

Continued

Table 15.15

Inducers or inhibitors of the cytochrome P450 isoenzymes—cont'd

CYP1A2	CYP2C9	CYP2C19	CYP2D6	CYP2E1	CYP3A3/4
Ketoconazole					Entacapone
Mexiletine					(high dose)
Norfloxacin					Erythromycin
Ritonavir					Ethynyl
Tacrine					oestradiol
Tertiary TCAs					Fluconazole
					(weak)
					Gestodene
					Grapefruit juice
					Haloperidol
					Indinavir
					Isoniazid
					Itraconazole
					Ketoconazole
					Metronidazole
					Miconazole
					Nefazadone
					Nelfinavir
					Nevirapine
					Omeprazole
					(weak)
					Propoxyphene
					Quinidine
					Quinine
					Ranitidine
					Ritonavir
					Saquinavir
					Sodium
					valproate
					Verapamil
					Zafirlukast

REFERENCES AND FURTHER READING

Aszalos, A., 2007. Drug–drug interactions affected by the transporter protein, P-glycoprotein (ABCB1, MDR1) II. Clinical Aspects Drug Discovery Today 12 (19/20).

Castle, D., Copolov, D., Wykes, T., Mueser, K., 2008. Pharmacological and psychosocial treatments in schizophrenia. Informa UK, London.

Maxmen, J.S., Kennedy, S.H., McIntyre, 2008. Psychotropic drugs fast facts. Norton and Co., New York.

Menon, S., 2008. Psychotropic medication during pregnancy and lactation. Archives of Gynaecology and Obstetrics 277 (1), 1–13.

Rosenbaum, J., Arana, G., Hyman, S., et al., 2005. Handbook of psychiatric drug therapy. Lippincott Williams and Wilkins, Philadelphia.

Schatzberg, A., Nemeroff, C., 2010. Essentials of clinical psychopharmacology. American Psychiatric Publishing, Washington.

Semkovska, M., McLoughlin, D., 2010. Objective cognitive performance associated with electroconvulsive therapy for depression: A systematic review and meta-analysis. Biological Psychiatry 68, 568–577.

Shiloh, R., Strjer, R., Weizman, A., Nutt, D., 2006. Essentials in clinical psychiatric pharmacotherapy. Taylor and Francis, London.

Stahl, S., 2008. Essential psychopharmacology. The prescriber's guide. Cambridge University Press, Cambridge.

Taylor, D., Paton, C., Kapur, S., 2009. The Maudsley prescribing guidelines. Informa Healthcare, London.

Tiller, J., Lyndon, R. (Eds.), 2003. Electroconvulsive therapy. An Australasian guide. Australian Postgraduate Medicine, Fitzroy.

Weiner, R., Fink, M., Hammersley, D., et al., 1990. The practice of electroconvulsive therapy: Recommendations for treatment, training and privileging task force. Report of American Psychiatric Association. American Psychiatric Association, Washington.

Wiznen, P., Op Den Buijsch, R., Drent, M., et al., 2007. Review article: the prevalence and clinical relevance of cytochrome P450 polymorphisms. Alimentary Pharmacology and Therapeutics 26 (Suppl 2), 211–219.

CHAPTER 15

A STORE MANAGER NAMED NEAL
CASE-BASED LEARNING

JOEL KING & ANDREW GLEASON

The following role-play requires two participants: one to play the GP registrar (candidate) and another to play the roles of the patient named Neal Darling and the examiner (actor).

OSCE Station Instructions

(Reading time: 2 minutes)

You are a GP registrar working in a metropolitan practice. You are asked to see Mr Neal Darling. Mr Darling is a 35-year-old who has a well-established diagnosis of bipolar I disorder, which is normally well-controlled with medication. He is concerned about increasing diarrhoea, nausea, and tremor.

Task (10 minutes)
- Please interview Mr Darling to establish the most likely reason(s) for his presenting problem. After 8 minutes you will be asked FOUR questions by the examiner.

Actor role: Neal Darling

You are Neal, a 35-year-old who lives in the suburbs. You bought your house five years ago. You work as a store manager of an office supply store. You have been employed there most of your adult life, starting as a shelving assistant at age 19, and working your way up. You manage a team of ten employees and are well-liked. You find your work satisfying and have no intentions of moving. You have a wide circle of friends and play golf on Saturdays with your best friend, Bill.

You are happily married to Elise (30 years old), whom you met at age 22. You have no children. You have bipolar I disorder, which was diagnosed at age 25. This is well-controlled on lithium.

You have come to your GP today because you have been experiencing nausea and vomiting, diarrhoea, dizziness, and tremor. These symptoms started three days ago and have been getting worse.

RECENT CHANGES TO OTHER MEDICATIONS IN THE LAST TWO WEEKS

Five days ago, you were helping your employees with a heavy box and sprained your lower back. When you came home, your wife saw you wincing in pain when you were trying to undo your shoelaces. She gave you a box of diclofenac and you have been taking three 50 mg tablets per day for the last five days.

If you are asked about whether you have any other medical conditions, state that you have high blood pressure and take a medication to lower this, called perindopril. Two weeks ago, your GP noted that your blood pressure was still raised and increased your dose from 5 mg to 10 mg daily. Other than the lithium, you take no other medications regularly.

FEATURES RELATING TO THE LAST THREE DAYS

If you are asked about the nausea, tell the candidate that this started three days ago and has been gradually getting worse. You have never had nausea like this. You have vomited twice in the last two days, expelling the contents of your last meal. There is no indication of blood or coffee grounds in your vomit. Your appetite has decreased considerably. You have not been travelling recently.

If asked about your bowel habit/motions or diarrhoea, tell the candidate that you have been having worsening diarrhoea over the last three days. You have no abdominal pain. It is more runny and more frequent. Yesterday, you opened your bowels five times. Your normal routine is once a day, in the morning. There is no blood, pus, mucus, or change in your stool colour. You have no abdominal pain. You have never had an episode like this before.

If asked about the tremor, tell the candidate, 'This is really weird because I've never had it before. It just started three days ago around the same time as my diarrhoea. It is getting worse. Both of your hands are affected. It's there all the time. Nothing seems to make it better or worse. It's difficult to hold a pen or do up buttons because your hands shake.' You are fatigued, your muscles feel weak and you have a few twitches in your arms. You feel a bit dizzy and unsteady on your feet.

OTHER NEUROLOGICAL SYMPTOMS IN THE LAST THREE DAYS

You may be asked about other neurological symptoms in the last three days. If asked about dizziness, state, 'Yeah, now that you mention it, I've been feeling dizzy over the last three days. That's also getting worse.' Deny headaches, trauma to the head, falling over, loss of consciousness, tingling sensations, numbness, and seizures. You have not experienced palpitations, changes in your pulse, changes in your breathing, or feelings of loss of control or impending doom.

IMPACT OF CURRENT SYMPTOMS ON YOUR PSYCHOSOCIAL FUNCTION

In the last three days, as the symptoms have become worse, you have been unable to go to work, due to the feeling of nausea and diarrhoea. The tremor has made it difficult to hold a pen, use the computer, and cook dinner with your wife. The diarrhoea and nausea keep you up at night and you have averaged four hours of sleep per night over the last three days.

Your wife, Elise, is very worried about you and has never seen you like this before. She has encouraged you to go to the GP practice.

PAST HISTORY OF BIPOLAR DISORDER

If asked about your bipolar disorder in general, say, 'My bipolar disorder has been very good and well-controlled. I last saw my psychiatrist, Professor Chamberlain, two weeks ago and he was happy with my progress. He stated that my lithium levels were good and that I should stay on 750 mg daily.'

If asked about Professor Chamberlain, state, 'I first met him when I was admitted to that private psychiatric hospital ten years ago and he's been my psychiatrist ever since. I see him in his rooms every month.'

If asked about the lithium level, state, 'Professor Chamberlain said it was 0.7 when I saw him two weeks ago. I get it checked every four to six months.'

If asked about the lithium dose, state, 'I've been taking 750 mg at night for the last year now. It's been pretty good.' You have perfect compliance with lithium because you and your wife are worried that if you miss a dose, you could become unwell and end up in hospital again.

If asked about previous adverse effects to lithium, state, 'I was pretty tired when I first got put on it, and this happens when the dose increases, but I get used to it over the next few days.' Previously, you have never had tremor, incoordination, nausea, vomiting, diarrhoea, arm and leg weakness, or changes in consciousness.

If asked about any admissions into hospital for bipolar disorder, state, 'I've been only admitted once. That was when I was 25. I wasn't sleeping for three weeks and thought I was a genius. My family got me into a private psychiatric hospital. That's where I met Professor Chamberlain, who has been my psychiatrist for ten years. He diagnosed me with a manic episode, which was part of bipolar disorder. He put me on lithium and I got better over the next month. I got discharged and have never been back to hospital.'

If asked about past manic episodes, state, 'Only the one when I was 25 and got hospitalised.' If asked about past hypomanic episodes, state: 'No. I haven't had those.'

If asked about past depressive episodes, state, 'I seem to get really depressed every three years. There doesn't seem to be a reason. My mood plummets, I get tired easily, I can't focus at work, I get irritable with my wife, and I don't enjoy playing golf. My appetite suffers. I've never been suicidal though. When this happens, I go see Professor Chamberlain, who usually increases my lithium for a little while until the depression goes, which is usually a few weeks. Then he slowly brings it back down. My last depressive episode was two years ago.'

If asked about other medications for bipolar disorder, state: 'No, just the lithium. Professor Chamberlain has mentioned others but I'd rather stick with lithium because it works for me.' If asked about ECT, state, 'No, I've never had that.'

If asked about psychological treatments, state, 'I see Professor Chamberlain every month and we usually have a fairly long chat. He sees me more frequently when I get depressed. Other than that, I haven't had any other psychotherapy. Is that what you're asking?'

If asked about your thyroid and kidney/renal function or blood tests that involve electrolytes, urea or creatinine, state, 'I get that checked here at this practice every six months. My GP checked it three months ago and said it was fine.'

CURRENT FEATURES OF BIPOLAR DISORDER

You have no current symptoms of mania, depression or psychosis.

FEATURES RELATING TO RISK

If asked about suicidal thoughts or thoughts of self-harm or harming others, state, 'No. I've never had those kinds of thoughts.'

DRUG AND ALCOHOL USE

If asked about alcohol use, say, 'I haven't had a drink since I was hospitalised ten years ago. Professor Chamberlain says that alcohol doesn't go well with lithium, so I avoid alcohol altogether.' If asked about other substance use, say, 'No, I've never taken any drugs'.

TIME COURSE OF SYMPTOMS

If asked when your current symptoms began, say, 'About three days ago'. If asked, you have never had an episode like this before. If asked about stressors, state, 'No, life's been pretty good. There have been no changes at home or work.'

OTHER MEDICAL HISTORY QUESTIONS

If asked about any medical conditions, state, 'Just high blood pressure.' The only regular medication you take is lithium carbonate 750 mg at night and perindopril, which was increased from 5 mg to 10 mg daily two weeks ago. You have never had surgery.

FAMILY HISTORY

You do not have a family history of medical or psychiatric disorders. Both your parents are alive and in their late seventies. They are in good health and do not require any community supports. You have a sister, Betty, who is a 30-year-old teacher and has no medical or psychiatric disorders.

FORENSIC HISTORY

You have never had any problems with the law.

HOW TO PLAY THE ROLE

You are polite to the candidate. You should look well-groomed. You have a noticeable coarse hand tremor in both hands. You are clearly not comfortable. You should answer any of the candidate's questions when asked.

Statements you must make:
If asked to talk about why you have come to the clinic today, state:

• 'I'm really glad you have time to see me.'

• 'I don't know what's going on.'

• 'I've been feeling really nauseous and have diarrhoea.'

• 'Also, I have this tremor.'

EXAMINER'S QUESTIONS

Ask the following four questions:

1 What is the most likely diagnosis?

2 List the two most likely precipitating factors to lithium toxicity in Mr Darling's case.

3 Please explain how diclofenac and perindopril contributed to lithium toxicity.

4 Lithium has a narrow therapeutic index. What does this mean?

Model Answer

There are three major tasks in this station: recognition of lithium toxicity, identification of causative factors to lithium toxicity, and the establishment of bipolar disorder in remission.

Students should ask about the symptoms of nausea, diarrhoea and tremor, particularly the nature, the duration, any precipitating or relieving factors, the severity and psychosocial impact, and any prior episodes. Better students may ask about other symptoms of lithium toxicity, including dizziness, changes in consciousness, thirst or polydipsia, muscle twitches and changes in speech (pages 241–242 of this chapter).

Students should recognise that these symptoms have all come on gradually over the last three days, following recent medication changes with an increase in perindopril and the addition of diclofenac. Students should explore the possibility of changes to lithium dosage specifically, ask about the most recent lithium level (which is normal in this case), and any previous adverse effects to lithium. Pre-existing renal disease is a predisposing risk factor for lithium toxicity.

The good student will also screen for manic or depressive symptoms, to ensure that the patient's bipolar disorder remains in remission (see Chapter 9).

In summary, the answers to the four questions at the end of this station are:

Answer 1: Lithium toxicity.

Answer 2: Addition of diclofenac, an NSAID, and increase in perindopril, an ACE inhibitor.

Answer 3: Lithium is renally cleared. Both NSAIDs and ACE inhibitors impair renal clearance.

Answer 4: The therapeutic blood level range is very close to the blood level range for toxicity.

Chapter 16

THE PSYCHOTHERAPIES

DARRYL BASSETT & DAVID J CASTLE

Psychotherapy is a broad term that encompasses everything from support of the individual through a time of personal turmoil, to daily psychoanalysis conducted over years. Indeed, the term is probably so broad that it has lost its usefulness, and requires a descriptor to specify what is meant. Box 16.1 outlines the major types of psychotherapy.

Common features of psychotherapies

All psychotherapies contain a number of common elements that are fundamental to their efficacy. Jerome Frank summarised these as:

- an intense, emotionally charged, confiding relationship with a helping person
- a rationale or myth that has face validity for the patient
- the provision of new information concerning the nature and the causes of a person's problems, and alternative ways of dealing with them
- strengthening the patient's expectations of help through the personal qualities of the therapist and his/her cultural recognition in this role
- the provision of success experiences that enhance hope, sense of mastery, interpersonal competence or sense of capability
- the facilitation of emotional arousal.

Box 16.1
Types of psychotherapy

- Supportive psychotherapy.
- Psychoeducation.
- Behavioural therapy.
- Cognitive therapy.
- Cognitive-behaviour therapy.
- Interpersonal psychotherapy.
- Interpersonal and social rhythms therapy.
- Family therapy and family-focused therapy.
- Dialectical behaviour therapy.
- Brief psychodynamic psychotherapy.
- Long-term psychodynamic psychotherapy (e.g. psychoanalysis).

Other important but more variable, commonly included elements are:
- reinforcement of desired behaviours and discouragement of undesired behaviours (operant conditioning)
- conscious examination of links in current thoughts and emotions to meaningful past experiences (prominent in psychodynamic therapies and cognitive therapies)
- exploration of family systems and interpersonal relationships (prominent in family therapy, family-focused therapy and interpersonal therapy).

Supportive psychotherapy

This term is applied to the most basic form of psychotherapy, which should comprise part of any therapeutic relationship. Arguably, other more specific forms of psychotherapy build onto a supportive framework.

Supportive psychotherapy entails:
- the provision of a supportive, caring and listening environment for the patient
- giving the patient an opportunity to ventilate their feelings (*catharsis*)
- discussion of the patient's strengths, vulnerabilities and current life stressors
- enhancement of the patient's coping skills to assist them to deal with life stressors
- the provision of a framework for monitoring clinical progress.

Management of grief

Bereavement and other forms of grief are common and frequently arise in clinical situations, with or without other forms of illness. Helping a person during such difficult times can be very relieving and help to prevent further deterioration into psychological illness. The initial response to grief in a person should be empathy expressed as regret and

Box 16.2

Management of grief and bereavement

- Empathy.
- Identify feelings.
- Practical and emotional assistance with living with the loss.
- Meaning in loss.
- Emotional incorporation of the loss.
- Time to grieve.
- Information about normal grieving and expectations.
- Explore coping strategies and emotional reactions to grief.
- CBT is helpful when grieving is becoming distorted and can help prevent depressive disorder.
- Identify pathological responses (denial of the loss, symptoms and signs of depressive illness, suicidal thoughts or plans, prolonged grieving, psychosis).
- Treat or refer as appropriate if psychopathology develops.

understanding. Just being with the person (or persons) is very helpful and silence should be tolerated, along with simple caring remarks. A gradual exploration of the person's feelings is helpful, but avoid any pressure to respond or continue if obviously distressed. Time and the supportive presence of a caring person are the most helpful interventions early on in grieving. The provision of assistance with the practical issues and emotional demands of daily living is very helpful (particularly when children are involved). Over time it is constructive to explore the meaning of the loss to the person and use this understanding to build a better understanding of how the loss can be processed. The nature of grieving is a process of incorporation of important elements of the lost person or object (e.g. a house), as a reassuring memory. This is achieved spontaneously in most people but is facilitated by the above process of exploration and empathy, amplified by the use of cognitive and behaviour therapy techniques when the process is not progressing. Allow time for this process and recognise that it is healthy to engage in the grieving process for at least 12 months after the loss. The first 'anniversary' is often very significant to the person as a point of conclusion. During the grief therapy process, information about normal grieving and what is happening will often be very relieving and constructive. Always be mindful of the possible development of psychological illness such as mood disorders, of varying severity and type. Treatment of psychological illness must not be delayed through misinterpretation of symptoms and signs as 'normal grief'. A summary of strategies to assist with grief are outlined in Box 16.2.

Psychoeducation

Broadly, psychoeducation refers to the provision by the therapist of general information to the patient (and their family and significant others, as indicated) regarding the nature of their mental illness and the potential therapeutic interventions available. There is also a more specific component, where the therapist addresses how this general knowledge applies to the particular individual. This process can also be an entry into a discussion about the impact of the illness on significant others, and lead to an understanding about how the patient can monitor their mental state and the specific steps they can take to help themselves get better.

For example, the patient with depression and alcohol abuse can be provided with information about the interaction between these and a discussion begun about how each set of problems can be addressed.

There are many useful resources that can assist in the process of psychoeducation. These include books, pamphlets, videos, DVDs, and myriad websites. It is best for the therapist to review such material before directing the patient to it. Also, some patients try to seek so much information that it becomes confusing and counterproductive. Thus, it is best to have a few good quality resources one can recommend.

Behavioural therapy

Behavioural therapy essentially encompasses techniques where a feared object or situation is faced rather than avoided. This can be done *in vivo* (i.e. in real life), or by imagining situations (i.e. the person summonses the image into their mind): the former is usually preferred, as it is easier to do and seems more powerful. Sometimes the feared situation is such that it is impossible to re-enact in vivo; for example, post-traumatic stress disorder after a horrific fire. In such cases imaginal exposure can be effective.

Behavioural therapy is usually undertaken in a step-wise manner, such that the patient constructs a *hierarchy* of fears and works at each step in an ongoing manner, akin to a runner getting fit according to a stepped exercise regimen. The 'least feared' object or situation is tackled first, consolidated, then the next task on the hierarchy attempted. The therapist acts much like a sports coach, guiding, supporting, encouraging the individual to take the next step, and providing useful tips about how to motivate oneself and overcome the barriers to 'getting fit' again. The actual 'work' has to be performed by the patient, and they need to 'stay with' the anxiety aroused by the situation or feared object until their anxiety abates to a substantial degree. This is done repeatedly until that fear step is conquered, and the next step can be taken. The process is also referred to as *exposure/response prevention (EX/RP)*, in that the patient 'exposes' themself to the feared situation, and does not give in to the urge to perform the usual 'response' (e.g. running away).

It can be useful to help the patient manage their overall anxiety, such that they employ, for example, slow breathing techniques and positive self-talk to help them through the tasks. However, they do need to experience some degree of discomfort and anxiety at each step, otherwise the step is not therapeutically useful. Some people employ techniques such as emotional withdrawal, asking others for reassurance, or resorting to alcohol or benzodiazepines to deal with anxiogenic situations: these can interfere with the therapeutic effect of behavioural therapy.

Case example: Behavioural therapy

A 35-year-old woman had severe agoraphobia and avoided any crowded situations. A major impediment to living her life to the full was her total avoidance of shops: this led to conflict with her husband because he had to do all the family shopping

Continued

Case example continued

and came to resent this. The patient constructed a hierarchy, with the most difficult task being supermarket shopping on a busy Saturday morning by herself. She was encouraged to start with small steps, including going to the local corner store with her husband during a time when no one else was around. Once she had conquered this she was encouraged to return to the store by herself, and then again at busier times of the day. She was also taught how she could reduce her anxiety and attenuate panic attacks through the use of slow breathing techniques. After some months of concerted work she felt able to tackle supermarket shopping: again, she first went with her husband, moving on to going by herself.

Occasionally, instead of a step-wise approach, the patient can be exposed in a single session to their most feared situation: for example, the spider phobic allowing a tarantula to crawl on them. This is known as *flooding*.

Behavioural therapy is also the primary therapeutic modality in obsessive-compulsive disorder. Here the individual 'faces' the fear associated with an obsessional thought, again in a hierarchical manner. For example, the patient who repeatedly checks electrical appliances is tasked with switching the toaster on, then off, and checking just thrice rather than 30 times, and 'stays with' the anxiety this arouses until it subsides. Again this task is repeated until conquered, whereafter the next step is embraced (e.g. check just twice, and then only once). The patient must be reminded not to seek reassurance from others, and their family members should be coached as supportive co-therapists rather than giving in to the reassurance-seeking of the patient, such as, for example, going and checking the toaster for them.

Cognitive therapy

The notion that un-useful cognitions drive depression and anxiety symptoms might seem obvious, but the utility of cognitive challenge in a therapeutic sense gained ascendancy only in the 1960s, with the work of, among others, Aaron T Beck. Beck postulated that people who are prone to depression (his initial focus) tend to see themselves, the world around them, and their future, in a negative way, and that they tend to have *negative automatic thoughts* in response to events in their world. He also identified a number of *thinking traps* that people with depression tend to fall into (see Box 16.3).

Cognitive therapy involves helping individuals identify and challenge negative automatic thoughts. They are also taught to recognise their own thinking traps, and use this knowledge to assist them to face the world in a more positive manner. The patient is encouraged to keep a diary of negative thoughts, including rating to what extent they believe them (usually as a percentage). They then try to challenge these, and then rate whether the intensity of the belief has been eroded, and to what extent. This is done in an iterative way, and therapy sessions include looking over the diaries with the therapist, and working through examples together. A further technique is the so-called *downward arrow*, which seeks to explore the underlying schemas held by the individual.

Box 16.3

Cognitive 'thinking traps'

- *Dichotomous thinking:* Seeing things as 'black-or-white'; all-or-nothing thinking, e.g. 'If I don't come first in the race, then I'm useless at running and might as well just give it up.' 'If I don't do it perfectly, then it will be no good at all.'
- *Overgeneralisation:* Concluding that if one thing goes wrong, then everything is going to go wrong, e.g. 'I didn't answer that interview question very well; I am sure they will think I am a moron and I won't get the job.'
- *Personalisation:* Jumping to an immediate conclusion that an event relates (usually negatively) to oneself, e.g. 'My colleague seemed grumpy in the morning staff meeting: I must have done something to offend him.'
- *Arbitrary inference:* Jumping to conclusions without weighing the evidence, e.g. 'I didn't manage to complete my homework properly; I will never get the hang of this therapy.'
- *Selective attention:* The tendency to 'filter in' only negatives, rather than giving equal weight to all sources, e.g. 'One person rated my lecture badly: I am a useless lecturer.'

Case example: Cognitive therapy

A 41-year-old woman presented with a recurrence of depression. She saw everything in a negative way, and talked about herself in a denigrating manner. Upon reflection, she reported that her childhood was dominated by highly critical and emotionally distant parents, who never saw anything worthwhile in her activities and were constantly finding fault. She had come to perceive herself as worthless and incapable of doing anything productive. The therapist challenged some of her *underlying assumptions*, including her lack of self-worth and her perceptions of incompetence, by encouraging her to identify her avoidance of anything good in herself and the achievements and abilities she has already demonstrated.

Cognitive-behaviour therapy

Cognitive-behaviour therapy (CBT) has become the ubiquitous approach to the management of many mental disorders. It integrates both behavioural and cognitive therapeutic techniques, and has proven to be of benefit for milder forms of depression, and many of the anxiety disorders. It has also been applied to bipolar disorder and to persistent delusions and hallucinations in people with schizophrenia.

Asking what is 'the worst possible' thing that might occur, can help place the patient's fears in some perspective. Helping the patient see themself more objectively can also be facilitated, for example, by asking them to imagine how they might respond to a friend who came to them with a problem similar to their own.

> ## Case example: Cognitive-behaviour therapy
>
> A 20-year-old student sought help because he was socially isolated and feared social situations. He wanted to socialise, but was terrified other people would think he was an 'idiot' and make fun of him. Working with the patient, the therapist set social interaction homework tasks, starting with going out to a restaurant with his sister. Incrementally he was encouraged to place himself in more challenging social situations. The therapist also *modelled* social interaction, taking the patient out for a coffee and encouraging him to go to the counter and order the coffee. The therapist also used cognitive challenge techniques, for example, asking: 'So, if you enter a room of strangers, what do you fear might occur?' 'I might blush.' 'So what if you blush, what does it matter?' 'Other people would think I am weak.' 'So, you are saying that anyone who blushes is weak?' 'Well, no, but that's what most people think when they see someone blushing.' 'And so, if you saw someone blush would you think they were weak and hopeless? Would you judge them negatively and not want anything to do with them?' 'No, I would probably feel sorry for them and try to help them.' 'And why, then, do you think other people will judge *you* negatively if *you* blush?'

Interpersonal psychotherapy

Interpersonal psychotherapy (IPT) has its origins on the one hand in the work of Adolph Meyer and Harry Stack Sullivan, who emphasised the role of *life events* in determining psychopathology; and on the other from John Bowlby's work on *attachment theory*, which emphasises the importance of the innate human drive for attachment, and that disrupted attachment in early life has consequences for later vulnerability to psychiatric problems such as depression. They recognised that early attachment experiences impact on adult relationship patterns, and these can be damaging for the individual and feed psychopathology.

Weissman and Klerman developed these principles into IPT as we know it today, emphasising that mood and life situation are related. It is a 'here and now' therapy, and addresses issues such as grief (e.g. loss events), role transitions (e.g. retirement), role disputes (conflictual relationships), major life change (e.g. migration) and interpersonal deficits (e.g. social isolation) on current psychopathology. The idea is that identification and resolution of interpersonal problems current at the time of onset of symptoms will lead to improved life circumstances and thus improved symptomatology. Initially used for depression, IPT has been modified for use in a range of circumstances including depression associated with HIV, depression in pregnancy and, in conjunction with *social rhythm therapy* (SRT), for bipolar disorder.

Dialectical behaviour therapy

Dialectical behaviour therapy (DBT) is a skills-based therapy that follows CBT principles, but with an emphasis upon acceptance of and by the person of their current maladaptive behaviours, combined with an expectation that these behaviours need to change. This combination creates a 'dialectical tension' (a concept drawn from philosophy) with the expectation of achieving a 'synthesis' that is more adaptive. This therapy was originally designed for the treatment of borderline personality disorder (Cluster B) but has application in other disorders such as eating disorders and other personality disorders.

DBT aims to address four specific goals:

- Reduce self-harming behaviours
- Reduce therapy sabotaging behaviours
- Reduce 'quality of life' self-sabotaging behaviours
- Develop constructive coping skills.

DBT encompasses *group therapy* aimed at developing 'core mindfulness skills' by increasing awareness of events, emotions and behaviours; and adopting a focused but non-judgemental attitude to these. The patient is also helped to develop 'interpersonal effectiveness skills' to enable effective communication and to manage conflict more constructively; 'emotional regulation skills' through increased understanding of emotions and strategies for emotional regulation; and 'distress tolerance skills' through accepting life for the moment and tolerating momentary distress.

Individual therapy is provided parallel to the group process, and aims to reinforce group therapy derived skills and awareness, with greater focus upon individual needs. Inter-session *telephone contact* is agreed upon as a strategy for contact between therapy sessions and needs to be established with clear but strict boundaries. The contact focuses upon crisis intervention and the application of the above skills to coping 'in the moment'. The patient is encouraged to tolerate the distress and to address this further in the next available therapy session.

Case example: Dialectical behaviour therapy

A 37-year-old married man presented with a history of a recurrent pattern at times of stress that included self-injury (burning his skin with cigarettes), self-disgust, explosive rage, derogatory and command auditory hallucinations (which were difficult to distinguish from prominent thoughts), and homicidal as well as suicidal thoughts. These episodes were highly distressing to his wife and on occasion he would leave home and stay on the farm of a relative to allow recovery from his distress and maladaptive behaviours. He exhibited strong motivation to change and considerable insight into his behaviour. However, he felt powerless to change. An important element of his history appeared to be violent sexual abuse as a child and the most potent life stresses appeared to relate to times of perceived loss of control, such as challenging times in his business.

He began DBT and found the group therapy plus homework self-monitoring particularly helpful. He felt understood and began to address the therapy approach with enthusiasm. Individual psychotherapy was more challenging as the intensity of emotion could be considerable at times and he appreciated having access to help between sessions. Over time he established better mood regulation, improved stress management and more effective communication of his needs with others. His therapy is still in progress and there have continued to be times when brief admissions to hospital at times of crisis have been required. However, the intensity of his symptoms and the severity of self-harm, as well as rage, have improved.

Box 16.4

Freud and the post-Freudians

Sigmund Freud: maintained that distortions in psychosexual development could be addressed by developing conscious awareness of their nature with the help of a therapist who repeatedly identified those distortions; the relationship with the therapist came to reflect the early powerful relationships of early childhood development (called *transference*) and this intensified the therapeutic experience.

Carl Jung: de-emphasised Freud's concentration on sexuality; introduced the notion of the *collective unconscious*, and explored dreams, myths and symbols.

Melanie Klein: concentrated attention on young children; used play techniques; postulated depressive and schizoid positions as a consequence of not negotiating certain early life hurdles adequately.

Erik Erikson: expanded Freud's concepts to a whole-of life series of 'hurdles' which were resolved by achieving a balance between opposing realities; for example the conundrum of 'trust versus mistrust' in early childhood.

John Bowlby: attachment theory; recognised the importance of very early attachment to parental figures and the distortions which followed serious disruption of these relationships.

Heinz Kohut: self-psychology; recognised the further importance of developmental relationships in the development of personality and placed emphasis upon the development of a cohesive and coherent sense of personal identity.

Eric Berne: transactional analysis; recognised that at different times a person's inner psychological experience could be conceptualised as taking either a 'parental' form (e.g. emphasis upon responsibility, control), an 'adult' form (e.g. an integrative and accepting approach to life) or a 'child' form (e.g. regressed, demanding); relationships reflected the interaction between these three states of mind.

Psychodynamic psychotherapy

This form of therapy owes much to Sigmund Freud, but subsequent workers refined, expanded upon, and/or challenged his original views, as outlined in Box 16.4.

Freud's original technique (*psychoanalysis*) involved asking the patient to 'free-associate', bringing to the session whatever came into their mind at the time. The therapist sat behind the patient, intervening only rarely and usually to suggest interpretations of what the patient had said. Freud also emphasised the importance of dreams, referring to them as 'the royal road to the unconscious', and offering interpretations thereof. Freud emphasised how the patient's interaction with the therapist was a recapitulation of earlier life interactions (*the transference*), and that the therapist also reacted to the patient according to the therapist's own earlier relationship experiences (*the countertransference*). A particular task of the therapist was to explore *resistance* on the part of the patient, to accepting the interpretations of the therapist.

Classical psychoanalysis is very time-consuming, entailing hourly sessions up to five times a week and conducted over months to years. Nowadays most psychodynamic psychotherapists would see the patient less often, sit facing them during the sessions, and be more 'active' during sessions. A shorter duration of therapy, with a more clearly defined end-point, is also more common now. The efficacy of psychodynamic therapy has been increasingly confirmed by a variety of studies.

> ### Case example: Psychodynamic psychotherapy
>
> A 38-year-old man presented with severe agoraphobia which prevented a wide range of life activities. For example, he worked at a city store and would drive as close as possible to the store before he parked the vehicle. He would then run to the store wearing dark glasses, but then feel calm and relaxed once he was inside the store. A behavioural program of graded exposure was introduced, starting with the removal of his dark glasses. When he began his exposure treatment, he realised as he was running to work without glasses that he had been afraid of being recognised by others as his father's son. He recalled that his father had been charged with a crime and sent to jail when the patient was a teenager. He had felt devastated by this event and progressively more anxious in public places because he felt he might be recognised and his embarrassment and shame exposed.
>
> The behaviour therapy continued successfully, and was facilitated by psychodynamic therapy which enabled him to explore his feelings about his father, the events that caused him so much shame, and the extent to which this had caused him to become crippled by unconscious defences such as denial (he had not been aware of the link to his father), reaction formation (he was a particularly upstanding member of the community) and projection (he perceived that others would be highly judgemental of him if they knew of his parentage). He responded to 20 sessions of psychodynamic psychotherapy and concurrent behaviour therapy.

Psychodynamic techniques are generally employed where the intention is to create lasting and profound change for the individual in terms of the way they see themselves. The patient needs to show some degree of *psychological mindedness*, a commitment to attending sessions regularly and the resilience (*ego strength*) to tolerate the feelings evoked through exploration of unconscious issues. It is not appropriate in the face of severe depression or psychosis.

Group therapy

Group therapy can utilise any of the therapeutic techniques outlined above, but with variation respectful of the group situation. The advantages of group therapy are shown in Box 16.6. Potential disadvantages include the logistics of bringing people together regularly; confidentiality issues; and the propensity for some members of the group to be (or perceive themselves as being) ostracised by the others (the skilled therapist can use this therapeutically, but it can be very difficult for the individual concerned).

Groups can be either *open*, where members can start and exit at pretty much any stage, or *closed*, where there is a set group of participants who make a commitment to the group, and no further members are allowed to join.

Family therapy

There are a number of ways in which families can be engaged in therapy. At its most basic, families with a member who has a psychiatric disorder can be brought together for the provision of psychoeducation; tips are given about how to recognise and effectively

Box 16.5

Defence mechanisms

In psychoanalytic theory, incorporated into psychodynamic psychotherapy, distressing thoughts and emotions provoked by the experiences of childhood development are frequently contained out of conscious awareness, by a mechanism called 'repression'. Repression serves to unconsciously (i.e. outside of ordinary awareness) prevent the person becoming aware of these very distressing and often unacceptable thoughts or feelings. However this is only partly effective and further avoidance of distress is achieved through the use of unconscious strategies called 'defence mechanisms'. Defence mechanisms provide relief from the immediate emotional distress, but create disruptions in everyday psychological functions which are often recognised as 'symptoms' of illness or maladaptive behaviours. Many of these labels have been adopted by other schools of thought regarding psychological illness. The essential meaning is the same, although the mechanism may be explained differently. Here are a few common examples of defence mechanisms and their relevance to psychological disorder.

More 'mature' defence mechanisms

Altruism: Behaviour which reflects high moral values and an effort to give for the benefit of others, as a way of coping with difficult emotions. Example: helping to detect and destroy land mines during times of peace after being a soldier in a related conflict.

Humour: Behaviour that evokes laughter and bemusement as a means of coping with distressing emotions. Example: relating amusing (but respectful) stories about the deceased at a funeral.

Sublimation: Redirection of intolerable thoughts or feelings into behaviour that is more acceptable. Example: keeping busy when distressed.

Compensation: Development of personal strengths to 'compensate' for perceived personal weaknesses. Example: trying hard at sport when academically weak.

Less 'mature' defence mechanisms

Reaction formation: Conversion of intolerable thoughts or feelings into their opposites, often expressed in behaviour. Example: excessive generosity when angry.

Rationalisation: Use of simplistic but unsupported logic to explain away or relieve intolerable thoughts or feelings. Example: claiming unreasonable provocation when violent.

Intellectualisation: Use of highly complex intellectual formulations to avoid being aware of intolerable thoughts or feelings. Example: long, tedious and convoluted responses to criticism.

Displacement: Shifting the focus of intolerable thoughts or feelings on to a person or thing, unconnected with those thoughts or feelings. Example: yelling at your children after a hard day with your boss.

Undoing: Behaviour that aims to reverse the effect of intolerable thoughts or feelings. Example: compulsive rituals with OCD.

Denial: Refusal to accept that a particular thought or feeling exists. The unacceptable experience is totally avoided. Example: refusal to recognise unacceptable behaviour.

Identification with the aggressor: Aggressive behaviour to others which is the same as behaviour shown to the person as a victim of abuse in the past. Example: an adult former victim of child sexual abuse now acting as an abuser to children.

More 'primitive' defence mechanisms

Regression: Return to an earlier stage of emotional development, in order to avoid recognition of difficult thoughts or feelings. Example: temper tantrums in adults.

Dissociation: Altered awareness of a situation which is considered intolerable. Example: 'dreamy states' associated with being the victim of violence.

Box 16.5 continued

Acting out: Relatively extreme behaviour which relieves the unconscious distress from intolerable thoughts or feelings, but is not recognised for its function. Example: promiscuous behaviour following sexual abuse.

Projection: Misattribution of intolerable thoughts, feelings or impulses towards another person, such that the other person is seen to be the source of those intolerable experiences. Example: 'You're angry with me!' (when the speaker is angry and the recipient has not shown any such emotion).

'Severely primitive' defence mechanisms

Idealisation and denigration: Unconscious failure to recognise any unpleasant aspects of another person ('idealisation') or failure to recognise any pleasant aspects of another person ('denigration'). The process is extreme and frequently moves from one extreme to the other, with regard to the same person. Example: often observed with patients suffering from borderline personality disorder.

Splitting: The application of 'idealisation and denigration' to two other people (or groups of people). One person or group is 'idealised' and the other is 'denigrated'. This defence often evokes powerful emotional reactions in the people involved, such that conflict may follow between the two people (or groups of people). Example: again common in patients with borderline personality disorder and highly disruptive in therapeutic environments.

Idealisation of self: An unconsciously maintained and impenetrable self-image and belief, in which a person considers themselves perfect and beyond reproach. Any challenge to this 'narcissistic' view of the self is rejected with intense rage and total disbelief. Example: narcissistic personality disorder.

Box 16.6

Advantages of group psychotherapy

- Cost effectiveness.
- A sense of *belonging* to the group.
- *Identification* with other members of the group, and a feeling of not being 'the only one' with a particular set of problems.
- Learning from other members of the group.
- A sense of *altruism* in helping others deal with their problems.
- The opportunity to *role-play* within the group, and/or perform exposure tasks (e.g. the patient with social phobia giving a presentation to other members of the group, and getting their feedback).

respond to symptoms and behaviours in the affected family member; suggestions are made about effective communication; and assistance is given with general problem solving.

Family therapy draws upon the principles of *systems theory*, which essentially recognises a system as a separate entity to its component parts. Thus, a family is seen as a new entity in itself and the members of the family are simply the components that make up this new structure and organisation. In family therapy there is no identified person who is considered to be the patient. Rather the family addresses the problems which exist as a whole. Everyone in the family is expected to contribute and to recognise the ways in which the operations of the family lead to certain problems arising, including emotional or behavioural problems in a particular family member.

There are a number of forms of family therapy which draw on different approaches. Generally, family therapists tend to use a combination of all of these models in different combinations for particular families. In some instances there will be an attempt to disrupt the structures that exist between individuals, with alterations in family alliances and activities together. Alternatively, it is sometimes very helpful to disrupt the family with a strategy that causes a substantial reorganisation of the family's approach to life activities and problems.

More specific forms of family therapy are employed where the family itself is the 'subject'. The *Milan school* approach uses *circular questioning*, reflecting family dynamics by asking one family member to conjecture how others might view a particular issue, whilst the others can be asked to comment or make suggestions for change. The *narrative approach* looks at the ways families see themselves and their history, and suggests that other, more adaptive 'stories' might be usefully integrated into the family's way of functioning.

The use of a one-way mirror, with the family and primary therapist on one side and the other members of the therapy team on the other, can be a useful tool for family therapy. The primary therapist can be prompted by other team members (through an earpiece) to ask or pose particular problems or scenarios to the family in question. After each session the team can jointly reflect upon the dynamics they have observed in the session, and suggest ways of taking the therapy forward in future sessions.

Couple therapy

There are a number of different approaches to helping couples as a dyad. These include behavioural, cognitive-behavioural and psychodynamic approaches. Systems theory, as used in family therapy groups, can also be employed. Skilled therapists can use a number of these different approaches in an integrated manner, depending upon the clinical problem and what the couple bring to the session. Couple therapy can be modified for specific situations, for example, sex therapy.

Case study: How different psychological approaches may be applied (supplied by Dr Ed Harari (EH), St. Vincent's Hospital Melbourne)

A 40-year-old hitherto successful professional man ('John') presented with a 6-month history of increasingly severe clinical features of depression, precipitated by his wife's discovery of his marital infidelities and the subsequent breakdown of his marriage. This had recently culminated in John being forcibly evicted from the family home by a court order sought by his wife. He rented a small flat where he sat alone most nights drinking heavily and refusing to answer phone calls from concerned family and friends. While he reluctantly went to work most days, he knew that his work performance was deteriorating. When interviewed he denied suicidal intent, but through tears and exclamations of distress he insisted that he had irreparably destroyed his wife's life, that he was condemned to be a social outcast and that his life was a failure.

A **psychodynamic approach** proceeded with the therapist empathising with John's obvious distress, then gently inquiring about the insistent, adamant manner with which he criticised himself, even though he was obviously suffering.

Case study continued

EH: John, such self-criticism feels to me that you are being harsh, almost cruel to yourself, even though you are in obvious emotional pain.

John: (*angrily*) I've always thought I was a weak bastard. (*Silence, then more softly*) Even when I was doing well, I always had this feeling that I didn't really have what it takes.

EH: Do you mean that despite your outer achievements you didn't feel very confident or worthwhile about yourself? (*Empathic comment*)

John nods, cries silently.

EH: You've doubted yourself? For a long time? That sounds very painful, and lonely. (*Empathic comment*)

John then began to speak about the shock of his mother's death when he was 6 years old; he described some of the confusion and feelings of helplessness he had at that time, and his father's expectations of him (in John's view) to be strong and stoical. John's voice rose angrily again as he declared how disgusted his father would have been at his recent infidelity.

EH: John, you seem to be saying that what you saw as your dad's expectations and judgements of you, especially when you were feeling small and alone and very sad, has something to do with how you criticise and judge yourself now. (*Interpretation*)

John: He was a man of his time. He became Director of ..... at the age of 37, but he didn't know much about fathering. His father had been in the war, and came back a changed man; that's what my mother told me about my grandfather. When my mother died, Dad remarried after a few months and went on as if nothing had happened. He expected me to do the same. (*Angrily, mockingly*) So tell me Doc, what do ya reckon, am I worth a bullet through the head? What do you do with weak bastards like me – give 'em shock treatment? You're a busy man, Doc. I don't think you'd want much to do with a failed Casanova.

EH: We will need to talk about your mum and how you lost her, and other things, including how you might have lost your wife. (*Allusion to a repetitive pattern in his life*) But I wonder if you are expecting me to criticise you when I ask you about your pain, in the same way you've taken on your father's judgements and criticise yourself? (*Interpretation of possible negative paternal transference to EH, as well as alluding to John identifying with his critical father*)

In subsequent therapy sessions the theme of John's life-long tendency to self-criticism was explored in great detail. His tendency to deny vulnerability in himself, but to perceive it in women, became clear. His tendency to scorn vulnerability in himself while wishing to protect the vulnerability in his wife emerged as a major unconscious conflict in his marriage, which had led him to feel resentful, discontented and to enact this in the occasional but recurring brief infidelities throughout his marriage. Psychodynamic psychotherapy aims to replace such emotionally-driven, often-rationalised enactments with self-understanding.

A cognitive-behaviour therapy (CBT) approach might respectfully invite John to examine his loudly proclaimed belief that his wife's life was irreparably damaged as a result of his infidelity. From what he had witnessed and others had told him, John knew that she was distressed and angry, but that she was receiving support from her family and friends. Did he believe that her distress would last forever? So John's *catastrophic thinking* could be challenged. He was invited to speculate about whether her obtaining a court order against him was the mark of an irreparably damaged woman or a very angry one. Furthermore, he knew that she had been out on a few occasions with some close (female) friends. Was this the sign of an irreparably damaged woman? What were the chances that if her friends

Continued

Case study continued

continued to support her in this way that eventually they might introduce her to an eligible man? Would she be 'too damaged' to accept his invitation for a date?

Similarly, his *overgeneralisation* and *black-or-white* style of thinking could be challenged when he concluded that his failure in marriage meant that he had failed in life. He was encouraged to list and describe some of his genuine achievements in his life, including professional, philanthropic and social. Without discounting the distress at his failed marriage, his complete negation of other areas of success could be presented as a distortion of reality.

An example of his tendency to *selective attention* centred on his conclusion following a rather mild expression of disappointment in him from his father-in-law that he (John) was viewed with contempt by others. This conclusion ignored the efforts of several concerned friends to contact him, and some obviously sad, but kindly words expressed by his mother-in-law. Even his father-in-law's comments could be viewed from the perspective of a father's protective concern for his daughter, rather than a final verdict about John.

If John's depression was judged to be severe enough to prevent him from genuine participation in psychotherapy, or if his condition deteriorated further, **antidepressant medication** would be indicated and **hospitalisation** considered. Therapy could resume when the depression had improved. If these measures did not reduce his misuse of alcohol, participation in an **alcohol detoxification** program could be advised.

If John had concerns about his children, either fearing for their emotional wellbeing or disturbed by what he believed might be their negative opinions of him, it might be possible, if his wife agreed, to arrange some **family therapy** in which John met with his children to discuss his concerns. **Marital therapy** would be relevant if the couple considered possible reconciliation, or were unable to agree on practical ways of arranging their lives as co-parents.

Armed with some of the insights from individual therapy about his anger at his own vulnerability and how he projected such vulnerability onto women, yet still unsure how to relate to women without becoming excessively solicitous and deferential, John might be offered **group therapy** in which he might learn more about his feelings as he interacted with other members of the group, the ways others viewed him and how they dealt with conflicts over loss and self-assertion in their own lives. This could also help to overcome John's feelings of isolation and of being uniquely flawed.

REFERENCES AND FURTHER READING

Bloch, S. (Ed.), 2006. An introduction to the psychotherapies, fourth ed. Oxford University Press, Oxford.

Brown, D., Pedder, J., 1989. Introduction to psychotherapy. Routledge, London.

Brown, J.A.C., 1987. Freud and the post-Freudians. Penguin Books, Middlesex.

Frank, J., 1978. Psychotherapy and the human predicament: a psychosocial approach. Scocken Books, New York.

Gabbard, G.O., 2000. Psychodynamic psychiatry in clinical practice, third ed. American Psychiatric Press Inc, Washington, DC.

Hawton, K., Salkovskis, P.M., Kirk, J., Clark, D.M., 1989. Cognitive behaviour therapy for psychiatric problems: A practical guide. Oxford Medical Publishing, Oxford.

Parker, G., Berk, M., 2009. Side effects of psychotherapy. The elephant on the couch. Australian and New Zealand Journal of Psychiatry 43 (9), 787–794.

Swales, M., Heard, H., Williams, M., 2002. Linehan's dialectical behaviour therapy (DBT) for borderline personality disorder: Overview and adaptation. Journal of Mental Health 9, 121–127.

Weissman, M.M., Markowitz, J.C., Klerman, G.L., 2007. Clinicians quick guide to interpersonal psychotherapy. Oxford University Press, New York.

STEPHEN RETURNS

CASE-BASED LEARNING

JOEL KING & ANDREW GLEASON

The following role-play should follow directly after the role-play scenario in Chapter 11. It requires two students: one to play a GP registrar (candidate) and another to play the role of a patient, Stephen (actor).

OSCE Station Instructions

(Reading time: 2 minutes)

You are a GP registrar working in a suburban practice. You have recently seen Stephen and made a diagnosis of OCD with secondary depression. You organised a second appointment for today to talk about treatment options. Stephen has excellent insight and has read about using CBT for OCD. He is interested in trying this for his OCD, which is predominantly around contamination obsessions and cleaning compulsions. He is not interested in medications at this stage.

Tasks (10 minutes)
• Discuss an appropriate CBT plan for Stephen and his OCD.

Actor role: Stephen

Please refer to the actor role in Chapter 11.

You are Stephen, a 20-year-old university student. You have only a bit of knowledge about CBT, mostly obtained from the Internet. You know that it involves talking to a trained professional in an office and there is apparently lots of evidence for its efficacy in OCD. You have never met anyone who has undertaken CBT.

HOW TO PLAY THE ROLE

You are very curious about CBT but don't know much about it. You are keen to try it. You would like to start straight away. You have no problems seeing the GP registrar for ongoing work or being referred to another professional. You are slightly concerned that it will cost you a lot of money, because you are on a tight budget. You are not interested in medications at this stage and would like to try the CBT first.

Statements you must make:
• 'I'm very interested in using CBT for the OCD.'
• 'How does the CBT work?'
• 'Will you do the CBT or do I have to go somewhere else?'
• 'How many sessions will this take?'
• 'Do I have to lie on a couch for this to work?'

Model Answer

The candidate should have a good understanding of CBT principles and be able to explain these in lay terms. Before any discussion of management can begin, there needs to be an effort to engage the patient. Better candidates will use an empathic approach throughout the station. This will include highlighting the patient's strengths and good prognostic factors, such as short duration of illness, lack of family history, good insight and strong motivation. This is an integral part of engagement and necessary in any form of CBT, which relies strongly upon patient participation. Candidates should explain technical terms clearly and slowly, frequently checking the patient's understanding. Using handouts and giving the patient further opportunities to ask questions, such as another appointment if necessary, are part of the engagement process.

The candidate should ask the patient's understanding of CBT and how he thinks it will help him with his OCD. This will provide a basis to begin education about the therapy. As the patient knows very little about CBT, the candidate should begin with a general overview. The candidate should agree that there is an excellent evidence base for the treatment of OCD with CBT. In lay terms, the candidate should explain that CBT is a time-limited, outpatient-based therapy that focuses on connections between underlying assumptions, conscious thoughts, and behaviours. It does not involve a couch and is most often performed in a standard office-based setting with both the practitioner and the patient sitting in chairs and facing each other. A CBT program usually runs for about 10 to 12 sessions conducted on a weekly basis. CBT can be performed by GPs, psychiatrists, clinical psychologists, and other allied health professionals.

Part of CBT involves looking at the evidence assumptions and thoughts (cognitive distortions or negative cognitions), and providing more adaptive alternatives (see Box 16.3, page 269). This is known as cognitive restructuring or challenging. CBT often involves 'homework' tasks and patients may be advised to keep an automatic thought record as part of the therapy.

The candidate should explain that cognitive restructuring is one component of CBT. Another component of CBT is learning relaxation techniques, such as deep breathing and progressive muscle relaxation. This should be taught and practised in the office, with handouts or tapes given for the patient to practise at home. Relaxation techniques provide patients a more adaptive option in their anxiety-provoking scenarios compared to less adaptive options, such as substance use or avoidance.

The candidate should explain that cognitive restructuring and relaxation techniques should be combined with another component of CBT called exposure/response prevention or graded exposure therapy, which is the main component of CBT for OCD (see pages 163–164 and 267–268). This involves establishing a threat hierarchy, which is an ascending list of anxiety-provoking scenarios, with expected subjective anxiety scores, and then gradually putting the person in these scenarios, starting with the least threatening. This may involve visualising or thinking about the scenario before actual physical exposure. In each case, the patient is asked to experience some of the anxiety in this attenuated form, learn to stay with it and reflect that the anxiety will not overwhelm them. Patients are then asked to compare the anxiety experienced to the level that they originally expected. They usually find that their expected score was much higher than the actual level of anxiety experienced.

Exposure/response prevention therapy may be performed as a homework task or in the office setting, depending on whether the patient requires someone to help them reflect upon the experience and guide them through cognitive rechallenging techniques or relaxation techniques. In Stephen's case, it would be useful involving his parents to assist him through this process, as they live in the same house.

FOR THE MORE ADVANCED LEARNER

The more advanced student may also address Stephen's secondary depression simultaneously and discuss using cognitive challenging, mood diaries and practical strategies, such as exercise. Students should also discuss the need for regular review and other options if this course of CBT does not work, such as starting an SSRI medication or adding or switching to another form of psychological therapy.

Chapter 17

DEALING WITH PSYCHIATRIC EMERGENCIES

DARRYL BASSETT & DAVID J CASTLE

An emergency in the context of this chapter is a clinical situation in which serious adverse consequences are likely to occur if a particular clinical problem concerning a sick person is not resolved quickly. First we address aggressive and violent behaviours, and then the management of the suicidal patient.

Aggression and violence

Aggression is behaviour which is intended to cause harm to another or self. *Violence* is the execution of the aggression through direct physical activity.

Aggression is a natural phenomenon which can be appropriate or inappropriate in execution (e.g. military force vs. criminal violence), driven by personal desire (e.g. to achieve a goal) or a response to intense fear (e.g. as a consequence of intense anxiety, depression or psychosis). *Reactive aggression* involves behaviour directed to the source of a perceived threat. This is the most common form of aggression associated with mental illness. *Instrumental aggression* involves behaviour that is purely goal directed and relevant in psychiatry mostly because of the legal implications of its distinction from reactive aggression driven by illness.

Neurobiology

Aggression is mediated by a circuit connecting the medial amygdala to the medial hypo-thalamus and the dorsal regions of the periaqueductal grey matter. This circuit is modu-lated by the orbital and prefrontal cortices, which introduce the elements of associative learning that accompanies development. Disruption of any of these may contribute to inappropriately aggressive behaviour.

Noradrenaline, serotonin, gamma-amino butyric acid (GABA), vasopressin (AVP), testosterone, oestrogens, progestogens, thyroxine and cortisol have been implicated in the production and modulation of aggression. Among these, serotonin appears to carry a particularly important inhibiting effect, which can be enhanced by medications that promote the action of this transmitter.

Psychosocial elements

Personality development is critically important as this establishes the patterns of behav-iour and internal experience that promote empathy, frustration tolerance and impulse control. The modulation of rage requires developmental experience that allows tolerance of emotional discomfort and learning of appropriate means to express such anger. Social context and cultural practices further affect the expression of rage and goal-directed aggressive behaviour.

Prediction of violence

The prediction of violence is an inexact science, but certain factors are important clinical pointers. These are shown in Box 17.1. The reader is also referred to Chapter 20 for a broader discussion of risk in the psychiatric context.

Management

It is important to gather as much information as possible from nurses, family, friends, and, where appropriate, other patients. Establish what led up to this event, and the imme-diate precipitant. Read past case notes and refer to any risk management plans for the patient. Remember that past violence is a good predictor of future violence and the *modus operandi* is often consistent.

Ensure your own safety. Remove any tie, scarf, necklace or similar item from around your neck, out of view of the patient, before approaching them. Remove any objects that might be used as weapons (e.g. mobile telephones, cutlery). Ensure a means of summon-ing help rapidly if required and agree upon signals in advance (e.g. 'If I say I need Mr Black's notes, it means I need help immediately.')

Avoid giving the patient the impression that they are trapped and allow yourself a route of escape, should it be needed. Unless the person is well known to you, address them formally and introduce yourself formally. If the patient has a weapon, suggest that they might put the weapon down, 'so that no-one will get hurt'. Never ask the patient to give you the weapon and do not accept it if offered. Optimally the weapon should be placed away from everyone present.

Try to limit conversation to one professional person. Establish the precipitating event (if any) and try to work through this. Question them slowly and allow time for responses: talk slow but think fast. Allow catharsis (release of emotion verbally). Maintain concerned

Box 17.1

Predictors of violence

Imminent predictors (minutes to hours)

- Increased restlessness or agitation.
- Hyperventilation.
- Increased volume of speech.
- Angry gestures.
- Verbal or non-verbal threats.
- Closing of personal space.
- Increased erratic movement.
- Hostile facial expression; fixed gaze or fixed avoidance of eye contact.
- Withdrawal and/or refusal to talk.
- Increased thought disorder.
- Increased impairment of concentration.
- Violent delusions and/or hallucinations.
- Current substance intoxication (particularly stimulants or alcohol).
- Current substance withdrawal (particularly alcohol).
- Recurrence of known violent *modus operandi.*

Medium-term predictors (hours to weeks)

- History of violence.
- Substance abuse (particularly stimulants or alcohol).
- Male gender.
- History of verbal threats of violence.
- Links with violent sub-culture.
- Active psychotic illness
  - delusions and/or hallucinations about a particular person
  - delusions of control (particularly violent)
  - agitation, excitement, overt hostility or suspiciousness
  - delirium.

Long-term predictors

- Organic brain disorders affecting frontal lobes (note: medial supra-orbital region and anterior cingulate gyrus), limbic structures (note: amygdala, hypothalamus, striatal nuclei) and thalamus.
- History of poor compliance with treatment.
- Explosive, impulsive or antisocial personality traits.
- Access to weapons.
- Poor social support and/or close relationship to potential victims.
- Early abuse; particularly physical and by father.
- Early emotional deprivation.

Box 17.2

A safe restraint method

- Six people to restrain one assaultive patient; prepare medications in advance of any physical action, as below.
- One person (leader) facing the patient and attempting to negotiate less intrusive care; often but not always, this will be a medical practitioner.
- One person opposite each leg.
- One person behind/slightly to side of each leg.
- When considered necessary, the leader gives a predetermined verbal signal and the others each grasp a corresponding limb (wrists/ankles).
- Those holding wrists pull down and forward.
- Those holding ankles pull back and up.
- Leader grasps the patient's head and guides it to the floor; maintaining airway.
- The movements must be simultaneous and rapid. Prior training is invaluable.
- The sixth person prepares an intramuscular/intravenous injection in advance of restraint and has monitoring equipment for vital signs ready. This person should also have ready access to a telephone or duress alarm.
- Immediately the restraint is performed, the sixth person administers the prepared medication, while the others restraining the patient talk with him/her to help calm and reassure the patient that they are safe and the treatment will help them.

attention, but avoid fixed or excessive eye contact. Perform a mental state examination as you can. Avoid writing notes until the situation is clarified and under control.

Time and the presence of trained staff are the best methods of management. Try to have an agreed means of assistance and ensure everyone knows what their expected role is going to be.

If at all possible, offer the person oral medication to help them *feel less distressed*. In some circumstances the patient may accept intramuscular medication and this has the advantage of rapid benefit.

Physical restraint

Physical restraint should be employed only if absolutely necessary for the safety of the patient and/or others. Always explain carefully what you are doing, and why. Reassure the patient that if they cooperate no-one will get hurt. Debrief with the patient once the crisis has passed and they are able to reflect meaningfully on their behaviour. Emphasise the therapeutic value of restraint in conversations with patients and family, and allow questions about its use. A safe restraint method is shown in Box 17.2.

Seclusion

Seclusion is the containment of a person in an enclosed space in which there is visibility through a window. The purpose is time-out for very severely ill patients and for staff to

Box 17.3

Notes regarding the safe use of medications in the acute setting

- Respiratory depression is possible and must be carefully monitored for in any patient given parenteral benzodiazepines.
- Dystonias can result from parenteral (more rarely with oral) antipsychotics, notably the typical agents; monitoring and immediate treatment with an anticholinergic agent (e.g. benztropine 2 mg intramuscularly or intravenously) is required. Laryngeal dystonias may be missed and can be fatal.
- An ECG is required in any patient receiving high doses of antipsychotics, especially if given over a short time-period.

facilitate calm and sometimes to give time for medication to take effect. It should offer a low stimulus setting and be used for the protection of professionals and the patient. Medication use should be minimal and reduced by this strategy. The duration of containment should as brief as possible. Regular physical observation and physical examination is required if the period of seclusion is extended. Debriefing for the patient at an appropriate time is essential, as the experience is potentially very traumatic.

Pharmacological management

The use of pharmacological agents in the management of the acutely aroused psychiatric patient should be judicious and carefully monitored (see Box 17.3 for important safety tips). Always check the patient's physical status as far as feasible, find out about any relevant medical conditions (e.g. cardiac conduction problems) and try to ascertain whether they have had any untoward reactions in the past to antipsychotics or benzodiazepines. Prescribing medications which nursing staff can use if necessary (PRN medications) can be very effective, but maximum doses must be noted and potential adverse effects considered.

Offer oral medication first, unless the situation is too volatile to allow this. Intramuscular administration has the virtue of more rapid onset of action, although some agents (e.g. clonazepam) are rather erratically absorbed via this route. Intravenous administration should be considered only in extreme circumstances and the patient must be carefully monitored (notably for cardiopulmonary problems). The exact choice of agent should be predicated by the underlying problem (e.g. an antipsychotic in the patient with schizophrenia who has suffered an acute relapse); the acuity; the manifest symptoms; and the prior experience of particular agents in the individual.

Oral medications

- Olanzapine (wafer or tablet) 5 to 10 mg *particularly useful*, or
- Risperidone (rapidly dispersing or regular tablet) 1 to 2 mg, or
- Haloperidol (liquid or tablet) 5 to 10 mg, or
- Chlorpromazine (liquid or tablet) 50 to 100 mg, or
- Lorazepam 1 to 2.5 mg, or
- Clonazepam 0.5 to 2 mg

Intramuscular preparations (most common initial doses)

- Midazolam 5 to 10 mg (about 0.1 mg/kg body weight) for immediate and ultra-short-term sedation (30 to 60 minutes); *particularly valuable for urgent restraint of dangerous behaviour;* larger doses may be required for stimulant intoxication; repeat at half-hourly intervals if needed; it is crucial to monitor respirations as these may be suppressed.
- Lorazepam 1 to 2.5 mg for rapid sedation and short-term sedation (up to 4 hours); repeat at half-hourly intervals if needed; *not usually available in Australia.*
- Clonazepam 1 to 2 mg may be useful for continuing management, but be aware of the relatively long duration of action and frequency of ataxia.
- Haloperidol 5 to 10 mg; *particularly useful and usually readily available;* may need higher doses for large males or intoxication states; monitor for extrapyramidal side effects.
- Olanzapine 5 to 10 mg; usually well tolerated and can be repeated half-hourly if needed; needs to be prepared from a powder, so access may be delayed.
- Ziprasidone 10 to 20 mg: 10 mg every 2 hours or 20 mg every 4 hours to a maximum of 40 mg in 24 hours; may not be available in many places.
- Zuclopenthixol acetate 100 mg as starting dose (may repeat once after 24 hours if tolerated and needed; monitor for extrapyramidal side effects carefully as duration of action lasts about 48 hours); 100–150 mg if tolerance has been established and high dose needed; a third dose should be given after a further 48 hours or more, if needed. *Note: Onset of action will take about 2 hours and rapidly acting medications will be required simultaneously. Benzodiazepines are preferable because of the risk of extrapyramidal side effects of Zuclopenthixol.* **Never use in a neuroleptic-naïve patient.**

Intramuscular and oral medications are often usefully combined, such as the combination of a benzodiazepine plus antipsychotic. The combination of a benzodiazepine (for sedation) and antipsychotic (for reduction of aggression and gradual alleviation of psychosis) is frequently helpful. *Beware, though, of the use of an intramuscular benzodiazepine and olanzapine, as there are potential dangerous interactions: a 2-hour gap should be left between such agents.*

Intravenous administration (most common initial doses)

- Haloperidol 0.5 to 5 mg
- Lorazepam 1 to 5 mg
- Midazolam 1 to 5 mg

Always give slowly with close monitoring of vital cardiopulmonary functions.

Compulsory treatment

Most countries have some form of legislation that allows compulsory treatment of persons who suffer serious mental illness, have insufficient insight to accept treatment and as a consequence, constitute a serious risk to themselves or others. The details of this legislation varies from country to country, and state to state in Australia. It is essential that all mental health practitioners are familiar with the legislation in their area of work and adhere to the guidelines regarding application of compulsory treatment. This facility for the care of the seriously mentally ill is vital for their appropriate care, and reflects proper consideration for their health needs and the safety of the community.

Clinician safety

The practice of psychiatry in any context carries a risk of injury to the clinician. The following principles are useful:

- recognise predictable risks and plan in advance the management strategies that could be employed to cope with aggression and violence. Duress alarms are frequently available in situations where violence is considered a likely occurrence and should be available at all times in such settings
- engage other professionals in this process of planning and preparation. Teamwork is essential
- avoid being alone with a potentially violent person wherever possible. This is critically important with home visits
- remember that the objective of the management of violence is for *everyone* involved to emerge unharmed. Taking unnecessary risks is not clever and bravado is foolish
- do not approach a patient who is carrying a weapon. Leave several metres distance between you and the patient, and have ready access to escape or help, if at all possible. Do not rush for a door, competing with the armed patient for escape. Often they will want to escape more than you do! Call the police and summon professional help
- after dealing with a violent patient, give yourself time to debrief with other professionals. This is an opportunity to share experiences, and to feel supported and safe. Fear in a clinician is a natural emotion and not a weakness.

Suicidality

Thoughts of suicide are ubiquitous when depressed, even if they are dismissed or resisted. The risk of suicide must *always* be considered in the assessment of anyone with a possible depressive disorder. Asking about thoughts of suicide, plans and preparations, reasons for avoiding suicide (e.g. to avoid hurt to family and friends), and any past history of suicidal or impulsive behaviour, will give a useful basis for determining the risk of suicidal behaviour (see Box 17.4). Particular factors associated with increased suicide risk are shown in Box 17.5.

The involvement of family, friends and other health professionals will also be invaluable in this assessment and intervention. The risk is markedly amplified by the presence of psychosis, substance abuse, severe physical disability and/or social isolation. Be aware of the risk during pregnancy and particularly the puerperium, where the context may *appear* to reduce the risk.

The risk of suicide in depressive disorders rises immediately before and after the introduction of any effective treatment (both pharmacological and psychotherapeutic) and may not fall until 1 or more weeks of treatment.

Box 17.4

Questions to assess suicidality

- Do you ever feel like giving up?
- Do these (your symptoms) ever become too much for you?
- Do you ever think that you will not get better?
- How does the future look for you?
- Do you ever think about suicide?
- Would you tell me if you thought about suicide?
- What stops you from committing suicide?
- Do you know anyone who has committed suicide?
- Have you thought of joining someone close to you who has died?
- Have you made plans for suicide? Do you have access to firearms?

Box 17.5

Risk factors for completed suicide

Static general factors
- Male gender.
- Late adolescence/early adulthood and elderly.
- Widowed, divorced.
- Social isolation.
- Unemployment.
- Certain professions (e.g. dentists, anaesthetists, psychiatrists).
- Family history of suicide.

Static psychiatric factors
- Depressive disorder.
- Bipolar disorder.
- Alcohol and substance dependence.
- Anxiety disorder (notably panic).
- Personality disorder (especially Cluster B).
- Schizophrenia.

Dynamic psychiatric factors
- Psychotic state.
- Exacerbation or recurrence of severe mood disorder.

Box 17.5 continued

- Prominent guilt.
- Persistent hopelessness.
- Severe agitation from any cause (including akathisia).
- Perceived 'entrapment' in life situation or illness.
- Anniversary of bereavement.
- Access to firearms.

Medical

- Chronic medical illness.
- Chronic pain.

Suicidal thoughts and impulses, particularly if accompanied by specific plans or actions, are best managed by the instillation of hope and the development of a caring relationship (see Box 17.6). Most depressed people will be ambivalent about suicide as an option, with the most important exception being those who are psychotic. Usually it is enough to provide specific reasons for hope and the consistent presence of caring people. If the person suffers from a psychotic depressive disorder, compulsory care in a secure, highly supervised environment may be appropriate. However, even in such intensive situations of care suicide can still occur because the drive is so overwhelming.

Box 17.6
Management of suicidality

- Ask the patient and you will usually be told.
- Offer understanding for the thoughts of desperation.
- Offer unequivocal hope that their distress can be relieved and a worthwhile future can follow.
- Ask what is keeping the patient alive, given their despair.
- Emphasise the distress significant others will experience if they suicide. This may seem to promote guilt, but the patient needs to be reminded that they are important to other people and their absence will always be emotionally painful.
- Ask them to make a specific commitment to stay alive until you can meet them again and while you introduce specific treatments aimed to help them.
- Try to ensure that they are not left alone.
- Often admission to hospital will be helpful as it will provide close support and psychological assistance, as well as supervision of treatment. 'Observing' the patient will not keep them alive. It will assist with assessment and management planning, but most importantly, personal contact will be highly therapeutic and protective.
- Compulsory treatment is rarely useful, unless the patient has a psychotic illness or has significantly compromised cognitive function (e.g. acquired brain injury, intellectual disability). Treatment is best negotiated whenever possible.

REFERENCES AND FURTHER READING

Bernstein, C. (Eds.), 1999. Emergency psychiatry. The Psychiatric Clinics of North America 22 (4). W.B. Saunders, Philadelphia.

Blair, R., 2009. The neurobiology of aggression. In: Charney, D., Nestler, E. (Eds.), Neurobiology of Mental Illness. Oxford University Press, New York, pp. 1307–1320.

Castle, DJ., Tran, N., Alderton, D., 2008. Management of acute behavioural disturbance in psychosis. In: Castle, D.J., Copolov, D.L., Wykes, T., Museser, K.T. (Eds.), Pharmacological and psychosocial treatments in schizophrenia, second ed. Informa Healthcare, London, pp. 111–128.

Dowden, J., Allardice, J., Ames, D., et al., 2008. Therapeutic guidelines: Psychotropic version. Therapeutic Guidelines, Melbourne.

Goldney, RD., 2008. Suicide prevention. Oxford University Press, Oxford.

Jamison, KR., 2000. Night falls fast. Vantage Books, New York.

Petit, J., 2005. Management of the acutely violent patient. In: Neuropsychiatry, Psychiatric Clinics of North America. W.B. Saunders, Philadelphia, pp. 701–712.

Tardiff, K. (Ed.), 1988. The violent patient. The Psychiatric Clinics of North America 11 (4). W.B. Saunders Company, Philadelphia.

Tardiff, K., 1992. The current state of psychiatry in the treatment of violent patients. Archives of General Psychiatry 49 (6), 493–499.

CHAPTER 17

A DIALYSIS PATIENT NAMED KEN

CASE-BASED LEARNING

JOEL KING & ANDREW GLEASON

The following role-play requires two students: one to play a renal resident (candidate) and another to play the roles of a patient named Ken Sutherland and the examiner (actor).

OSCE Station Instructions

(Reading time: 2 minutes)

You are the renal resident working in a city hospital. The nurse unit manager, Gwen, has called you to the dialysis unit because a patient, Mr Ken Sutherland, arrived today and has refused his usual twice-weekly dialysis. He told Gwen that he no longer wanted to receive dialysis and was going home to die. He gave Gwen a thank you note for her support and wished her well. Gwen convinced him to stay in her office until you arrived to speak to him.

Task (10 minutes)

- Take a history from Mr. Sutherland (8 minutes).
- After 8 minutes you must terminate the interview and discuss Mr Sutherland's risk factors for suicide with the examiner (2 minutes).
- In this station the role of the patient and the examiner will be played by the same actor.

Actor role: Ken Sutherland

You are Ken Sutherland, a 58-year-old divorced man. You live in public housing and have no social supports. You have poorly controlled Type 2 diabetes mellitus that has led to chronic renal failure and twice-weekly dialysis. You have no past psychiatric history.

Your Type 2 diabetes was diagnosed at age 45 by your GP, who referred you to the diabetes clinic at the local hospital. You found it difficult to stick to the recommended diet and engage in exercise. You were placed on oral hypoglycaemic agents and insulin two years later. Your diabetes has gradually become worse. By age 52 you began to experience shooting and burning pain down your legs which was diagnosed as neuropathic pain by the endocrinologist. You were placed on lots of medications that you can't remember the names of, but nothing helped with the pain. Six months ago you began to experience increasing lethargy, weakness and shortness of breath. You were diagnosed with chronic renal failure and started on twice weekly haemodialysis. You have never experienced a heart attack, stroke, or problems with your eyes.

Your son, Paul (25 years old), died in a car accident two years ago. Paul was your only child whom you loved dearly and you were shattered by his death. You could not see the point of life, although you had no suicidal ideation at this time. Overcome with grief, you started to drink to the point that you were consuming six beers a day and your work performance as an automobile salesman suffered. Your wife, Laura, disapproved of your drinking and the effect it was having on your diabetes. This led to frequent arguments and long periods of not talking. When your company went bankrupt and you lost your job, you sat at home and did not bother looking for more work. By this point you had stopped seeing friends and socialising. Laura became tired of you doing nothing and asked for a divorce. You moved into a public housing apartment one year ago. You spend most of your time at the pub, playing pokies or drinking when you can afford it. You have no friends or community supports.

You grew up as an only child in a small country town. Your father hanged himself when he was 30 and you were 5, leaving your mother to raise you on her own. Your mother died from cancer when you were 35. You do not consider yourself religious. You were teased at school for having a 'crazy' dad and you had few friends. You never got into trouble and were an average student. You dropped out of secondary school at age 17 and came to the city. You found work as a car salesman at a small dealership, where you stayed until it went out of business. At age 28 you met Laura through friends and got married a year later. Your marriage was always conflictual. Laura would often say that you lacked confidence and never had any ambition. She tended to take the lead when it came to decision-making, including raising Paul, whom you thought was the highlight of your life. You had a very close relationship and were very proud of him, especially when he went to university and became a civil engineer. You talked to him on the phone nearly every night and were devastated when he died.

In the last year you have experienced increasing depressive symptoms, such as a negative view of self, others and the world, anhedonia, passive suicidal ideation, and feelings of guilt and worthlessness. This is the first time you have experienced these symptoms. This has been accompanied by a loss of appetite, weight loss, initial insomnia, and poor concentration. You have never experienced psychotic or manic symptoms. As you rarely speak to anyone, apart from exchanging pleasantries with Gwen and the dialysis staff, no-one has noticed you becoming depressed.

It was the second anniversary of your son's death two weeks ago. Out of loneliness you called Laura on the anniversary. She told you that she was getting married to another man and could not talk to you for long on the phone. Since then, you have thought more and more about how your son was the only good thing in your life and now there is nothing really to live for. You do not see any point in living anymore. You do not think things will get better for you.

You have devised a plan to drive your car off a deserted cliff to kill yourself, while avoiding harm to other people, and believe that there would be a sense of connection dying in a similar way to your son. You have found a cliff near where you grew up and plan on going there after you say your goodbyes. You have written a letter to Laura. You went to deliver your note to Gwen in person, as she has been the most consistent and supportive person to you over the last six months. When you thanked Gwen and told her that you no longer needed dialysis and were going home to die, she looked very distressed and upset, and asked you to sit in her office near the main reception while she got a doctor. You felt sorry for her and guilty for making her so upset, so you agreed.

HOW TO PLAY THE ROLE

You are a depressed and forlorn man. Your eye contact is poor. You should move slowly, like everything is an effort. You should answer all the questions honestly, but not volunteer information unless asked.

EXAMINER'S QUESTION

Please list FIVE risk factors for suicide in Mr Sutherland's case.

Model Answer

This station focuses on assessment of suicidality, including risk factors for suicide. Although it is tempting to begin by asking about his thoughts of suicide, this is not necessarily the best approach. The candidate should employ a calm and confident approach to the situation. In real life, there should be an initial assessment of immediate risks to the clinician and others, such as a highly agitated patient or a small room with only one door (see pages 284–286 and 289).

The candidate should explain their role clearly to the patient: 'Hello, Mr Sutherland. My name is _____ and I'm a doctor in this hospital. Gwen has asked me to see you because she is very concerned about your safety.' This may prompt the patient to speak freely about their current situation, in which case the candidate should allow the patient to speak, offering occasional encouragements such as 'Go on' or 'Hmm hmm'. If the patient does not speak freely, the candidate may use a more structured approach (see Chapter 3), starting with the demographics and working through a psychiatric history and a mental state examination. By doing so, the candidate will cover most of the risk factors for suicide (see Box 17.5, pages 290–291).

Particular attention should be paid to the presence and severity of Mr Sutherland's depressive symptoms. The better student will recognise that patients with chronic medical illnesses, such as renal failure, often have symptoms that mimic the neurovegetative symptoms of depression. As such, students should focus more on the negative cognitions, such as feelings of hopelessness and guilt, and a negative view of oneself, others and the world (see Chapter 8).

Students should be aware of the possibility of psychotic features. These can occur in severely depressed individuals and may involve command auditory hallucinations to harm or kill oneself. Mr. Sutherland's alcohol dependence is important in that he is at increased suicidal risk due to increased impulsivity and impaired cognition and judgement while intoxicated or withdrawing from alcohol.

The student should enquire about the current level of suicidality (see Box 17.4, page 290). Students should establish any precipitants to the suicidal ideation, the presence and feasibility of a suicide plan, any protective factors, any past attempts, and the time course of the current suicidal ideation to clarify acute versus chronic suicidal ideation. Patients with a change from chronic suicidal ideation to acute suicidal ideation, such as a change in suicidal behaviour, planning, or the loss of protective factors, require special attention.

In answer to the examiner's question, Mr Sutherland has numerous risk factors for suicide, including:
• male gender
• divorce
• social isolation
• unemployment
• family history of suicide
• depression
• alcohol abuse
• chronic medical illness (Type 2 diabetes, chronic renal failure)
• chronic pain (neuropathic pain).

Part 4

SPECIAL GROUPS

Chapter 18

CHILD AND ADOLESCENT PSYCHIATRY

ALESSANDRA RADOVINI

About one in ten young people suffer from mental symptoms sufficiently distressing to justify seeking professional help. Australian studies suggest that as many as one in seven (14%) have symptoms of emotional and behavioural disturbance.

Mental heath problems and disorders in children and young people can damage self-esteem, impede relationships with peers, decrease school performance and impact on the quality of life of the child, parents/carers and families.

This chapter provides an overview of psychiatric disorders in childhood and adolescence. We begin with a general overview of aetiology, and then turn to general principles of assessment and management. We then give consideration to specific disorders that afflict young people.

Aetiology

Mental illnesses in children and adolescents share many aetiological factors with those that pertain to adults. However, there are unique factors that impact on the young person and their world and these can of themselves, or through interaction effects, lead to the manifestation and perpetuation of emotional and behavioural problems. Such factors encompass biological, psychological, social and developmental factors in the context of the child's family and school environment.

Genetic factors

Increasingly, research is discovering the role of genetic factors in the aetiology of several disorders such as autism, intellectual disability, attention deficit hyperactivity disorder (ADHD), conduct disorder, anxiety and depression. This may result from the influence of single or multiple gene abnormalities or the complex interaction between genes, brain function and environment.

Trauma

An alarming number of children are direct victims of abuse and neglect, or witness domestic violence. Research has established the direct deleterious effect of child abuse and neglect on the growth and development of the brain. This impacts on the child's sense of self, ability to develop trust, ability to form relationships and ability to learn. All of these can have long-term consequences.

Educational factors

The school environment is an important influence on children. Normal transition points and multiple school changes can be stressful. Poor peer relationships, bullying, and under-achievement in academic or sporting areas, can cause significant stress/distress for children, leading to behavioural or emotional difficulties. Further, children with disruptive behaviours and/or unrecognised learning difficulties may end up in a negative cycle of conflict and punishment, making school an aversive experience.

Family factors

Family factors include parental separation and divorce, parental mental illness, and social and economic hardship.

Parental separation and divorce

In many Western cultures, around one in two marriages ends in divorce. The impact on children can be significant, including fear and confusion regarding the threat to their security; the actual or perceived loss of a parent; self-blame and feeling responsible for the parental conflict; the deleterious effect of exposure to ongoing conflict; and the ongoing uncertainty of long custody disputes.

Parental mental illness

This can adversely impact on a child, not only in relation to inherited genetic vulnerability, but also through modelling behaviours and learnt maladaptive strategies for dealing with stress, in addition to the impact of mental illness on the availability and ability of the adult to parent adequately.

Social and economic hardship

Many families struggle with a variety of challenges such as poverty, unemployment and unstable housing. These challenges place significant stress on the family unit and family wellbeing.

Box 18.1

Aims of psychiatric assessment in children and adolescents

- *Understanding the presenting problems*. The predisposing, precipitating and perpetuating factors and family beliefs need to be understood.
- *Assessing the impact on functioning at home and school*. Relationships with others, academic performance and social functioning need to be assessed.
- *Assessing the development of the child*. Particular note should be paid to early infancy and the quality of the bond between infant and mother, any disruptions in primary caregiver, attainment of milestones, transitions to preschool and primary school, cognitive and physical development, and medical history.
- *Understanding the family context, the stresses and strengths*. This includes understanding the relationship with siblings, the parental and marital relationship, the parental medical, psychiatric, drug and alcohol history, and the influence of significant others (e.g. grandparents).

Assessment

The main aims of the psychiatric assessment of children and adolescents are shown in Box 18.1. Assessment of young people differs from that of adults in a number of ways, including:

- children are not usually help-seeking, but are brought to attention by others
- parents rather than children are often the primary source of information. Collateral history from other professionals such as teachers and school counsellors is vital in understanding the overall functioning of the child
- the presenting problem needs to be understood in the context of the expected developmental level of the child
- assessment of the child and the family and school situation takes longer
- psychiatric comorbidity is common (around 50% of those referred to mental health services). This needs to be both thought of and looked for when children present to services.

Clinicians vary in who they see at the first appointment. It is often the parents and the child, but during the course of the assessment the clinician will commonly meet with the child separately, with the parents (together and individually), and with the family unit as a whole. In some circumstances this does not occur (e.g. during a crisis assessment or single session therapy). Also, older adolescents may not wish to involve their parents.

Assessing children

The interview needs to be adjusted, taking into account the appropriate developmental and cognitive level of the child. Younger children will be assessed by observation of their play and interactions, and less so via language. From about the age of 7 or 8 children can be directly interviewed in addition to engaging them in play. They can be asked questions such as whether they know why they have been brought to the appointment, their likes and dislikes regarding school, their friends and interests. They can be asked about things that make them sad, happy, worried or angry. Asking children to draw themselves, their family, a happy and sad/scary dream, or three wishes they would make, can offer further insights into a child's world. A playful and curious approach to the child and their world is helpful. Children are usually initially seen with their parents and then on their own.

Assessing adolescents

Adolescence is a time of increasing independence, moving towards adult functioning. Adolescents are often seen by themselves first, to obtain a history directly from them and to begin to form a therapeutic relationship directly with the young person by demonstrating that the clinician is interested in their point of view as well as that of parents. Parents are then asked to join the interview, or joint sessions are separately arranged. Engagement with an adolescent is facilitated by being transparent and clear about the limits of confidentiality and issues of safety and risk (where appropriate) and how the clinician will deal with these. A collaborative stance where the adolescent is given some choice where possible and appropriate (e.g. appointment times or venues) is helpful.

Physical examination and investigations

Conducting physical examinations and the extent of investigations will vary depending on the clinical context, the presenting problem and who else is involved (e.g. a paediatrician). The use of laboratory investigations depends on the nature of the problem. Specific testing, such as cognitive, speech and language, and occupational therapy assessments, is commonly requested where there are any concerns regarding a child's attainments.

Formulation and feedback

The formulation seeks to answer the question: 'Why does this child present with these problems at this time?' The task is to synthesise the wealth of information from various sources and to provide feedback and recommendations for treatment to the child and family. This is sometimes done in written format as well as in discussion.

Management

The management plan needs to identify and prioritise the areas of possible intervention. An agreed initial focus of intervention needs to be established with both the family and the child/adolescent. Families especially are the agents of change for younger children and need to be actively involved in the treatment plan. The management plan is often multimodal (individual, family and system work), reflecting the need to intervene at a number of levels when working with children, adolescents and families, who often present with multiple and complex needs.

Medication

While the use of psychotropic medication has increased for children and adolescents, this needs to be done with due caution and as part of a broader management plan. Relatively few drug trials exist for this population and much less is known about the metabolism, efficacy and long-term side effects than in adults. Information regarding medication needs

Table 18.1

Classification of psychiatric disorders of childhood and adolescence

Disturbance of	Group	Specific disorders
Normal development	Developmental disorders	Intellectual disability Autism Asperger's disorder
Function	Elimination disorders	Enuresis Encopresis
Learning	Learning disorders	Speech disorders Motor skills disorders Specific learning disorders (e.g. reading, maths)
Emotions	Internalising disorders	Anxiety Depression
Behaviour	Disruptive disorders	Attention deficit hyperactivity disorder (ADHD) Oppositional defiant disorder (ODD) Conduct disorder

to be provided to families, together with careful ongoing monitoring. Where a risk of overdose exists, issues of supervision and access to medication need to be addressed.

Specific disorders

Psychiatric disorders of childhood and adolescence can be grouped into a number of broad categories. They can be thought of as disturbances of normal development, aspects of functional mastery, learning, emotions and behaviour (see Table 18.1).

It is further useful to group disorders that commonly present at particular developmental stages. This is to be taken as a rough guide as there is, of course, significant overlap between these groupings. Children with any of these disorders can first present to services at any time (e.g. Asperger's disorder diagnosed in late adolescence) or the disorder can arise at any age (e.g. anxiety and depression). Onset of 'adult-like disorders' such as psychosis, schizophrenia, bipolar disorder, eating disorders and personality disorders can also emerge, particularly in mid to late adolescence. The reader is referred to disorder-specific chapters for details.

Detailed below are the individual disorders according to developmental life phase.

Infancy and early childhood: 0–5 years

Disorders of infancy and early childhood are listed in Box 18.2.

Intellectual disability

Intellectual disability is defined as below average intelligence (IQ < 70), together with significant problems in everyday functioning. It usually presents in young children as a global delay in milestones (i.e. delays in motor skills, language, social skills or play).

Box 18.2
Disorders of infancy and early childhood

Disorders of infancy and early childhood include:
- intellectual disability
- autism
- Asperger's disorder, and
- elimination disorders.

A comprehensive multidisciplinary evaluation is required, including general physical, neurological, hearing, vision, psychological/psychiatric and need for special education. Particular attention should be given to emotional, behavioural and psychiatric comorbidities, as these are common and need to be addressed in their own right.

A multidisciplinary approach to treatment is essential to address the multiple disabilities and complications. This will include medical and psychiatric interventions, parental support and education, behavioural management, educational evaluation and planning, and the standard therapies for comorbid psychiatric disorders. Medical and psychiatric comorbidities are often missed as any changes are all too often attributed to 'behavioural problems'. For more information on intellectual disability, see Chapter 21.

Pervasive developmental disorders (autism and Asperger's disorder)

Autism and Asperger's disorder share similarities as well as differences, as shown in Table 18.2.

Management requires a multidisciplinary approach, as for children with intellectual disability. Medication may be useful to target problematic behaviours (e.g. repetitive head banging), particular symptoms (e.g. poor sleep) or comorbid psychiatric disorders; however, they need to be used with care and as part of a holistic package of care.

Case example: Autism

A 4-year-old boy was brought by his parents because they were concerned about his very limited speech and odd use of language (including pronoun reversal and echolalia). They also reported that he did not like being cuddled and ignored other children, preferring to spend hours lining up his collection of toy trucks and tractors. He also did not respond when he was called. He would wear only Thomas the Tank Engine long-sleeve tops regardless of the weather. He hated the feel of water on his head and washing his hair resulted in a major tantrum. He repeated phrases from a *Thomas the Tank Engine* DVD and became extremely upset if this was interrupted. Diagnosis was of autism and moderate intellectual disability. Management included enrolment in an early childhood intervention program to assist with improving social interactions and communication, parenting strategies for managing difficult behaviours, and advice regarding educational needs. The latter are probably best met in a specialist school setting.

Table 18.2

Comparison of autism and Asperger's disorder

Problems with	Autism	Asperger's

Communication	Speech delay
	Poor non-verbal and verbal
	Echolalia, perseveration
		No delay
		Pragmatic language
		  difficulties (social use of
		  language)
		Odd use of language

Social interaction	Gaze avoidant
	Aloof/withdrawn, no interest
	  in others
	Preferring solitary activities
	Does not respond to others
		Odd/awkward manner
		Difficult peer relationships
		Only one or two friends
		No understanding of social
		  norms

Repetitive, restrictive
  interests and
  activities
	Repetitive activities (e.g.
	  rocking)
	Restricted range or odd
	  interests
	Fixed adherence to routines,
	  difficulties with change
		As for autism, but fewer
		  motor mannerisms

Cognitive functioning	70% associated with intellectual disability	Normal range of IQ
Onset of problems	Before 3 years of age	Usually later (i.e. present in primary school)

Comorbidities	Significant behavioural and
	  learning difficulties
		Increased risk of
		  psychological/psychiatric
		  difficulties, especially
		  adolescents

Elimination disorders

Bowel and bladder control are usually achieved by the age of 4 years. Enuresis and encop-resis (respectively wetting and soiling not due to a physical cause) may be part of matu-rational delay, a response to transient stress in the child's life (e.g. change of school or birth of a sibling), or a sign of more significant emotional difficulties (e.g. anxiety).

Management

- Exclude a physical cause.
- Evaluate the home and school environment to identify possible precipitants (e.g. marital discord or bullying).
- Provide psychoeducation for parents.
- Implement non-punitive strategies to assist the child with toileting (i.e. reminders, limit fluids in the evenings and assist child to get up at night to go to the toilet for nocturnal enuresis).
- Use operant conditioning; using a 'bell and pad' can be very effective.
- Address the underlying cause, if 'secondary'.

Box 18.3

Disorders of primary school children

Disorders in this age group include:

- anxiety disorders
- learning disorders
- disruptive disorders such as attention deficit hyperactivity disorder (ADHD)
- oppositional defiant disorder (ODD) and conduct disorder.

Primary school children: 5–13 years

Box 18.3 lists disorders of primary school children.

Anxiety disorders

Anxiety is expected and normal at specific times in development (e.g. distress in a preschooler separated from their parents). Many children have short-lived fears such as the dark, storms or animals.

Anxious children are often overly tense, but they can also be quiet and compliant and therefore not diagnosed.

For it to be a disorder, the level of anxiety must interfere with the child's usual activities. Common childhood anxiety disorders are shown in Table 18.3. For more information on anxiety disorders, see Chapters 10 and 11.

Management

- Evaluate the child, family and environment to identify possible precipitating, contributing and perpetuating factors.
- Interventions are a combination of individual and family strategies. Involving parents is critical to the success of the management plan.

Case example: Anxiety disorder

A 10-year-old girl presented with a number of somatic complaints and was refusing to go to school. She had been described as always being a 'worrier', but this had intensified following the death of her grandmother 4 months previously. She had become increasingly clingy and irritable and was having difficulty getting off to sleep. Specifically, she was worried that something might happen to her parents. Management included individual work, including relaxation techniques and exploration of loss and grief issues. Psychoeducation and parenting strategies were provided to assist her parents to reassure her appropriately and help manage her anxiety and minimise avoidance. Liaison with her teacher regarding her return to school and managing her somatic complaints were also important.

Table 18.3

Childhood anxiety disorders

Disorder	Core features
Separation anxiety	Constant fears about the safety of parents/carers
	Frequent stomach aches/physical complaints
	Distress at times of separation from parents; overly clingy
	Trouble sleeping or nightmares; extreme worry about sleeping away from home
	School refusal
Specific phobia	Extreme fear of a specific thing or situation
	Fears interfere with usual activities
Social anxiety	Fear of meeting or talking to people
	Avoidance of social situations
	Few friends outside the family
Generalised anxiety	Worries about things before they happen
	Constant worries about family, school, friends and activities
	Fear of embarrassment or making mistakes
	Low self-esteem; lacking in self-confidence
Obsessive-compulsive disorder (OCD)	Commonly begins in childhood and has a waxing and waning course
	Symptoms are often not experienced by the child as ego-dystonic
	Unwanted thoughts (obsessions); repetitive actions (compulsions)

Learning disorders

Parents are often worried when their child has learning difficulties at school. There are many reasons for school failure, but a common one is a specific learning disability. This affects about 1 in 10 children, often runs in families and is often not recognised. They are believed to be caused by perturbations of brain functioning that affects receiving, processing and communicating information. Commonly, a child will fail to master reading, spelling, writing and or maths skills, despite trying hard to learn, or will have problems with language or motor skills (see Table 18.4). This needs to be distinguished from school underachievement due to other factors, such as non-attendance or depression.

Secondary problems of poor self-esteem, misbehaviour and school refusal may arise if the difficulties are not identified and specific interventions put in place. Co-occurring ADHD and learning disorders are common. Diagnosis is made on the basis of standardised assessments of speech, educational attainments or coordination (occupational therapy assessment). The diagnosis can be easily missed if not thought about. Specific interventions to address these difficulties are required in addition to psychoeducation for parents and teachers.

Attention deficit hyperactivity disorder (ADHD)

The main features of ADHD are shown in Table 18.5. Difficulties are present from early childhood, are more severe and frequent than other children of the same age or developmental level, and present in multiple settings (i.e. home and school).

Table 18.4

Learning disorders of childhood

Disorder	Features
Communication disorders	Expressive language disorder
	Receptive language disorder
	Mixed expressive/receptive language disorder
Motor skills disorder	Slow to develop motor coordination
	Overly clumsy; poor hand writing
Specific learning disorders (academic skills)	Reading disorder
	Mathematics disorder
	Written language disorder

Table 18.5

The main features of ADHD

Feature	Characterised by
Hyperactivity	'On the go' all the time
	Fidgets and squirms
	Runs around or climbs excessively
Impulsivity	Blurts out answers; talks too much
	Has trouble taking turns
	Interrupts others
Inattention	Easily distracted; has trouble listening
	Inattention to details; makes careless mistakes
	Loses things
	Has trouble finishing tasks

Secondary problems of poor self-esteem, poor peer relationships and school failure are common. Comorbid disorders might include anxiety, depression, conduct disorder and learning disorders. In the differential diagnosis, consider 'normal' behaviour, parenting issues and attitudes, and trauma or neglect, as traumatised children can be hypervigilant, reactive to the environment and have poor concentration.

Management

Management is multimodal, including parenting techniques (clear instructions, consistency, appropriate praise and reward), classroom strategies (sitting close to the teacher, information in small amounts, short breaks) and medications to reduce the target symptoms. In addition, remedial teaching, identification of and interventions for specific learning disorders, and addressing issues of poor self-esteem and social difficulties are crucial.

Box 18.4
Symptoms of ODD

Symptoms of ODD include:
- frequent temper tantrums
- arguing with adults
- refusal to comply with adult requests or rules
- deliberately annoying others
- blaming others for their mistakes.

Oppositional defiant disorder (ODD)

These children demonstrate a persistent pattern of uncooperative, defiant and hostile behaviour towards authority figures, which affects their social, family and academic life (see Box 18.4). These behaviours are seen in multiple settings, including at home and at school.

Such behaviours may be part of normal development for a 2- or 3-year-old, and adolescents tend sometimes to be oppositional, disobedient and uncooperative. Thus, labelling a child as 'oppositional defiant' needs to be done according to the developmental context. Some children with ODD go on to develop conduct disorder.

Management

Management includes parenting skills training and the identification and treatment of comorbid conditions such as anxiety, depression and ADHD. The family environment and parenting issues should also be addressed, and specific interventions provided, should the child have been the victim of trauma.

Conduct disorder

Children with conduct disorder show serious difficulty following rules and behaving in socially acceptable ways (see Table 18.6). Onset may be in childhood or adolescence, and these children are often viewed by others as 'bad' or delinquent rather than mentally unwell. The behaviours often lead to school expulsion, out-of-home care and involvement of the youth justice system.

The aetiology is multifactorial, including brain damage, child abuse, genetic vulnerability and traumatic life experiences. Comorbidity is common and includes mood disorders, anxiety, post-traumatic stress disorder (PTSD) and substance abuse.

Management

Management can be difficult, and early identification and treatment is likely to have the best results. Interventions need to target the child, the family and the system, encompassing:
- identifying underlying factors (e.g. child abuse)
- parenting strategies and family work
- problem-solving strategies
- identification and intervention for comorbid conditions.

Table 18.6

Features of conduct disorder

Feature	Characterised by
Aggression to people and animals	Bullying, threatening or intimidating behaviour Initiating fights; has used a weapon Physical cruelty to people or animals Forcing someone into sexual activity Stealing from a victim while confronting them
Destruction of property	Deliberately engaging in fire setting with the intention to cause damage Deliberately destroying others' property
Deceitfulness, lying, stealing	Breaking into houses/cars Lying to obtain goods/favours or to avoid obligations Stealing items without confronting a victim
Serious violation of rules	Often staying out at night Running away from home Being truant from school

Case example: Disruptive behaviours in a teenager

A 13-year-old boy was referred by the juvenile justice system following being charged with car theft. He had been a client of the child protection system for 2 years and had been placed in 'out-of-home care' because of inadequate parental supervision at home. He had a long history of getting into fights and being verbally aggressive, and had been expelled from two schools. Since being in foster care, he had started using inhalants and smoking marijuana. He frequently absconded from his placement and went home to his mother's house or simply went missing. He had a long history of academic difficulties and his IQ was in the borderline range. Management was multimodal and incorporated interventions at the child, family and system levels. These included mental state and risk assessment, including addressing the substance use. Appropriate school placement, involvement in suitable activities, and support for both his mother and foster parents were addressed. This included appropriate limit setting and the building in of consequences for errant behaviours.

Adolescents and young adults: > 13 years

Box 18.5 lists disorders of adolescence and young adulthood.

Depression

Depression affects about 5% of children and adolescents in the general population, with a higher risk for those with comorbid attentional, learning, conduct or anxiety disorders,

Box 18.5
Disorders of adolescence and young adulthood

Disorders of adolescence and young adulthood include:

- depression
- deliberate self-harm
- substance use (see Chapter 22).

Table 18.7
Features of depression in adolescence and young adulthood

Feature	Characterised by
Mood changes	May be sad, tearful and anxious, or irritable and angry (especially adolescents)
	Extreme sensitivity to perceived rejection or failure
Cognitive changes	Poor concentration
	Overwhelmingly negative thoughts
	Thoughts of hopelessness, guilt, low self-worth and low self-esteem
	Thoughts of 'not wanting to be around', self-harm or suicide
Functional/ behavioural changes	Disruptive behaviour at home or school
	Decreased interest/pleasure in usual activities
	Social isolation, no longer playing/spending time with friends
	Relationship difficulties
	Decreased school performance
	Deliberate self-harm
Physiological changes	Changes in appetite or sleeping patterns
	Low energy levels
	Frequent physical complaints (especially younger children)

substance abuse or those who experience loss or ongoing stress. Changes in behaviour may be the first sign, rather than mood difficulties (see Table 18.7). There may be associated reckless behaviours, deliberate self-harm or suicide attempts (expressly in adolescents). For more information on depression, see Chapter 8.

Management

- Address the risk issues and implement a safety plan.
- Identify stresses, such as school, peers and family relationships.
- Use non-pharmacological modalities, such as cognitive-behaviour therapy (CBT), problem-solving skills and family work.

Table 18.8

Factors that might contribute to self-harm

Factor	Reason
Part of subculture	To take risks, rebel, reject parental values To be accepted
As a form of self-soothing/distraction	To cope with emotional distress
As a communication	To convey emotional distress, pain, low self-esteem To get help
Symptom of psychiatric illness	Increased risk of deliberate self-harm with depression, psychosis, substance abuse May be seen in children with intellectual disability, autism and abused children
Emerging personality difficulties	Increased risk of deliberate self-harm with emerging borderline personality disorder

- Use medications with caution. There is little evidence for the efficacy of antidepressants in adolescents.
- Monitor carefully, especially mental state, risk, response and side effects.
- Address comorbid conditions (e.g. drug and alcohol use).

Deliberate self-harm

Self-injury is a complex behaviour that results from a variety of factors, including those shown in Table 18.8. Self-harm can take many forms, including minor skin scratching, marking, picking, burning, overdose of prescribed and non-prescribed substances, head banging, bruising and reckless behaviour. The behaviours may overlap with thoughts of wanting to die or suicide.

Management

- All self-harm should be taken seriously and requires a thorough assessment.
- Risk evaluation should assess the ongoing risk of self-harm, of suicide, of accidental injury or death, and implementation of a safety plan (strategies for keeping safe, such as distraction, self-soothing, identifying supports, who will assist and how).
- Static risk factors (e.g. history of impulsivity or previous self-harm) and dynamic risk factors (e.g. times of conflict or drug use resulting in increased risk) need to be identified.
- Any underlying mental illness needs to be treated.

Case example: Depression in an adolescent

A 17-year-old student in her final year at school, usually a grade A student, was starting to struggle to complete her assignments, and had done very poorly in her exams. She was considering dropping out of school. She had become increasingly distressed and had begun cutting herself and become increasingly preoccupied by thoughts of death. She disclosed to the school counsellor that she had been raped on her way home from school some 6 months previously. Management included a risk assessment and safety plan. Psychoeducation was provided for both her and her parents regarding the links between trauma and depression. Liaison with the school included discussions regarding the safety plan and a variation of workload, with special consideration for exams. Individual work focused on teaching strategies
for managing low mood, thoughts of self-harm and traumatic memories. Antidepressant medication was introduced only after she had not responded fully to the psychosocial interventions.

REFERENCES AND FURTHER READING

American Academy of Child and Adolescent Psychiatry website, Practice parameters: guidelines for the management of psychiatric disorders in child and adolescent psychiatry. Online. Available: www.aacap.org/cs/root/publication_store/practice_parameters_and_guidelines. Accessed 10 December 2012..

Attwood, T., 1997. Aspergers?': a guide for parents and professionals. Jessica Kingley, London.

Barkley, R., 2006. Attention deficit hyperactivity disorder: a handbook for diagnosis and treatment. Guilford Press, New York.

Frith, U., 2003. Autism: explaining the enigma. Blackwell, Oxford.

Martin, A., Volkmar, F., 2007. Lewis's child and adolescent psychiatry. Lippincott Williams and Wilkins, Philadelphia.

Rutter, M., 2008. Rutter's child and adolescent psychiatry. Blackwell, Oxford.

Werry Centre for Child and Adolescent Mental Health, New Zealand 2008 Evidence-based age appropriate interventions: a guide for Child and Adolescent Mental Health Services (CAMHS). Online. Available: www.werrycentre.org.nz/site_resources/library/Workforce_Development_Publications/Evidence_Based_Intervention_Final_Doc.pdf. Accessed 10 December 2012.

CHAPTER 18

A MOTHER NAMED KATE

CASE-BASED LEARNING

JOEL KING & ANDREW GLEASON

The following role-play requires two students: one to play a GP registrar (candidate) and another to play a patient named Kate Taylor and the examiner (actor).

OSCE Station Instructions

(Reading time: 2 minutes)

You are working as a GP registrar at a suburban clinic. Kate Taylor, a 33-year-old mother, has come to the clinic because she is very concerned about the behaviour of her 3-year-old son, Peter.

Tasks (10 minutes)

- Take a history from Kate about her son, Peter (8 minutes).
- After 8 minutes, you must terminate the interview and discuss with the examiner the most likely diagnosis for Peter and discuss the next step in management (2 minutes).
- Peter will not be present in this station.

Actor role: Kate Taylor

You are Kate Taylor, a 33-year-old woman. You live with your husband, Alex, who is 39 and works as a partner at a major accounting firm, and your son, Peter, who is 3. You have been married for eight years. You work as a book editor for a publishing house. You enjoy this job immensely, both intellectually and socially. You don't really do it for the money. Your work colleagues and boss are very supportive. Your work colleagues and friends consider you a kind person who wouldn't hurt a fly, although they do state that you're often very serious and find it hard to relax.

You met Alex when you were 23 through mutual friends. He was completing an MBA. You and Alex married when you were 25 and you moved out of your parents' house. Your marriage is stable, but Alex is often away at work. Unfortunately, since he was made partner in his firm one year ago, he has worked even longer hours, including weekends and interstate travel. As such, you do most of the child-rearing by yourself.

You are very concerned about Peter, your son. He was a planned and much wanted baby. The pregnancy was normal. He was born in hospital at 38 weeks via normal vaginal delivery. The Apgar score was 9 at birth. He did not spend any time in a neonatal intensive care unit. You were discharged home a few days later. Peter was a fussy baby who did not sleep or attach to the breast very well. This frustrated you and you blamed yourself for these problems. You switched Peter to bottle-feeding and this went well. You became a stay-at-home mother.

Peter sat up at 5 months and walked at 14. He started using single words at age 18 months and uses a maximum of three words together. He stopped using words he had previously learned between 18 and 24 months, but has now regained most of these words. He does use words to request and he points at objects, but does not look at his parents when he does this. He has difficulty with pronouns. For example, he might point at his father while saying, 'me'. Yesterday, he pointed at himself and said, 'You hungry'. He plays with toys but prefers to play alone. His favourite toys are trains, which he tends to connect and reconnect in a slow, monotonous manner. He repeatedly counts the car windows, saying 'One window, two window. One window, two window.' He enjoys lining things up on the floor, such as objects in the pantry, and goes into a rage when his lines of objects are disturbed.

He plays with you, but only does this when you bring toys or books to him. He usually points at the object he wants, rather than asking for it. You often try to hold him in your lap and read to him, but he screams and struggles to get out of your embrace. You find this very hurtful.

There is very little eye contact with you when he does play and you are the one who has to make eye contact with him. Often you have to get in his field of view and then he looks away. He rarely smiles when you smile, despite your most animated attempts at doing so. He screams when taken to the supermarket and doesn't like noisy environments. He tends to flap his hands at times and he often stares at the ceiling lights for 10 to 20 minutes at a time, despite your attempts to distract him. He is a fussy eater and hates being messy. He does not like different foods that you introduce to him. He likes pasta and this is essentially all you can feed him. This upsets you as you enjoy cooking. His physical health is otherwise well and he is up-to-date with immunisations. Past testing of his hearing and vision has been normal.

You find it very exhausting looking after him and a friend suggested going back to work for a few days a week to get back to adult company. You placed Peter in a child care centre a month ago and returned to your old workplace. You were surprised when the child care centre's manager said that Peter showed little interest in other children. When he does play with children, he prefers those younger than himself and tends to treat them as objects, pushing them around the room. He does not share and takes toys from other children, even when they are playing with them. He never initiates play with others and keeps to himself or copies other children from the other side of the room. The child care staff report that he seems to have no idea that they are children like himself.

You have taken this very personally and feel that you have somehow failed Peter as a mother. You try your best, but you fear that your own 'failings' – switching Peter to bottle-feeding, not wanting another baby because you found having Peter such an ordeal – have led to Peter being a social misfit and developing abnormally. You tried to explain your frustration to Alex, who told you that you were a great mother and Peter will grow out of it. You stopped discussing the issue with Alex after that.

You have no history of a psychiatric disorder. There is no family history of mental illness, developmental delay, intellectual disability, or a pervasive developmental disorder.

Statements you must make:
- 'Thank you for seeing me, Doctor. I'm very worried about my son, Peter.'
- 'The staff at the child care centre tell me that Peter doesn't socialise like the other children.'
- 'Peter doesn't like playing with other children.'
- 'Peter doesn't look at me. Am I doing something wrong?'

Model Answer

This case is an almost classic description of a 3-year-old boy with autistic behaviour (see pages 303–304 of this chapter and Chapter 21, pages 346–348). The candidate must provide appropriate reassurance to the mother, take a history about her son's abnormal development, show an understanding of the most probable diagnosis of autism, and suggest options for appropriate further assessment to the examiner.

There are obvious limitations in this station, namely that the child and the other primary caregiver, the father, are not present. This is important in assessing not only the child, but also the parental dynamics and the parental-child attachment. Parental discord and poor attachment between the child and parents play a major role in a developing child's behaviour and must be considered simultaneously with more biological issues (see page 299).

The candidate will take a developmental history. This is best done chronologically, starting with conception, pregnancy, and delivery. Difficulties with pregnancy, such as infections, and delivery, such as obstructed labour, foetal distress, and time spent in a neonatal intensive care unit may indicate prenatal and perinatal insults to the child's brain. Poor sleep and eating and failure to gain weight appropriately may suggest an underlying medical disorder, such as coeliac disease.

The famous paediatrician-turned-child psychoanalyst, D.W. Winnicott, said, 'There is no such thing as a baby.' While the candidate gathers information about the child, the candidate must keep asking about the interactions and the reciprocal impact between the child and caregiver. A baby who does not accept being cuddled by the mother or look at the mother may lead to the mother feeling rejected or a failure as a caregiver. This in turn may lead to the mother giving up on the child, blaming the child, or becoming depressed. Parental discord is not uncommon in these situations. In these situations, children can fail to receive the appropriate environmental stimulation to develop proper language and communicative skills and can thus appear to be autistic or intellectually disabled.

The astute candidate should recognise that autism tends to manifest itself usually from age 3 onwards, with the child usually being described as 'odd.' The candidate should narrow this description down and ask specifically about impairments in the three key areas associated with autism, namely social interactions, communicative functioning, and restricted, repetitive and stereotyped patterns of behaviour, interests and activities. This is described in more depth in pages 303–304 of this chapter and Chapter 21, pages 346–348. Candidates should enquire about the pragmatics of language, which relates to how words are sequenced together to communicate a concept. Candidates should also ask about whether the child engages in age-appropriate imaginative play and reciprocal social interactions, such as eye contact with parents, mirroring the parents' facial expressions, and interest in other children.

At the end of the interview the candidate should arrive at an appropriate list of differential diagnoses while acknowledging the limitations of the interview, such as not seeing the child or having the necessary expertise. The differential diagnoses include autism (the most likely diagnosis), speech and learning difficulties, intellectual disability, medical disorders including vision or hearing impairment, or issues relating to attachment or the care-giving environment.

The next step in management is a longer assessment session with the child and both parents, and collateral history from the father and child care centre.

FOR THE MORE ADVANCED LEARNER

Good students may suggest some of the following:
- a review of the child's developmental milestones records (which is often completed by a maternal child nurse)
- appropriate physical examination and investigations to look for medical causes for Peter's behaviour
- referral to a psychologist for assessment of IQ (although this may be easier to do when Peter is slightly older)
- speech pathology assessment
- vision and hearing assessment
- referral to specialist services.

Specialist referral options include a paediatrician, a private child psychiatrist, or a public child psychiatry service with an autism assessment team.

Chapter 19

OLD AGE PSYCHIATRY

DAVID AMES, SAMANTHA LOI,
NICOLA LAUTENSCHLAGER & DANIEL O'CONNOR

The world's population is ageing. The proportion of
Australians aged 65 and over is expected to double from
13% to 25% of the total population between 2007 and 2051.
Past high birth and immigration rates, which then fell
dramatically from the 1970s, are the main reasons for this
demographic change. Older people form a smaller
proportion of the population in developing countries, but
their numbers are growing rapidly. The median age of
people in China will rise from 30 to 45 years by 2050, when
over a third will be aged above 60.

Population ageing leads to more people being affected by disorders whose prevalence rises
with age. *Dementia,* for example, becomes twice as common for every 5 years of increase
in age from age 60 to 90. Over 27 million people are affected by dementia in our current
world, and this number is projected to double every 20 years, surpassing 100 million by
2050. Most new cases will appear in developing countries, but Australia will experience
a big rise from 266,574 (1% of the population) in 2011 to 942,624 (2.8%) by 2050.

Although most elderly Australians are well and have a good quality of life, it is not
unusual for very old people to be widowed, to live alone and to have health problems that
limit independence. Over half eventually enter residential care.

The specialty of old age psychiatry offers assessment and treatment to older people with
mental disorders. Old age psychiatry is a multidisciplinary specialty and requires teamwork. All doctors need to display patience and compassion, especially when dealing with
the old and frail.

Table 19.1

Causes of dementia in Australia

Cause	Percentage of cases
Alzheimer's disease (AD)	50
Mixed AD and cerebrovascular disease	20
Pure vascular dementia	5
Dementia with Lewy bodies and Parkinson's disease dementia	10
Primary frontotemporal dementias	5
Alcohol induced dementia	5
Other rare dementias	5

Dementia

Dementia is an acquired decline in higher mental functioning (especially memory, intellect and personality) occurring in an alert individual (to distinguish it from delirium) that affects multiple cognitive functions (not just memory) and interferes significantly with everyday function. Most dementias are irreversible and progressive.

After age 60 the prevalence rate doubles every 5 years, rising from 1.8% at 65 to 25.5% at 85 (see Table 19.1 for the main causes of dementia in Australia). In 2009 some 1500 Australians were newly diagnosed as having dementia each week, but by 2050 this will increase to 7400 new cases each week.

Clinical presentation

Dementias affect memory, intellect, behaviour and personality. Usually loss of insight causes problems to be brought to medical attention by relatives. Dementia often leads to poor hygiene and diet, unsafe use of appliances, failure to pay bills and getting lost. Repetitive questioning, night-time disturbance and challenging behaviours can distress family members.

The array of symptoms listed in Box 19.1 are referred to as 'behavioural and psychological' or 'neuropsychiatric' symptoms of dementia. Some are common (60% of people with dementia living at home exhibit one or more of these symptoms); most upset either the person with dementia or those around them; and they may lead to the prescription of psychotropic medication.

Assessment of the person with suspected dementia

History

To ascertain the nature and extent of cognitive deficits and establish their cause, to determine their impact on function, to diagnose comorbid delirium or depression and to check the available supports, a good history is needed. Information should also be obtained from someone who knows the patient well, as the individual's own account may be inaccurate.

The history should cover the patient's life experiences and premorbid personality; assess function; enquire about mood symptoms, unusual ideas or challenging behaviours; and

Box 19.1

Behavioural and psychological symptoms of dementia

- Mood changes (depression or euphoria)
- Delusions
- Misidentifications of familiar people and places
- Hallucinations
- Personality change (especially apathy)
- Excessive motor behaviour (pacing, agitation)
- Noisiness
- Resistance to care interventions
- Aggression
- Sexual disinhibition.

take note of possible causes of dementia. Any personal or family psychiatric history should also be recorded.

One must distinguish between cognitive changes that develop slowly, due to dementia, and those that develop acutely because of delirium. Since delirium, when it occurs, is more often than not superimposed onto dementia, it is vital to enquire about recent changes in physical health or medication use.

Mental state examination

People with advanced dementia who live alone often look neglected, but those living with a relative may be neat and well nourished. Patients' cognitive deficits often remain unsuspected and undetected for long periods. Given the high likelihood of dementia being complicated by delirium, it is important to note evidence of physical illness and gauge the capacity to sustain attention. Patients with uncomplicated mild to moderate dementia can attend to questions. Patients with delirium look unwell, are either hyperaroused or drowsy, and are easily distracted.

Disorientation to time is common. Orientation to place is usually well preserved when patients have lived in the same home for years, but may be poor if in hospital or a recent change in the living arrangements has occurred.

Demands that exceed a patient's capacity to cope may lead to anxiety, agitation and even extreme emotional disturbance. Up to 5% of people with dementia have a major depressive disorder and many more have milder depressive symptoms. Social withdrawal, agitation, tearfulness, insomnia and anorexia suggest comorbid depression.

Language abnormalities range from mild word-finding difficulty to aphasia. Thinking becomes repetitive and simple. Up to half of all dementias are accompanied by misinterpretations, delusions or hallucinations for at least some portion of the illness. Loss of insight is evident early on. Many patients insist that they are coping well when they are not.

Cognitive testing

Cognitive testing is essential. Mildly affected articulate people hide their deficits easily. Short instruments like the Mini-Mental State Examination (MMSE) are useful, but screening tests should not be used to make a diagnosis without additional information, as a poor performance may be due to deafness, poor vision, depression, lack of cooperation, lack of fluency in English or limited education. Such tests provide little information on frontal lobe function and are insensitive in people of above average intelligence with early dementia. Test scores should be *interpreted* in the light of other information obtained from the patient and informants. When available, neuropsychological testing often yields useful results and helps to identify the underlying type of dementia.

Physical examination and investigations

Physical examination and selected investigations must be performed. Dementia is rarely reversible, but subdural haematomas, cerebral tumours and 'normal pressure' hydrocephalus must be excluded, as must anaemia, diabetes mellitus, hypothyroidism, vitamin B12 deficiency and drug toxicity. Standard investigations include a full blood count, B12, folate, liver function tests (LFTs), erythrocyte sedimentation rate (ESR), glucose, urea, calcium and electrolytes (UEC), thyroid function and urine microscopy and culture. Others (e.g. syphilis and HIV serology and C-reactive protein (CRP)) may be indicated. *Structural brain imaging* has a high yield in the detection of treatable neurological diseases when dementia presents with a history of less than 1 year's duration, focal neurological signs are present, symptoms are not typical of Alzheimer's disease, or the patient is aged less than 65, but has a low yield in other circumstances.

Management

Medical issues

Tasks include establishing a diagnosis of dementia and its most likely aetiology; excluding treatable causes, including depression and delirium as sole or contributing precipitants of confusion; and ensuring optimal physical health. The latter is important because patients with dementia often forget to mention symptoms, fail to attend appointments for investigations and do not take medications reliably. Incidental physical pathology is common, so doctors should look for it. Attention should be paid to the effects of the dementia or other mental disorder on family members who care for the affected person. Many carers are anxious, depressed or grieving, and may experience 'carer burnout'.

Cholinesterase inhibitors (donepezil, galantamine, rivastigmine) can improve the cognitive symptoms of Alzheimer's disease and slow its progression a little. Some treated patients become more alert and function better, but not all patients benefit. However, some patients worsen notably when medication is stopped, even in later stages. Cholinesterase inhibitors can cause nausea, vomiting, diarrhoea, vivid dreams and muscle cramps, but most patients do not develop these side effects if the dose is titrated up slowly. Rivastigmine is also available as a transdermal patch. *Memantine*, an NMDA receptor blocker, may be of modest benefit when patients cannot tolerate or fail to benefit from a cholinesterase inhibitor.

Psychotropic drugs have a limited role in dementia management. *Antipsychotic medications* are used when delusions, hallucinations, misidentifications or aggression distress the patient or others. Evidence for efficacy is limited. Risperidone (up to 2 mg daily) is the drug of choice because it has been tested most thoroughly in this population, but it (and other antipsychotics) may raise the risk of stroke and should be avoided in patients with poorly controlled atrial fibrillation, hypertension, diabetes mellitus, or previous stroke. These drugs can also contribute to Parkinsonism, weight gain and falls in some patients. If prescribed, drugs must be reviewed regularly, tapered and then ceased when the symptoms that prompted the prescription have remitted.

Antidepressants are used to treat comorbid major depression, but recent research has cast doubt on their efficacy in patients with dementia. Selective serotonin reuptake inhibitors (SSRIs) are the drugs of first choice.

Personal and family issues

People with mild dementia can express preferences about future care, assign enduring power of attorney and sometimes can make a will. The diagnosis should be explained with sensitivity and hope, given the availability of medications and excellent support services.

Assessment of activities of daily living is important. Are there difficulties with dressing, washing, toileting and bathing, or with cooking, housekeeping, shopping and handling money? How much help is needed and who gives it? What services are in place? Are relatives distressed by challenging or dangerous behaviours?

A diagnosis should be accompanied by advice to carers about strategies to minimise conflict. Argumentative patients should be humoured rather than challenged. Those who resist dressing or bathing should not be forced to conform to a timetable. Distraction, music and touch sometimes help. Carers need to ventilate concerns and have chances to rest. Home help, meals on wheels, day care, respite care, dosette boxes to organise medications, help with bathing, and carer support groups are often helpful. Patients and carers should be referred to Alzheimer's Australia for education, advice and carer support. Carers experience high rates of depression, anxiety, distress, isolation, physical ill health and financial hardship. These problems can be ameliorated by education, advice and support, and by treating any manifest psychiatric disorder.

Admission to a residential facility comes sooner for those who live alone or whose carer is frail, but a move from familiar surroundings can worsen confusion. Any such shift should be carefully planned.

Case example: Dementia

A 75-year-old woman was referred to an old age psychiatrist by her GP since the family was concerned regarding her progressive memory problems and irritability during the previous 6–12 months. She had been leaving the tap running and had burnt cooking pots on the stove several times. She was having trouble remembering familiar recipes despite having cooked them from memory for decades. During the previous 2 months she got lost several times and had to stop playing bridge because she was forgetting to count the cards and could no longer remember all the rules. She herself was annoyed at her family for insisting on an assessment since she felt her memory was no worse than that of her friends. *Assessment* revealed the presence of a mild dementia syndrome and *diagnostic work up* suggested late onset Alzheimer's disease as the most likely cause. *Treatment* included a trial of a cholinesterase inhibitor, and education and support for the family, including referral to Alzheimer's Australia.

Delirium

Delirium is characterised by acute onset of fluctuating cognitive impairment and diminished attention. It affects at least 20% of patients aged over 65 who enter a general hospital. It is often unrecognised. If a proper history is taken, a story of recent abrupt cognitive decline with a fluctuating mental state over hours or days, will emerge.

Prevention strategies should focus on orientation; early mobilisation; minimising the use of psychotropic drugs; preventing sleep deprivation; attention to hearing aids and spectacles; and prevention or treatment of dehydration.

Management of delirium involves treatment of its causes, supportive care, prevention of complications and treatment of behavioural symptoms. Adequate lighting and a quiet environment are preferred. Prevention of pressure sores and deep vein thrombosis, ensuring night-time sleep and encouraging day-time wakefulness, close supervision and clear communication to both patient and family are vital. *Psychotropic drugs* should be used only when symptoms are causing marked distress, threaten safety, or interrupt life-saving treatment. Haloperidol (0.5 to 1.0 mg two to three times daily) has been the traditional agent of choice in these circumstances, but olanzapine and risperidone are used increasingly, as haloperidol can produce marked extrapyramidal effects and can affect cardiac conduction.

Delirium can be frightening and bewildering. Families need support and information so that they can understand the changes seen in their relative. Recovered patients often need repeated reassurance and explanation of frightening memories of the delirious episode.

Case example: Delirium

A GP received a phone call from a hostel (low level aged care facility) regarding an 85-year-old female resident who had been her patient for some years. She was usually a very pleasant and quiet person. The staff reported that during the previous 3 days she had become increasingly irritable and agitated, showing fluctuating levels of confusion, more pronounced in the evening and at night. *Assessment* revealed the presence of a hyperactive delirium and *diagnostic work up* identified a urinary tract infection as the most likely cause. *Treatment* involved treating the underlying cause of her delirium with fluids and an antibiotic, as well as ensuring the safety of the patient and educating the staff.

Depression

(see also Chapter 8)

About 1% of older people fulfil criteria for a major depressive disorder and up to 20% have mild but significant depressive symptoms. Risk factors include female sex, previous depression, pain, physical or sensory handicap, personality disorder, adverse life events, lack of a confiding relationship and poverty. Depression can be triggered by physical conditions (e.g. cancer, stroke and degenerative neurological disorders) or medications (e.g. corticosteroids, L-Dopa, methyldopa). Cerebrovascular disease is an important contributing factor in some late-life depressions.

Suicide rates are quite high among older men. Those who commit suicide often live alone and have serious, disabling, painful physical illnesses. Manipulative overdoses are uncommon in old age; any expression of suicidal intent must be taken seriously.

Clinical features

Symptoms of depression are outlined in Chapter 8 and are similar in both older and younger patients. Psychotic features (delusions of poverty, disease or guilt) and hallucinations can occur but are uncommon. Depressed older people may be reluctant to admit to low mood even when other symptoms are prominent. Around two-thirds of depressed elderly people presenting for psychiatric treatment have had a previous episode.

Major depression can be hard to detect in people with serious physical illness. Somatic complaints may stem from new or pre-existing physical pathology or depression or both. Depression is likely if physical symptoms are out of keeping with physical signs, but heart failure, respiratory disease, renal failure and cancer also precipitate anorexia, insomnia and fatigue. The presence of severe anhedonia can be a useful diagnostic symptom when the clinical presentation of depression in the elderly is uncertain.

Late-life depression has a significant mortality because of its association with serious physical illness. Otherwise, prognosis is similar to that of younger age groups. Around 80% to 90% of patients recover or show significant improvement with treatment, but relapse rates are high. Usually continuing antidepressant treatment is required, especially if there is a past history of depressive relapses.

Assessment

Patients may believe that depression is a normal part of ageing. In some cultures emotional distress is expressed in somatic terms. Enquiries about mood and other relevant symptoms are necessary when depression is suspected.

Relevant elements of the history and mental state examination include questions about persistence and severity of depression, appetite, food and fluid intake, weight, sleep, energy and suicidal ideas. A physical examination and investigations (e.g. full blood count, UEC, LFTs, CRP, ESR, clinical chemistry including calcium, B12, folate and thyroid function tests, chest X-ray) can exclude physical causes.

Management

Social and psychological therapies

Supportive psychotherapy is useful. Family counselling may assist in improving relationships. Cognitive-behaviour therapy has a useful role in people with a practical outlook, and includes recording a schedule of pleasurable activities and positive reinforcement for tasks performed. Grief therapy is often useful and some patients appear to benefit from psychodynamic psychotherapy. Other strategies include attention to nutrition, regular exercise and social interaction.

Physical treatments

SSRIs and other modern antidepressants are the drugs of choice for moderate to severe depression. Starting doses are halved for old, frail people, but many require a standard adult dose. Electroconvulsive therapy (ECT) is indicated for marked psychomotor retardation or psychotic symptoms, in those who will not eat or drink and where there is a high risk of suicide.

A 72-year-old retired school teacher was referred by his GP to an old age psychiatry service, since treatment for his depression (the third episode he had experienced in 20 years) had been unsuccessful so far, and during his last visit he mentioned feeling himself to be a burden to his family and wanting to die. *Assessment* revealed the presence of sleep problems, marked depressed mood and anhedonia, especially during the morning, mood-congruent delusions (he was convinced that his family had been financially ruined because of him, although this was not true), loss of appetite and weight, and prominent suicidal ideation. *Diagnostic work up* indicated a major depressive episode, with mood-congruent delusions (psychotic depression) as the most likely diagnosis. *Treatment* involved admission to a psychiatric ward because of the severity of his illness and the risk of suicide. After unsuccessful treatment with a series of different antidepressants combined with antipsychotics, a course of 16 ECTs resulted in significant improvement. He was discharged on combined prophylactic antidepressant and low-dose antipsychotic medication with regular follow-up visits from members of the old age psychiatry treatment team.

Bipolar disorder

(see also Chapter 9)

Mania and bipolar disorder arising after age 50 should be presumed to be organic in origin until proven otherwise. Potential precipitants include antidepressants, ECT, stroke, head injury and medications such as corticosteroids and L-Dopa.

Elderly manic patients are overactive and show pressure of speech, flight of ideas, insomnia, disinhibition and poor judgement. Mood is often irritable and in some elderly patients manic and depressive symptoms coexist. Delusions and hallucinations can occur. Patients may be so pressured in thought and speech that they appear to have delirium or dementia.

Usually, admission to hospital is necessary. Atypical antipsychotics are indicated. Mood stabilisers are used acutely and in prophylaxis. Lithium is the treatment of choice, but has a low therapeutic index, and substantial side effects. In frail older people, ideal plasma levels are 0.4–0.6 mmol/L for treatment and prophylaxis. Sodium valproate is better tolerated, but evidence for its efficacy is less well established.

A 68-year-old man was admitted to a psychiatric ward after he had been brought to hospital by his case manager from the local Aged Psychiatry Assessment and Treatment team. The patient had been diagnosed with bipolar disorder in his early 20s and had had several episodes of both depression and mania throughout his life, with prolonged periods of inter-current normal functioning between these episodes. However, over the previous 4 weeks he showed increasing symptoms of mania with disinhibition, insomnia and euphoria, after his lithium medication had been stopped in hospital 6 weeks earlier when he was treated for kidney disease. Acutely he developed grandiose delusions, believing he had supernatural powers. *Assessment* and *diagnostic work up* revealed the presence of a manic episode in the context of bipolar disorder. *Treatment* involved atypical antipsychotics, sodium valproate, psychoeducation and social support.

Anxiety disorders

(see also Chapter 10)

Around 10% of the elderly experience significant symptoms of anxiety. Half of them have always been anxious, but anxiety disorders can arise following physical illness, bereavement, burglary, and other adverse events. Panic attacks can simulate angina or myocardial infarction. Many anxious people have a comorbid physical disease. Anxiety can lead to avoidance behaviour; for example, an accidental fall may be followed by reluctance to go out.

Anxious patients need reassurance. Mild episodes often remit spontaneously, but conditions associated with avoidance or panic merit intervention. Anxiolytic medications should be avoided to prevent falls and dependence. Better options include an explanation of the nature of anxiety symptoms, relaxation training and graded exposure to stressors. Cognitive-behaviour therapy is effective, but underused due to a lack of trained practitioners. If non-drug treatments fail, a medium-acting benzodiazepine may be warranted for a few days (e.g. oxazepam 7.5 mg twice daily). Some anxious patients, even those in whom depression is not prominent, are helped by the regular prescription of an SSRI antidepressant.

Case example: Anxiety

An 80-year-old woman visited her doctor asking for medication to help her sleep. She had recently been widowed after 50 years of marriage and felt unsafe alone in the house. After her neighbour experienced a home invasion she felt anxious all day, but especially at night. *Assessment and diagnostic work up* revealed significant symptoms of anxiety in the context of recent bereavement. Physical examination was normal and investigation revealed normal thyroid function. *Treatment* focused on grief-focused cognitive-behaviour therapy and avoiding benzodiazepine dependency.

Schizophrenia and delusional disorder

(see also Chapter 7)

Schizophrenia is described in Chapter 7. It can arise for the first time in old age and is then more likely to affect women than men. In such cases organic causes should be considered. Delirium, dementia and mood disorder are differential diagnoses; all may present with delusions, hallucinations and disturbed behaviour.

Most older people with schizophrenia have had it for decades. Some remain psychotic, but negative symptoms tend to predominate. Patients who spent years in old psychiatric hospitals have few social and personal care skills. Complications include susceptibility to the side effects of antipsychotics, polypharmacy and the loss of caring relatives. Isolation, poverty and sub-standard accommodation are common.

Delusional disorder is uncommon, tending to develop over months or years. Delusions are banal and unsystematised: neighbours are accused of banging on walls and throwing rubbish over fences. Less often, patients are convinced that malign entities tap their telephones or irradiate them. Risk factors include female sex, a suspicious personality and a family history of psychosis.

Management

Some patients are so frightened that help is gladly received. Others refuse help and insist that treatment is unwarranted. Involuntary hospital admission may be necessary. Physical examination and laboratory tests are required. Atypical antipsychotics are better tolerated than the older (i.e. first generation) ones. Treatment is long-term.

Case example: Schizophrenia

A 65-year-old woman, living alone, was visited at home by the local Aged Psychiatry Assessment and Treatment team. The neighbourhood police station had contacted the team after she had repeatedly visited the police station (several times every day) complaining that her neighbour was trying to poison her. She had been visiting the police station with these claims occasionally over the previous 3 years, but in the past the police had been able to reassure and calm her. She now stated that she could hear her neighbour pumping poisonous gas through the walls and she was convinced that he observed her via her television. Despite the police having investigated these claims and finding no evidence for them, she had increased the frequency of her visits to the police station, often appearing very distressed. *Assessment and diagnostic work up* revealed the presence of psychotic symptoms (delusions and hallucinations, as well as ideas of reference), suggesting schizophrenia as the likely underlying cause of her symptoms. *Treatment* included atypical antipsychotics, psychoeducation and social support.

REFERENCES AND FURTHER READING

Access Economics 2009 The dementia epidemic: economic impact and positive solutions for Australia. Available online at www.alzheimers.org.au.

Ames, D., Chiu, E., Lindesay, J., Shulman, K. (Eds.), 2010. Guide to the psychiatry of old age. Cambridge Medicine, Cambridge.

Folstein, M., Folstein, S., McHugh, P., 1975. The Mini Mental State: a practical method for grading to cognitive state of patients for the clinician. Journal of Psychiatric Research 12, 189–198.

Inouye, SK., 2006. Delirium in older persons. New England Journal of Medicine 354, 1157–1165.

Jacoby, R., Oppenheimer, C., Dening, T., Thomas, A. (Eds.), 2007. Oxford textbook of old age psychiatry. Oxford University Press, Oxford.

A DAUGHTER NAMED SOPHIA

CASE-BASED LEARNING

ANDREW GLEASON & JOEL KING

The following role-play requires two participants: one to play an intern (candidate) and another to play a patient's daughter named Sophia (actor).

OSCE Station Instructions

(Reading time: 2 minutes)

You are an intern working in the emergency department. Your consultant asks you to see Mrs Gladys Elder, a 67-year-old lady who has been brought in by her daughter, Sophia, who can no longer cope with Mrs Elder at home. Sophia would like to talk with you before you see her mother.

Task (10 minutes)

- Take a collateral history from Sophia (8 minutes).
- Towards the end of the interview Sophia will ask you what you think is wrong with her mother, and what you plan to do. Tell her your main differential diagnoses and explain your short-term management plan.

Actor role: Sophia Elder

You are 38 years old and live with your husband, Rick, in your mother's house. Rick runs a very busy hardware store. You have two children, aged 2 and 4. You work two days a week in the local newsagency.

Four years ago your father died of a sudden heart attack. He was 15 years older than your mother. You were worried that your mum would be lonely living on her own, so you and Rick moved in with her. You were pregnant with your first child at the time, which meant your mum would be able to help out with your new child. Your mum is now 67 years old.

HISTORY OF PRESENTING ILLNESS

You are really worried because last night Mum barricaded herself in the house while you were at work. When you got home it took you 45 minutes to convince her to let you in. She insisted that she had seen a burglar in the yard, so she bolted the doors and put chairs against them. Mum couldn't explain why she wouldn't let you in. She settled down pretty quickly after you came inside. You weren't really sure what to do but in the morning it occurred to you that maybe she had suffered a stroke because you had read in a magazine that strokes can cause funny behaviour, so you called your GP. He told you to take Mum to hospital.

Mum's behaviour has been changing for a while now. You are not sure exactly when it all started. Your mum did a few odd things after you all moved in together, but you figured this was because she was grieving for your dad. For example, Mum took a wrong turn walking to the local grocery store six months after you moved in. This seemed really odd because she has been walking that same route for 35 years. Most of the change has been over the last two years or so, but it has become more noticeable over the last six months.

The main problem is that she is becoming muddled and forgetful of new information. This seems to be gradually progressing. Mum will clean the kitchen, and then go back and do it again an hour later. You have to tell her things over and over again, and she still doesn't seem to get it. She sometimes puts her clothes on the wrong way, for example, putting on her cardigan inside out or putting buttons of her blouse in the wrong holes. She has developed problems organising and preparing meals. A few times she has left the stove on. There are some circular burn marks on the kitchen floor, and you think that your mum must have put pots on the floor when they were still hot. She also sometimes uses the wrong word for things. For example, she couldn't seem to remember the word for 'remote control' the other day and called it the 'TV thingy'. She also gets your children's names mixed up.

You are worried about Mum's weight. She has lost 10 kg over the last six months. Her intake has decreased, but you aren't sure if this is enough to explain the weight loss.

Mum's mood has been okay overall, but sometimes she gets really anxious. This seems to happen when she has recently forgotten something. She will get really agitated for about 30 minutes and then settle down. She is sleeping well.

If the doctor asks you about whether your mother has seen or heard things that aren't there, think about this, and say that maybe she hallucinated the burglar in the yard, but otherwise she hasn't done or said anything that would suggest a hallucination.

Mum's walking seems slightly slower, but otherwise you haven't noticed any changes in her movements. She hasn't had any falls. You are not aware of any incontinence. You are not aware of any symptoms suggestive of acute neurological deficits such as sensory loss, weakness, headaches, etc.

In terms of day-to-day function your mum has trouble cooking and you do need to help her at times when she gets her clothes on the wrong way. She can wash herself and eat without any assistance. Your mum does go shopping on her own occasionally, but you are worried about this, so usually you shop together. Your husband has managed all of the finances since you moved in with your mother. Your mum hasn't driven a car for years.

PAST MEDICAL HISTORY

Your mum has a history of high blood pressure and cholesterol. She had gallstones a few years ago.

PAST PSYCHIATRIC HISTORY

You have heard that Mum had a period of post-natal depression after your brother was born but you don't know any details about it.

MEDICATIONS

Mum takes a blood pressure tablet and a cholesterol tablet. You had seen her take the tablets twice on a few occasions, so you asked the pharmacist to put the medications in one of those blister packs. This has worked well.

DRUG AND ALCOHOL HISTORY

Mum often has a small glass of sherry in the evening, but never more than this. She has smoked since she was in her twenties. You really wish she would stop, but she has cut down from a pack per day to ten per day since your dad died.

SOCIAL HISTORY

You don't know anything about your mum's early development but guess that it was normal. Your mum did well in school and left at the age of 18. She worked as a seamstress for two years before getting married to your father, who was a civil engineer. They met at church. She had two children, your brother, David (now aged 43) and you. She had David when she was 24. David is an accountant for a large firm and currently lives overseas. Your mum spent most of her life doing domestic duties, but she was actively involved in local church charities. Now she spends her time helping look after your children.

Statements you must make:

- Open with 'Doctor, you have to help me with my mum. You see, I have two young children of my own and I can't look after them and Mum any more.'
- 'Do you think that maybe she hasn't gotten over Dad's death? Could depression be causing all of this?'
- 'My neighbour said that this could be dementia. What do you think? But she's only 67, I thought dementia happened when people are in their late seventies or eighties.'

Model Answer

Sophia asks what the cause of her mother's condition might be. Although the history is suggestive of a dementia such as Alzheimer's disease, this cannot be determined on collateral history alone. It would be reasonable to say to Sophia that some of the things she has thought about, such as dementia and depression, are possibilities, but further investigation is needed to determine the cause.

In the short term it is essential to investigate for a reversible dementia (see Box 19.2, below) as well as a delirium, either as the sole condition or superimposed on a dementia. The time course of this vignette is not suggestive of a delirium as the sole causative condition, but this cannot be excluded on history alone. Delirium is common and should be part of the differential diagnosis of any behavioural change in older people. Some of the features that commonly distinguish delirium, dementia, and depression are listed in Table 19.2 (page 331; also see Chapter 6). In delirium, attention is usually impaired and sleep-wake cycle is frequently altered. Dementia may affect various domains of cognitive function, such as praxis and language, depending on the anatomical distribution of pathology and the type of dementia. Behavioural and psychological symptoms also occur (see Box 19.1, page 319).

The candidate will explain that they need to take a history from, and perform cognitive and physical examinations on Mrs Elder. A standardised cognitive

Box 19.2
Some reversible causes of dementia

- Structural causes (subdural haematoma, hydrocephalus)
- Substance induced (alcohol, anticholinergics, hypnotics)
- Malignancy (primary CNS, metastases, paraneoplastic syndromes)
- Infection (encephalitis, HIV, syphilis)
- Vitamin deficiency (B12, folate, niacin)
- Inflammatory conditions (vasculitis)
- Endocrine disease (hypothyroidism)
- Obstructive sleep apnoea
- Depression (i.e. depressive pseudodementia).

Table 19.2

Common features that help distinguish delirium, dementia, and depression

Features	Delirium	Dementia	Depression
Onset	Rapid	Insidious	Varies
Course	Fluctuating	Progressive	Often episodic
Duration	Days to weeks	Months to years	Weeks to months
Consciousness	Clouded	Clear	Varies
Mood	May fluctuate	May fluctuate	Pervasively low

screening instrument, such as the Mini-Mental State Examination, should form part of the cognitive examination. A thorough physical examination is necessary to look for treatable or comorbid conditions. Blood tests also assist with this, and might include full blood count, urea, creatinine, electrolytes, liver function tests, calcium, thyroid function tests, vitamin B12 and folate (see page 320 and Table 19.2 above). Cerebral imaging needs to be performed. As a minimum, computerised tomography should be done to look for evidence of a cerebrovascular or neoplastic cause for her symptoms. Magnetic resonance imaging may also be helpful in ruling in a dementia as well as ruling out other causes, although this does not necessarily need to be done in the emergency department. Other tests may be indicated depending on the history and examination findings. For example, Mrs Elder might need urine microscopy and culture, and a chest roentgenogram. Mrs Elder may also require further investigations to seek the cause of her weight loss. Collateral history should be obtained from her GP.

From a practical point of view, Mrs Elder will probably need a hospital admission, partly for the purpose of investigation, and also because Sophia is finding it difficult to manage her mother at home. As an intern in the emergency department, the candidate should seek an admission under the geriatrics, psychogeriatrics, or general medical unit.

A medical student performing this station will recognise that while dementia is the most likely diagnosis, this cannot be determined on the history alone. A reasonable list of differential diagnoses, including reversible causes of dementia, should be given. A medical student should also recognise the need for a cognitive examination and thorough physical examination and propose suitable investigations, including blood tests and cerebral imaging.

Chapter 20

FORENSIC PSYCHIATRY AND RISK ASSESSMENT

DANNY SULLIVAN

Forensic psychiatry is the specialty that deals with the interface between law and mental health. Thus, forensic psychiatrists work in prisons, community clinics and secure hospitals. They may give evidence in court or be involved in advising lawyers and judges on the relationship between psychiatric disorders and legal issues, such as offending, compensation and decision-making capacity. This involves the assessment and treatment of a range of different conditions, the provision of medico-legal reports and the giving of evidence in courts and tribunals.

The core skills of a forensic psychiatrist are not inherently different from those of the general adult psychiatrist (or in some situations, child and adolescent or old age psychiatrist): what differs is an understanding of the legal and ethical context in which their skills are used. In addition, some specialised areas of practice may be developed (e.g. in the assessment and management of sexual offenders).

Areas of work for the forensic psychiatrist

Civil arena

Many forensic psychiatrists work in the private sector and provide medico-legal opinions, predominantly relating to civil matters. These include insurance – mainly workers'

Box 20.1

Psychiatric diagnoses commonly encountered in civil forensic practice

Diagnoses include:

- acquired brain injury (head trauma)
- organic mental disorder (toxin exposure)
- depressive syndromes
- anxiety syndromes
- post-traumatic stress disorder (PTSD)
- pain disorders
- protracted adjustment disorders
- malingering/factitious disorder.

compensation and traffic accidents – as well as providing psychiatric reports for other jurisdictions such as professional registration boards.

There are a range of psychiatric consequences that may develop from workplace or traffic accidents (see Box 20.1). But moreover, premorbid personality and mental disorder may affect the development of psychiatric illness, and forensic psychiatrists are involved in assisting the trier of fact (court, tribunal or insurer) to determine what was pre-existing and what someone else is liable for.

Note, however, there are many other pre-existing diagnoses that may impact upon the development of psychiatric disorders that may be attributed to a traumatic event.

Children and family

Issues of child sexual abuse, neglected children and psychiatric issues related to the break-down of relationships are the specialty of some forensic psychiatrists, often with child and adolescent psychiatric training. They provide opinions to assist the court in determining how to regulate relationship breakdowns and look after the welfare of children.

Criminal jurisdictions

Most people think of forensic psychiatrists as working in criminal jurisdictions. In these areas, forensic mental health services are involved in many stages of the care of mentally disordered offenders. Such offenders may be diverted from police custody into psychiatric units. The prevalence of mental disorder in people remanded in custody is greatly increased compared to the general community, as is the proportion of people with troublesome substance use. Court liaison services assess and divert some mentally disordered offenders.

Once imprisoned, individuals with mental disorders are assessed and managed by forensic mental health staff, although it should be noted that compulsory treatment is not permitted in prisons. Mental disorders are overrepresented in the prison system. Overall, well over half of all people remanded in custody have significant substance abuse problems; personality disorders are massively increased; and the prevalence of psychotic illnesses is approximately eight times that of the general population and possibly more for women. In the United States, some prisons have so many mentally disordered people that they qualify as the largest psychiatric institutions in the country.

Some people with mental disorder are not able to be managed in the prison system. Typically, they have severe mental health problems and refuse treatment. Most mental health legislation provides for the involuntary transfer of prisoners to secure psychiatric facilities for treatment.

Secure psychiatric units

Secure units are classified as *high, medium* and *low* secure. High secure units generally have a perimeter wall and complex security arrangements, including biometric scanning, registration of visitors, and a range of processes to maintain security in the unit. Medium secure units may not have a perimeter wall, but are locked. Low secure units do not provide the same level of security and are used for patients who have community access, although with conditions.

Secure psychiatric units are designed to meet the treatment and rehabilitation needs of mentally disordered offenders who may pose a significant risk to the community. The length of stay is much longer than in general psychiatric units, and staffing levels are often much higher.

The courts and fitness to plead

The expert opinions of forensic psychiatrists, who give evidence in court and are available to be examined and cross-examined by barristers, is integral to the use of so-called mental state defences.

When a person is considered to have offended while mentally ill, legal systems take this into account. In some cases insanity or mental impairment provisions exist which enable a person to be found 'not guilty by reason of insanity' or to be similarly acquitted, if at the time of offending their mental disorder interfered grossly with their reasoning. However, despite acquittal, the person is likely to be detained thereafter in hospital or subject to treatment provisions to reduce the risk to the community.

At the stage of a trial, some accused people are psychiatrically unwell or have significant cognitive impairment, which prevents them from fairly participating in a trial. When the question is raised, the court may engage in a formal process to determine whether or not the person is fit to stand trial. This involves assessment, expert evidence and a determination of whether or not the person is able to understand and follow legal proceedings. In the event that they are not, the person may be directed to remain in prison or hospital for an indefinite term: the trial does not proceed.

Case example: Fitness to plead

A 52-year-old man was charged with sexual offences against his children, alleged to have occurred 10 years previously. Since then he had been in a car accident and sustained a severe brain injury. A recent neuropsychological assessment demonstrated impairments of memory and attention, and significant frontal lobe

Continued

Case example continued

injury. The injury was documented and the cognitive assessment was consistent with neuroimaging scans.

Both the prosecution and defence arranged forensic psychiatrist assessments. The psychiatrists reviewed the documentation, assessed the defendant and provided reports to court. Instead of hearing the criminal allegations, the court conducted a special hearing into the issue of fitness to be tried. Both psychiatrists gave evidence and were cross-examined in front of a jury. They stated that his brain injury meant that he could not understand the evidence and would not be able to follow a trial or instruct his lawyer in order to participate meaningfully in a trial. The jury found that he was not fit to be tried.

As a result, no criminal trial proceeded, and he returned to live in a residential facility in the community, with conditions of psychiatric supervision.

Box 20.2
Particular risk markers in schizophrenia

Risk markers include:

- persecutory delusions that a person is under threat
- passivity phenomena (the experience that one's thoughts, actions or moods are taken over by others)
- delusional jealousy
- delusional beliefs specifically targeted upon one Individual.

Risk assessment

Forensic mental health expertise is frequently used in the prediction of risk, the management of high-risk patients, and formal assessments of people who might pose a risk. Risk assessment is integrated with risk management, as there is little benefit in defining risk without determining how to intervene to diminish it!

Risk can be defined as the likelihood of a chosen outcome. In forensic practice, the likelihood is strongly associated with the outcome of concern. For example, an exhibitionist may expose himself to hundreds of women, but the harm may not be significant, whereas a single episode of penetrative sexual abuse against a child is more likely to have significant and lasting consequences. Thus, the risk posed by the latter offender is much greater.

Schizophrenia is associated with violent offending, although for some years this association was discounted. Rates of violence are two to five times greater, and around tenfold increased for homicide. Some violence is situational and difficult to predict. It is, however, clear that associated substance abuse and specific difficult personality traits may amplify this risk. Certain specific symptoms or behaviours may accentuate risk in schizophrenia: these are shown in Box 20.2.

Risk factors are *static* or *dynamic*. The former consist of historical or demographic variables such as gender or a history of serious violence. The factors are immutable, although other counterfactual factors may alter the risk. For example, a man with a long history of violence who is 60 and has had a stroke may register as high risk on historical analysis, but the counterfactual element of a severe physical disability reduces his ability to be aggressive.

Dynamic risk factors are changeable variables. Some are rapidly variable, such as intoxication; others act over the longer term, such as unstable accommodation.

Risk assessment involves a variety of methods, including:

- clinical judgement
- actuarial prediction
- adjusted actuarial assessment
- structured professional judgement.

Initially, risk assessment was historically conflated with dangerousness prediction. At that time, the prevailing thought was that violence was inherently unpredictable, and not strongly associated with psychotic illness. In addition, dangerousness was described as a trait inherent in certain individuals, rather than the effect of a range of different factors pertaining to an individual.

Clinical judgement of risk may be unstructured, involving intuition or 'clinical experience'. However, research has demonstrated that clinical judgement is rarely better than chance at predicting which patients will act violently.

In some cases, clinical judgement includes a functional analysis of behaviours (see Box 20.3). This permits an examination of the problem behaviour or historical event, and will generate both hypotheses about the behaviour and ideas about how best to reduce its recurrence.

Actuarial prediction has focused upon analysing data about past violent offenders to generate probabilistic algorithms and translate them into useful instruments to predict future risk. The evidence from large surveys supports the improved prediction characteristics of actuarial instruments. *Adjusted actuarial assessment* involves modifying the result of actuarial prediction by considering idiosyncratic features of the individual being assessed and tweaking the result accordingly.

More recently, these have been combined with the current preferred approach to risk assessment: *structured professional judgement*. This involves the use of (preferably multiple) empirically derived risk assessment instruments that address both static and dynamic risk factors. The ratings obtained from these instruments are used in subsequent case-specific modification of the resultant risk estimate, to reflect the individual characteristics of the specific person (as the risk instruments are based upon categories or groups, rather than the unique characteristics of the specific offender being considered). The structured professional judgement method is current best practice in risk assessment.

Box 20.3

Functional analysis of behaviours: A–B–C

Functional analysis comprises clinical judgements about:

- **A**ntecedent thoughts, emotions and circumstances
- the actual concerning **B**ehaviours, and
- consideration of the **C**onsequences of the behaviour and their effects on the protagonist.

Box 20.4

The HCR–20

Historical items

H1.   Previous violence

H2.   Young age at first violent incident

H3.   Relationship problems

H4.   Employment problems

H5.   Substance use problems

H6.   Major mental illness

H7.   Psychopathy

H8.   Early maladjustment

H9.   Personality disorder

H10. Prior release or detention failure

Clinical items

C1.   Lack of insight

C2.   Negative attitudes

C3.   Active symptoms of major mental illness

C4.   Impulsivity

C5.   Unresponsive to treatment

Risk items

R1.   Plans lack feasibility

R2.   Exposure to destabilisers

R3.   Lack of personal support

R4.   Non-compliance with remediation attempts

R5.   Stress

(Webster et al 1997)

Risk assessment instruments

Risk assessment instruments have a variety of acronym-based names. The most commonly used is the HCR–20 (see Box 20.4), which is a structured instrument to predict violence based on historical, clinical and risk variables spread across 20 domains. It is reliable, valid and easy to use. Each item is marked 0, 1 or 2 (corresponding to absent, partially present or uncertain, and definitely present). The score is less important than the spread of scores, and the HCR–20 presents targets for intervention which may reduce risk.

There are strong arguments to use this instrument in routine psychiatric practice, based in part upon the fact that the prediction of violence is so difficult (as serious violence is relatively rare) and its consequences are so dire.

Other instruments, such as the STATIC–99, are of use for the prediction of future risk in convicted sexual offenders. The plethora of risk assessment instruments available reflects that an instrument must be applicable to the category of person being assessed, and thus instruments may not apply to different samples such as women, youth or people with intellectual disability.

A concept known as *psychopathy* is often invoked. This pejorative term is based upon a particular assessment, the Psychopathy Checklist. Psychopathy is an individual risk factor and is also enmeshed with other risk factors, but is robustly associated with increased rates of offending behaviours, particularly when associated with mental disorder and substance use.

The current trend in risk assessment is increasingly to focus upon the dynamic variables that may indicate concurrent instability and increase the risk of imminent serious violence.

REFERENCES AND FURTHER READING

Bronitt, S., McSherry, B., 2005. Principles of criminal law, 2nd ed. Lawbook Co, Sydney.

Gilligan, J., 2001. Preventing violence. Thames & Hudson, London.

Hollin, C., 2004. The essential handbook of offender assessment and treatment. Wiley, Chichester.

Laws, D.R., O'Donohue, W.T., 2008. Sexual deviance: theory, assessment and treatment, 2nd ed. Guildford Press, New York.

Maden, A., 2007. Treating violence. Oxford University Press, Oxford.

Mullen, P.E., 2000. Dangerousness, risk and the prediction of probability. In: Gelder, M.G., López-Ibor, J., Andreasen, N.C. (Eds.), New Oxford textbook of psychiatry. Oxford University Press, Oxford.

Soothill, K., Rogers, P., Dolan, M., 2008. Handbook of forensic mental health. Willan Publishing, Devon.

Wallace, C., Mullen, P.E., Burgess, P., 2004. Criminal offending in schizophrenia over a 25-year period marked by deinstitutionalization and increasing prevalence of comorbid substance use disorders. American Journal of Psychiatry 161, 716–727.

Webster, C.D., Douglas, K.S., Eaves, D., et al., 1997. Assessing risk for violence, version 2. Simon Fraser University, British Columbia.

CHAPTER 20

AN ACADEMIC NAMED ALI
CASE-BASED LEARNING

ANDREW GLEASON & JOEL KING

The following role-play requires two participants: one to play an emergency department resident (candidate) and another to play both the role of a patient, Ali Husain, and the examiner (actor).

OSCE Station Instructions

(Reading time: 2 minutes)

You are a resident working in a metropolitan emergency department. Your next patient is Mr Ali Husain, who is 26 years old. He has been brought into emergency by the police, who say he tried to jump out of a window at the university after breaking into his PhD supervisor's office. The police say he has been behaving strangely and are afraid that he is suicidal. They do not want to press charges because they believe he is mentally unwell.

Tasks (10 minutes)

- Take a history from Mr Husain, including a risk assessment.
- After 8 minutes you must terminate the interview and present your differential diagnoses and immediate management plan to the examiner. The examiner will ask you questions about managing the risks in this case (2 minutes).

Actor role: Ali Husain

You are a 26-year-old, originally from the United Arab Emirates. You moved to this country two years ago to undertake a PhD in electrical engineering. You live in a single room in university housing.

Over the last few weeks you have developed a brilliant design for a new type of microchip which is smaller and faster than any developed to date. The chip also has embedded radio frequency technology that will transmit very large amounts of data much faster than current wired technology, obviating the need for cables to connect to monitors. Last Tuesday a page of the blueprints went missing from your office at the university. You searched everywhere for the page, to no avail. The next day you saw your PhD supervisor, Professor Flavia. You knew that he had taken it the moment he said hello. There was something about the tone of his voice, and the expression on his face, that confirmed your suspicions. He has also managed to impersonate several other students in the lab so that he can more closely monitor your activities. You believe that Professor Flavia recognises your superior intelligence, and has been trying to stimulate and support you just long enough for you to produce the device. He is secretly working with some executives from a microchip company based in Mumbai.

This morning, you noticed a slightly metallic taste in your coffee. You are afraid that Professor Flavia placed arsenic in it in an attempt to poison you. One of the other PhD students in the lab, whom Professor Flavia is impersonating, was looking at you when you took a sip. You realised that you had to escape immediately. The only safe place for you to go is Silicon Valley where a friend will help you finish developing the chip. You sneaked into Professor Flavia's office to take one last look for the blueprints before you left for the airport. You turned the office upside down but the blueprints were nowhere to be found. When you opened the office door, you saw some police officers at the other end of the hallway. Professor Flavia had sent them to kill you. They must have been employees of the microchip company masquerading as police. The only choice you had was to jump out the window, because the police were going to torture you until you revealed your plans for the chip in full detail. You bolted the door and opened the window. The police broke down the door and grabbed you just before you were able to climb through the window. You realised you might die or be injured if you jumped but figured this was better than capture and regarded climbing through the window as your only possible means of escape.

You think that you have been taken to hospital so that Professor Flavia can sedate you and extract the remaining plans for the microchip from your brain before he kills you.

If asked about other suicidal thoughts, you saw a man outside the window of your room two days ago wearing a suit. You recognised that he was sent by the microchip company. You thought about grabbing a knife from the kitchen to slit your throat before he got you, but you hesitated, and he disappeared shortly after.

You have not had any violent or homicidal thoughts, but if you were cornered by Professor Flavia or anyone in cahoots with him, you would do whatever is necessary to protect your life and escape. You have been carrying a knife in your bag just in case you need it.

Your mood has been in the normal range recently (say 'fine'). You have not experienced any hallucinations.

PAST HISTORY

You have no past psychiatric history. You had an appendectomy at the age of 22.

DRUG AND ALCOHOL HISTORY

Three months ago you began to take small quantities of speed intranasally (but not intravenously) in order to help you stay up longer. When you developed the idea for the microchip you wanted to stay up as long as possible so that you could complete the design while the ideas were still fresh. You have needed to increase your use in order to stay awake, and you are now taking about one to three grams most days. You have not slept for three days. You used very small quantities of speed in the past when taking exams in your bachelor's degree. Until recently, you had never taken more than one line in an evening because you were very cautious about maintaining your ability to work. You have never driven while intoxicated or used it in situations where it is physically hazardous. You do not have symptoms of amphetamine dependence, such as tolerance, withdrawal, using more than intended, or unsuccessful attempts to cut down. You have not experienced any physical adverse effects from amphetamines aside from mild bruxism. You buy the speed from another student.

You drink two to five cups of coffee most days. You do not drink alcohol or use any other drugs. You do not smoke cigarettes.

FORENSIC HISTORY

You have no forensic history.

FAMILY HISTORY

You have no family history of psychiatric conditions or substance abuse. Your father has eczema and your maternal grandfather died of a stroke at the age of 64.

PERSONAL AND DEVELOPMENTAL HISTORY

Your early development is unremarkable. You always did well in school. Your father is on the board of directors for a large international company. You went to boarding school in Switzerland. You completed a bachelor's degree with a double major in electrical engineering and information technology at a prestigious university in the United States. You then worked for a computer firm in Boston for one year before winning a scholarship to do your PhD.

You had a girlfriend for two years while in the United States. You are friends with some other PhD students. You have meals or watch movies together on occasion.

HOW TO PLAY THE ROLE

You talk enthusiastically about your plans for the new microchip to the doctor. Somehow, you don't seem to realise that openly discussing these ideas is discordant with your paranoid fears. If the doctor talks about admitting you to hospital, explain that you must leave so that you can fly to Silicon Valley. If the doctor asks for your knife, it is in your bag that you gave to the nurse.

Statements you must make:

- 'You have to help me escape before Professor Flavia kills me. I need to get on a plane to San Francisco tonight.'
- 'I hope you're not planning on admitting me to hospital, Doctor. This is part of Professor Flavia's plan. He wants to have me sedated so that he can extract the remaining information about the chip design from my brain. He's going to kill me.'

Actor role: examiner

You do not need to interrupt the presentation, but if the risk assessment is cursory you may ask for further detail. If the candidate does not mention the need to do a physical examination or order investigations, you should ask them what they would look for on physical examination and/or what investigations they wish to order.

Questions you must ask:

- 'Please list at least four risks in this scenario.'
- 'How would you manage these risks?'

Model Answer

This is a case of amphetamine-induced psychosis. Differential diagnoses with respect to the patient's psychotic symptoms include schizophrenia, a brief psychotic disorder, a manic episode, and a psychotic disorder due to a general medical condition. Amphetamine abuse and dependence are also differential diagnoses.

There are many risks in this case. For example, Mr Husain is a risk to his personal and professional reputation. He is at risk of injury (e.g. if he had jumped out of the window, or if he had got into a fight in response to his delusional beliefs) and of suicide. He is at risk of misadventure and financial loss, e.g. if he had purchased a ticket overseas and flown to the United States. He is at risk of an undiagnosed medical condition, either causing his psychotic symptoms or as a consequence of them. People with psychotic conditions and mood disorders are also often at risk through impaired self-care, such as dehydration or malnutrition. There are also risks to others, including a risk of injury or even death to Professor Flavia. There is a risk of damage to Professor Flavia's property, as a consequence of Mr Husain's delusional beliefs. There is a potential risk to staff in the emergency department if Mr Husain were to become aggressive or incorporate them into his delusional system.

The medical resident and other staff should consider their own safety when interacting with Mr Husain. It would be wise for the initial interview to take place with a second staff member present. Interacting in a calm and empathic manner will help Mr Husain feel at ease. He is most likely confused and frightened.

Immediate management in the emergency department will include consideration of a one-to-one nurse, given that Mr Husain is fearful and may abscond. If he remains settled, he may be manageable in a cubicle, but many emergency departments have special rooms for agitated or aggressive patients.

The management plan should include a thorough physical examination, looking for consequences of the psychotic symptoms, such as physical injury or dehydration, as well as for medical causes of psychosis and comorbid medical conditions. Physical sequelae of substance use should also be sought (e.g. track marks). It is important to also note that comorbid medical conditions are not uncommon in people with psychotic conditions and in substance users, and are often not adequately screened for on physical examination. Basic blood tests should be performed as a screen for a medical cause or comorbid condition, and also to establish a baseline prior to the use of any pharmacotherapy (e.g. full blood examination, electrolytes, creatinine, liver function tests, and thyroid function tests). There should be a low threshold for neuroimaging if there is any suggestion of a neurological cause or comorbidity.

If he is significantly anxious or agitated, Mr Husain may require an anxiolytic such as a benzodiazepine. There are some situations where highly agitated patients require restraint, but this is very rare and best avoided if at all possible – coercive management of an already fearful and anxious patient will often exacerbate the situation.

A resident working in the emergency department should discuss the case with their supervising registrar or consultant if they have any uncertainties about the work-up or management plan. They should request a psychiatry consult. Usually, the decision about whether to use antipsychotics would be made by the psychiatry team. Some cases of drug-induced psychosis will settle after a period of abstinence without the use of antipsychotics.

The Mental Health Act may need to be used if the patient wants to leave hospital, though it may also be possible to manage Mr Husain on a voluntary basis if he is agreeable. It would be sensible for the emergency resident to discuss the use of the Mental Health Act with the psychiatry registrar if any concerns arise prior to the registrar seeing the patient. In many jurisdictions, mental health paperwork can be initiated by any medical practitioner, but if there is any uncertainty about whether this should be done it is best discussed with the psychiatry team first.

The advanced candidate will be aware of duty-to-warn issues, though the decision to warn or act to protect others at risk would usually lie with seniors rather than a junior doctor. The most famous legal precedent is Tarasoff v. Regents of the University of California, where it was determined that health professionals in the state of California have a duty to protect an intended victim (see Chapter 2, pages 30–31).

Chapter 21

DUAL DISABILITY

CHAD BENNETT

Dual disability refers to the coexistence of an intellectual disability (ID) or autism with mental health problems. Both ID and autism are classified as developmental disorders and require evidence of their presence in the first 18 years of life for a diagnosis to be made. However, the manifestations of these disorders extend into adulthood and the field of dual disability is concerned with the mental health of adults with either ID or autism. The need for this specialty arises because the presence of a developmental disorder both increases the risk of comorbid mental disorders, and complicates their assessment and management.

This chapter provides a brief overview of ID and autism, before concentrating on dual disability.

Intellectual disability

The concept of an intellectual disability (ID) is that some people have difficulty in caring for themselves due to deficits in intelligence. The current DSM–IV–TR uses the term 'mental retardation'. The criteria are shown in Box 21.1. DSM–5 proposes to use the term *intellectual developmental disorder*, as this is thought to be more descriptive of the actual problem and is more consistent with international usage.

Box 21.1
DSM–IV–TR criteria for mental retardation (synopsis)

DSM–IV–TR criteria are:

A significantly sub-average intellectual functioning: an IQ of 70 or below (for infants, a clinical judgement of significantly sub-average intellectual functioning)

B concurrent deficits or impairments in adaptive functioning in at least two of the following areas: communication, self-care, home living, social/interpersonal skills, use of community resources, self-direction, functional academic skills, work, leisure, health and safety

C onset before age 18 years.

This is further sub-categorised based on the degree of severity of intellectual impairment, as follows:

* mild: IQ level 50–55 to approximately 70
* moderate: IQ level 35–40 to 50–55
* severe: IQ level 20–25 to 35–40
* profound: IQ level below 20.

In making a diagnosis, a person's culture needs to be considered as a reference point in deciding if function is significantly impaired, and less emphasis will be placed on IQ scores in coding.

The number of *adaptive functioning domains* is reduced in DSM-5 and is now based on factor analytic studies of adaptive behaviour that best determine impairments and level of overall functioning leading to a restriction in participation and performance in one or more aspects of daily life activities, such as communication, social participation, functioning at school or at work, or personal independence at home or in community settings.

Population surveys usually find that about 2% of the population have an ID. People with severe ID are more likely to be identified early in life , as well as an identifiable aetiology. Below the age of 6, the diagnosis is based on delay in achieving developmental milestones. Those with less severe ID may not be identified until they start school when poor academic performance becomes evident. Some may not be identified until secondary school and may present with oppositional behaviours and truancy due to their inability to meet the intellectual demands placed on them. The diagnosis is confirmed by demonstrating the IQ and functional deficits. At any age it is important to exclude medical problems that may be contributing to impaired intellectual function (e.g. hypothyroidism).

Aetiology

There are over 300 identified causes of ID and more are being identified as technology becomes more advanced, particularly in the field of genetics. In clinical populations the cause will be identified in about 10–15% of cases, but with more intensive investigation it is possible to determine the aetiology in up to a third of cases. Understanding aetiology is useful for the following purposes:

- in the development of preventative strategies
- in predicting the health needs of people with specific syndromes, including targeted screening and intervention programs
- in understanding certain behavioural patterns and the development of particular psychiatric disorders associated with specific syndromes.

Management

The underpinning philosophy of management is to assist people with an ID to lead as normal lives as possible. This means that the role of staff is to attempt to compensate for the functions that the person cannot complete independently. This can range from full assistance with dressing, toileting and eating in those with a severe ID, to occasional help with issues such as budgeting or a weekly shop for a person with a mild ID.

Many people with an ID live with their families. Those accommodated by services usually live in small groups of four to six people in residential houses, although some live independently and others remain in institutional settings. There is an expectation that whenever possible people with an ID should access the same facilities as the rest of the population, including schools, recreational, health and social services.

Autism and autism spectrum disorders

In the 1940s Kanner initially described autism as a condition characterised by a lack of verbal development, significant cognitive impairment, and a characteristic lack of interest in interacting with other people. Over time, the concept of a spectrum of autistic disorders evolved, to refer to a group of disorders with impairments of varying severity in three major areas, namely *social interaction, communicative functioning* and *imagination*. In DSM–IV–TR, the term *pervasive developmental disorders* (PDD) has been used as the overarching term that covers the five types of autism spectrum disorder (ASD) (autism, Asperger's disorder, Rett syndrome, disintegrative disorder and pervasive developmental disorder not otherwise specified). However, the distinctions between disorders have been found to be inconsistent over time, variable across sites and often associated with severity, language level or intelligence rather than features of specific disorders. This has resulted in DSM-5 proposing to unite the different disorders into a single diagnostic category being *autism spectrum disorders*, concluding that 'a single spectrum disorder is a better reflection of the state of knowledge about pathology and clinical presentation'. It is proposed that clinical specifiers such as severity, verbal abilities and associated features (e.g. known genetic disorders, epilepsy, intellectual disability) will allow clinicians to account for individual variation in presentation.

DSM-5 also proposes to combine the social and communication deficits into a single factor so that the original three domains become two. The rationale behind this is that deficits in communication and social behaviours are so intertwined that they are inseparable for practical purposes. In DSM-5, language delay will be considered as a factor that influences the clinical symptoms of ASD, rather than defining the ASD diagnosis. The proposed DSM-5 criteria are shown in Box 21.2.

Although there are many standardised tools to explore the symptoms and behaviours associated with PDD, the diagnosis is a clinical one and consists of gathering evidence of impairments. The manifestations of these deficits are broadly covered in the diagnostic criteria (see above), but can present in many different ways depending on age, sex, IQ,

Box 21.2

Proposed DSM-5 criteria for pervasive developmental disorders Autism spectrum disorders

Must meet criteria A, B, C and D:

A Persistent deficits in social communication and social interaction across contexts, not accounted for by general developmental delays, and manifest by all three of the following:

   1 Deficits in social-emotional reciprocity; ranging from abnormal social approach and failure of normal back and forth conversation through reduced sharing of interests, emotions, and affect and response, to total lack of initiation of social interaction

   2 Deficits in non-verbal communicative behaviours used for social interaction; ranging from poorly integrated verbal and nonverbal communication, through abnormalities in eye contact and body language, or deficits in understanding and use of nonverbal communication, to a total lack of facial expression or gestures.

   3 Deficits in developing and maintaining relationships, appropriate to developmental level (beyond those with caregivers); ranging from difficulties adjusting behaviour to suit different social contexts through to difficulties in sharing imaginative play and in making friends to an apparent absence of interest in people.

B Restricted, repetitive patterns of behaviour, interests, or activities as manifested by at least two of the following:

   1 Stereotyped or repetitive speech, motor movements, or use of objects (such as simple motor stereotypies, echolalia, repetitive use of objects, or idiosyncratic phrases)

   2 Excessive adherence to routines, ritualised patterns of verbal or nonverbal behaviour, or excessive resistance to change (such as motoric rituals, insistence on same route or food, repetitive questioning or extreme distress at small changes)

   3 Highly restricted, fixated interests that are abnormal in intensity or focus (such as strong attachment to or preoccupation with unusual objects, excessively circumscribed or perseverative interests)

   4 Hyper- or hypo-reactivity to sensory input or unusual interest in sensory aspects of environment (such as apparent indifference to pain/heat/cold, adverse response to specific sounds or textures, excessive smelling or touching of objects, fascination with lights or spinning objects).

C Symptoms must be present in early childhood (but may not become fully manifest until social demands exceed limited capacities)

D Symptoms together limit and impair everyday functioning.

personality and situational context. The more severe the autism, the earlier the diagnosis. The more subtle variations may never be formally identified. In addition to the classic triad, there are some other features that are common but not essential for the diagnosis. These include abnormalities of mood and of biological functions (e.g. eating, drinking and sleeping). Physical disabilities such as epilepsy and sensory impairments are common.

The earliest epidemiological studies used Kanner's very narrow criteria and found a prevalence rate for autism of around 0.05%. Much higher rates (around 1%) have been recorded using current broader diagnostic criteria for ASDs.

Aetiology

A range of factors have been implicated in causing ASDs. Genetic factors seem to predominate, although no simple pattern of inheritance has been identified and there are thought to be a range of genes that contribute to risk with recent research suggesting that most individuals with autism are actually probably genetically unique, each having their own genetic form of autism. Some specific genetic disorders are also associated with a higher risk of developing autism; these include fragile X syndrome.

Management

There is no known cure for autism, but appropriate management can ameliorate the impact. There is an emphasis on early intervention focusing on building communication skills using an educational approach. Operant-based behavioural techniques can enhance basic learning skills. Less conventional medical approaches include specific diets, supplements and medications, although there is no consistent evidence for any effect on the core features of autism. The outcome of any approach depends on the needs of the individual, which vary greatly, and on the appropriate application of the intervention itself.

Comorbidity and developmental disorders

Comorbidity is seen both between the developmental disorders themselves, as well as with other psychiatric disorders. Thus, around 20% of people with an ID have autism, while about 70% of people with autism have an ID. Around a third of people with developmental disorders have a comorbid mental disorder, with the risk increasing with the more severe levels of disability. The higher rates of comorbidity are thought to be due to exposure to risk factors, encompassing those factors shown in Box 21.3.

Assessment issues

There are a number of issues that complicate the assessment of a person with a dual disability. These may be considered in terms of the diagnostic process itself, as well as in terms of the classification of these disorders.

Process issues

- People with developmental disorders are often brought to treatment by carers and it can be they, rather than the patient, who is experiencing the distress.
- Psychiatric symptoms may be attributed to the ID itself; this is called *diagnostic overshadowing*. It must be remembered that the only 'symptoms' of ID are deficits in intelligence and functional impairment.
- Psychiatric illness commonly presents with difficult behaviour and is treated as a behavioural problem.

Box 21.3

Factors underpinning comorbidity between ID and psychiatric symptoms

Biological factors

- Some genetic syndromes are linked both with ID and psychiatric illness (e.g. Down syndrome and dementia; fragile X syndrome and attention deficit hyperactivity disorder (ADHD)).
- Brain damage associated with an ID may give rise to problems of arousal, and difficulties in emotion regulation that can present as a psychiatric disorder.
- Certain genes lead to an ID and can be associated with specific behavioural problems called behavioural phenotypes (e.g. Lesch-Nyhan syndrome and severe self-harming behaviour).
- People with an ID often have problems with hearing and vision, which is associated with increased risk for psychotic illnesses.
- Epilepsy occurs in 20% of people with an ID and is associated with depression and psychotic illnesses.
- Up to 30% of people with an ID are prescribed psychotropic medication, which can have a number of behavioural and cognitive side effects.

Psychological factors

- People with an ID may be less able to develop effective coping strategies to deal with life stressors.
- People with an ID experience higher rates of stressful life events that are not explained to them (such as bereavement).
- Many people with developmental disorders have been teased and insulted from an early age and suffer from the effects of stigma and labelling.
- Low self-esteem and self-image may result from having an ID.
- Lack of verbal skills may result in an inability to tell carers about problems and to make use of advice.
- Both psychiatric and physical symptoms may be modified by the presence of an ID, making their recognition and treatment less likely.

Social factors

- People with an ID often have few meaningful social supports.
- The family of origin may have unresolved grief issues.
- There are often high levels of expressed emotion in families and residential units.
- People with an ID may be living with people who have behavioural problems that may include aggression.
- Abuse of all types is common and often unrecognised.
- People with an ID are reliant on carers who may lack the skills to assess and manage the issues they present with.
- People with an ID lack choice and live a lifestyle of 'bureaucratic convenience'.
- The sexual needs of people with an ID are infantilised and treated as deviant and troublesome.

- Concrete thinking, an inability to understand abstract concepts, such as emotions or time, and poor communication skills, can lead to difficulties in understanding the person's internal experiences.
- The impoverished social and life experiences can lead to the unsophisticated presentation of symptoms which are then not recognised (*psychosocial masking*).
- Stress-induced disruption of information-processing can present as bizarre behaviour and thought disorder (*cognitive disintegration*).
- People with a severe ID have a limited range of responses and illness can present as a change in the frequency of certain behaviours that may be difficult to recognise as the manifestation of a psychiatric illness.
- Stigma means many people with an ID try to appear 'normal' and symptoms may be denied.
- People with an ID are suggestible and may not provide accurate information.

Diagnostic and classification issues

People with developmental disorders were largely excluded from the research used in the development of modern classification systems. This has given rise to the following problems:

- People with an ID may not have developed the ability to experience the normal range of thoughts and emotions required to meet diagnostic thresholds.
- Behavioural presentations of psychiatric illness have not been operationalised.
- Some behaviours that may be troublesome in some people with developmental disorders have not been included in the classifications for mental illness (e.g. faecal smearing, wandering, shouting or undressing).
- Some specific causes of an ID are associated with certain behaviours which have not been accounted for in the classification system (e.g. the overeating evident in Prader-Willi syndrome).
- The types of problems presented do not fit neatly into a classification system based on mental disorders alone and may be due to social factors such as changes in staff at the residential unit or physical factors such as pain.
- Psychiatric disorder may present in an altered form, such as regression and loss of skills.

To account for these difficulties, the assessment process needs to be modified. It is important to determine who the main stakeholders are, as they may have different perceptions as to what constitutes the reason for assessment and treatment. There is increased reliance on observation and collateral history and a large part of the work often involves reviewing previous reports and file notes. It is important to establish the person's best level of functioning, as this forms a point of comparison to judge the impact of any illness. The ability of the person to understand and report on their internal mental state needs to be assessed and the mental state examination modified accordingly. It is important to assess cognitive, emotional, physical and social developmental levels, as problems can arise from unrealistic expectations or mismatches between levels. Box 21.4 provides some clinical tips in the assessment of dual disability.

Box 21.4

Clinical tips in the assessment of people with dual disability

- The assessment process is prolonged and cannot be completed within the usual single 1-hour session. It is important to allow adequate time, and often assessments consist of many interviews over several weeks.

- Beware of excessive compliance and scripted answers as people with an ID have often been interviewed many times and just want to say the 'right' thing.

- Do not mistake self-talk for hallucinations or imaginary friends for delusions. This can be normal depending on the person's developmental level.

- Good interview technique is crucial, as unlike the normal population this group will need guidance and support to tell their story and it is important to avoid leading questions ('Were you feeling depressed?') or multiple questions ('How are you sleeping and eating?').

- People with developmental disorders may have difficulty answering open-ended questions ('How are you feeling?'). Multiple-choice questions may have to be used ('Are you feeling sad or happy?'). The answers should be cross-checked by asking the question in different ways and reversing the order of choices ('Are you feeling good or bad?').

- People with developmental disorders may have difficulties with abstract concepts, including time. It is sometimes useful to use anchor events ('How were you feeling at Christmas?'). They may also have difficulty in putting events in the correct time sequence to make a coherent history and you may have to make the links for them.

- Seeing the person in their own environment usually gives a much more accurate picture of how they are, as much behaviour is specific to a situation or environment.

- The person's appearance is more a reflection of the quality of care they receive than a measure of their ability.

- It may not be possible to interview people with severe developmental disorders, although they may be engaged in activities such as going for a walk, drawing or playing a game, and this can provide useful information about their ability to interact with others.

Case examples: Dual disability

- A 21-year-old man with an IQ of 40 lived with his Italian Catholic family. He had started to rub his erect penis against other people, irrespective of age or gender. The possibility of a manic illness was considered, but the problem was thought to be because he had never had any sex education, nor did he have any outlets to express his sexuality as his family did not think this was appropriate due to his intellectual impairment. In this case, his physical development was out of synchrony with his cognitive level.

- A 24-year-old man with a mild ID and cerebral palsy became increasingly agitated over a period of months and lost a considerable amount of weight

Continued

Case examples continued

before making several serious suicide attempts. He complained of hearing the voice of a man telling him to do things. He was diagnosed with depression and treated with electroconvulsive therapy (ECT), making some improvement. Some weeks later he was able to disclose to his case manager that he had been sexually abused over a period of months at his day placement by his care worker, who had also been telling him what to do and say. The diagnosis was revised to post-traumatic stress disorder (PTSD).

- A 32-year-old woman with a mild ID had not left her room for several months and had been spending all her time lying on her bed. She had attracted a previous diagnosis of borderline personality disorder on the basis of aggressive behaviour and transient paranoia and hallucinations. On review, her parents reported a much wider range of psychotic symptoms that they had attributed to her ID. Her diagnosis was revised to schizophrenia and with appropriate treatment she was able to return to her day placement.

Specific psychiatric disorders

In people with intellectual disability, comorbid disorders are well recognised in research settings, but often underreported and undiagnosed in clinical practice. Specific clinical scenarios include those described below.

Dementia and delirium

People with an ID are more likely to develop delirium in response to factors affecting brain function, such as infection, trauma, and illicit and prescribed drugs. People with Down syndrome are at a very high risk of developing Alzheimer's dementia and from age 40 onwards almost all will have pathological changes (although only a third will have clinical signs). The rest of the ID population seem to dement in the same way as the non-ID population, although it may be evident at a younger age due to the lower cognitive reserves. Problems can occur in making the diagnosis if the level of premorbid cognitive function is unknown.

Schizophrenia

Developmental disorders are risk factors for the development of schizophrenia and herald a poorer prognosis. Schizophrenia occurs at high rates in people with an ID (2–3%). The symptom profile in people with ID is similar to that described in Chapter 7, but the disorder can present with aggression, disturbed behaviour or poor self-care.

Negative symptoms can exacerbate skill loss and cognitive changes can impair the ability to learn new skills. Schizophrenia cannot be reliably diagnosed in people with an IQ lower than about 50.

Mood disorders

Depression has a high prevalence in people with an ID. It may present with classical features such as tearfulness, lack of interest, social withdrawal and psychomotor retardation.

However, some patients present with aggression, acting out or self-harming behaviour, or simply a loss of skills and social withdrawal. *Mania* presents with an increase in activity, intrusive behaviour, destructiveness, irritability and sometimes self-abusive behaviour.

Anxiety disorders

As in the normal population, anxiety may present with repetitive worrying thoughts, fear and, in extreme instances, panic. However, people with an ID may have difficulty communicating their fears, and physiological manifestations such as flushing, sweating, pallor, tremor, hyperventilation and insomnia can be useful clues. Avoidance is a common behavioural manifestation of anxiety. Relatively greater emphasis is placed on phenomena such as agitation, screaming, crying, withdrawal, regressive/clingy behaviour or freezing.

Personality disorders

Many patients with an ID have a background of abuse, neglect, poor parenting, inadequate education, and poor social and coping skills, coupled with a low tolerance of frustration with impaired impulse control. A personality disorder can often present with a range of unacceptable behaviours such as aggression or inappropriate sexual activity, but is often labelled a behaviour disorder. The prevalence is thought to be about 20% among those with an ID.

Behaviour disorders

People with an ID can present with behaviours that can be dangerous to themselves or others and limit their opportunities to lead a normal life. The current term to describe these is *challenging behaviours*, although the term *behaviours of concern* is coming into vogue. In some cases these behaviours are secondary to an underlying illness, which may be medical or psychiatric, and it is important to exclude these before adopting a behavioural framework. A behavioural framework assumes the behaviour has a function for the individual. In this situation an intensive process is undertaken to record the situations leading to the behaviour, and what happens afterwards. This information can be analysed with a view to understanding the underlying motivation; this is termed a *functional (or applied) behavioural analysis*. Interventions are based on helping the person to communicate and to learn skills that help them meet their needs, in addition to adjusting the environment to encourage appropriate behaviour.

Mental health in the severely disabled

This group often has multiple handicaps, including epilepsy, sensory deficits and limited mobility and communication. They have a restricted range of responses, and the bulk of pathology consists of behaviour disorders, with an unclear relationship to other forms of psychiatric illness. Impulsive, explosive and sexually inappropriate behaviours are common. Repetitive stereotyped movements often occur and connections to obsessive-compulsive disorder and to schizophrenia have been suggested.

Case examples: Manifestations of dual disability

- A 40-year-old man with Down syndrome abruptly started running up to people and hitting them at the factory where he worked packing tins into boxes. Dementia was considered but there was no loss of skills. It was thought that he might be responding to hallucinations, but the behaviour was specific to his workplace. A behaviour analysis over several weeks revealed that the only time staff interacted with him was following an assault. It was established that since a new particularly disabled client had started at the workplace, staff had had significantly less time to interact with the patient. Increasing the staffing levels to deal with the new client resolved the issues.

- A 20-year-old man with a moderate ID exhibited a deterioration in behaviour over a period of 6 months. He was pacing while mumbling 'bad boy', 'don't do that' and 'shush', and engaging in severe self-harming behaviour by charging at walls and banging his head. As his mother had treatment-resistant schizophrenia, it was thought he had become psychotic and was responding to hallucinations. On assessment it was determined that he had autism and the self-talk was usual when he was agitated. On physical review it was noted that he had pus in his left ear. Otitis media was diagnosed and treated, after which his behaviour returned to base line.

- A 60-year-old man with a mild ID was taken to the hospital emergency department after making suicidal threats. This was in the context of his having been evicted from his shared accommodation after he had attempted to set fire to the house using petrol. There was concern that he had a depressive illness. However, on review of his file it was evident that he had a long history of offences with repeated threats of suicide when confronted with the consequences of his actions. He met the criteria for antisocial personality disorder with significant borderline traits. It was recommended that he be charged with arson.

Management

There is little research specifically on the treatment of mental disorders in people with developmental disorders, and treatments broadly parallel those used for the rest of the population. However, a number of specific issues need to be borne in mind when articulating a treatment plan in those with a developmental disorder. One particular issue is that of *consent to treatment*. Although in common law an adult is presumed to have capacity to give or withhold consent until proved otherwise, developmental disorders impair some of the abilities required for decision-making, leading to a lack of capacity. Although mental health Acts usually provide a legal framework to enable individuals who lack capacity to be treated, there is often no equivalent power in disability legislation. In general, it would be appropriate to use mental health legislation when the person is being treated for a mental illness and to use guardianship powers for other decisions involving health and lifestyle problems.

Pharmacotherapy in people with a developmental disorder should be directed at specific diagnostic hypotheses using the same principles as for the general population. There is some evidence that drugs take longer to work and that lower doses are required in those with developmental disorders. Objective measures of response and side effects should be implemented.

Psychological treatments have general applicability in the developmental disorders population, but modifications may be required to ensure the individual can understand the intent and process. Behavioural treatments have ascendency, although cognitive approaches can be used in those of higher intellectual functioning. People with ID often take longer to respond to psychological treatments, and may need lots of real-life practice to understand some of the techniques. This often works best if the person's social network is involved in the treatment program.

Social interventions are a critical component of comprehensively caring for the individual with a developmental disorder. These encompass provision of pleasant living situations, opportunities for meaningful recreational and vocational activities, and opportunities to develop satisfying relationships. Regrettably, these aims are often difficult to achieve.

Table 21.1

Roles of members of the multidisciplinary and extended team in the management of the person with dual disability

Profession/ position	Role
Disability case manager	Identify the person's needs and broker other services to provide these. Sometimes this role itself is undertaken by another agency
Mental health case manager	Monitoring and delivering therapeutic interventions
Psychiatrist	Assessment and treatment of mental disorders
General practitioner	Provision of general health care and screening
Psychologist	Assessment of IQ and neuropsychological function
Behaviour intervention and support practitioner	Undertake a functional behaviour analysis with the aim of developing a behaviour management plan
Carers and families	Carers may be paid or unpaid family members. They will often assist the person with day-to-day function, as well as implement strategies devised with the assistance of other professionals (e.g. administer medication and behaviour interventions)
Guardian	A guardian is often needed to make decisions on behalf of the person, including consenting to treatment. They may be formally appointed through a court process or a family member may often informally adopt this role
Other	There is a range of other people with significant roles who may be involved, including the house supervisor or manager in shared accommodation facilities, house staff, teachers, one-to-one workers (often employed to supervise the person for several hours at a time), counsellors, employers, trainers/ educators at day placements and also peers with whom they may have significant relationships

It usually is not possible for one service provider to meet the complex needs of this population and there are often several services involved with a multitude of different professionals and carers. Table 21.1 provides a guide to the different activities undertaken by the more commonly involved service providers.

REFERENCES AND FURTHER READING

Bouras, N. (Ed.), 2007. Psychiatric and behavioural disorders in intellectual and developmental disabilities, second ed. Cambridge University Press, Cambridge.

Deb, S., Matthews, T., Holt, G., Bouras, N. (Eds.), 2001. Practice guidelines for the assessment and diagnosis of mental health problems in adults with intellectual disability. Pavilion Publishing. Online. Available at: www.estiacentre.org/docs/PracticeGuidelines.pdf.

Dosen, A., Day, K. (Eds.), 2005. Treating mental illness and behavior disorders in children and adults with mental retardation. American Psychiatric Press, Washington, DC.

Fraser, W.I., Kerr, M.P., 2003. Seminars in the psychiatry of learning disabilities, second ed. Gaskell, London.

Griffiths, D., Stravrakaki, C., Summers, J. (Eds.), 2002. Dual diagnosis: an introduction to the mental health needs of persons with developmental disabilities. Habilitative Mental Health Resource Network. Online. Available at: www.naddontario.org/.

Roy, A., Meera, R., Clarke, D. (Eds.), 2006. The psychiatry of intellectual disability. Radcliffe Publishing, Oxford.

Royal College of Psychiatrists, 2001. DC-LD: diagnostic criteria for psychiatric disorders for use with adults with learning disabilities/mental retardation. Royal College of Psychiatrists' Occasional Paper OP48. Gaskell, London.

A MAN NAMED MICHAEL

CASE-BASED LEARNING

ANDREW GLEASON & JOEL KING

The following role-play requires two participants: one to play a GP registrar (candidate) and another to play the role of a patient named Michael O'Donnell and an examiner (actor).

OSCE Station Instructions

(Reading time: 2 minutes)

You are a first-year GP registrar working in a suburban practice. The secretary asks you if you can see Mike O'Donnell. Mr O'Donnell is a regular patient of Dr Lee, one of the GPs at the practice, but Dr Lee is away today and all of the other GPs are fully booked. Mr O'Donnell is saying that he needs to see a doctor urgently.

You review his file. Mr O'Donnell is 40 years old and has a mild intellectual disability of unknown aetiology. He had psychometric testing many years ago, which showed an IQ of 65. He has a history of gastro-oesophageal reflux, treated with omeprazole 40 mg daily, cholecystectomy, and migraines. He sees Dr Lee every few months, usually with minor complaints such as upper respiratory tract infections, or to have his omeprazole script renewed.

Task (10 minutes)

- Take a history from Mr O'Donnell (8 minutes).
- After 8 minutes you must terminate the interview and present the most likely diagnosis and pharmacological and psychological treatment options to the examiner (2 minutes).
- You do not need to physically examine the patient at this stage.

Actor role: Michael O'Donnell

You are 40 years old and live on your own in a flat that your parents bought for you in a suburban area. You receive a disability pension and work part-time packing boxes in Fraser House, a sheltered workshop for people with disabilities. You are mostly independent, but receive some help from your parents. You manage your own finances with minimal assistance from your parents, get around using public transport, and do your own shopping and cooking.

HISTORY OF PRESENTING COMPLAINT

You have come to see the doctor because you are worried that you might be having heart attacks. You think that the first one happened two months ago when heard that your mother had fallen and broken her ankle. You were at work at the time, and Cathy told you that she had received a telephone call that your mother was in hospital. If asked who Cathy is, say, 'She is my friend'. With further prompting, explain that she is a supervisor at Fraser House. If the doctor asks what Fraser House is, say it is where you work. You can elaborate that it is a place for people with disabilities if you are specifically asked for more information.

When Cathy told you your mother was in hospital, you suddenly felt like you were going to die. Your heart was going really, really fast, and you couldn't breathe. You felt dizzy. Your hands were tingling, and you were sweaty and nauseous. Things didn't seem real. You asked Cathy to call an ambulance. She took you to the office, but by the time you got there, you were okay. You're not sure how long you felt unwell for.

After this episode, you have had attacks about once a week. Most often, they come on when you worry about your parents. Be vague about the precipitants, but if the doctor gently continues to ask simple direct questions, provide more and more information about your parents' declining health as detailed below.

You have not had any fears about having an attack in a public place, nor have public or enclosed spaces brought on an attack. You have not had any chest pain. If asked about chest pain, answer both yes and no to this, but finish with 'no'.

You thought the episodes could be heart attacks because you have heard that people get short of breath and get numb in their arm when they have a heart attack. You had a really bad attack yesterday when Cherie told you that she likes Dimitri. If asked who Cherie is, say, 'She's my girlfriend.' Dimitri and Cherie also work at Fraser House. You don't like Dimitri very much because he is not very nice. You will admit that you would like to punch him if the doctor asks about physical violence, but you have never hurt anyone and would not do this.

PAST HISTORY

If the doctor asks if you have had any health problems in the past, say 'No, I'm very healthy, except I sometimes get reflux. Dr Lee says I have too much acid in my stomach.' You have also had migraines in the past, but not for a long time. You take a reflux tablet every morning that you get from Dr Lee. You have no past psychiatric history.

FAMILY HISTORY

Your mother has 'weak bones'. She broke her ankle on the stairs at home and spent a week in hospital. You are really worried that this will happen again, and that she won't be able to look after your dad anymore. Your dad is 'very sick', and you think this is from smoking cigarettes. He has a breathing tank at home and your mum has to do everything for him. You aren't sure how old your parents are. You think that they are 70 or 75.

While you can't readily articulate this, you are very worried about your parents getting old and dying. You don't think you would be able to look after your dad if something happened to your mum, and you don't think your younger sister, Karen, who is 33, could manage it either. If the doctor asks if Karen has medical problems say, 'She is fat, so she will never get married.' If asked what your grandparents died of, say, 'Old age.'

DRUG AND ALCOHOL HISTORY

You think that drugs are bad. You have one glass of wine on festive holidays with your parents, but never drink otherwise. You don't drink coffee because it's 'yucky'. You do have a soft drink sometimes, but not more than once a day.

PERSONAL AND DEVELOPMENTAL HISTORY

You don't know anything about your birth. You had trouble learning in school. You had extra help in primary school, and went to a special secondary school for people with learning problems. You have worked at Fraser House for about ten years and really enjoy it. Be vague about what you do, but say you pack boxes and 'make things'. You get on well with the other people who work at Fraser House (except for Dimitri), and like the staff. You live in your own flat, which your parents bought for you ten years ago. Before this, you lived with your parents. You are proud of the fact that you work, get around on your own, and live independently. You clean your flat on your own. Your parents help you with bills a bit, but you usually pay them yourself. You think your sister is lazy because she doesn't have a job, but you don't know why this is the case. She was living on her own but moved back in with your parents about a year ago. You have dinner with your family every Sunday evening, and often go shopping or have lunch with your mum during the week. Cherie has been your girlfriend for six months. You hold hands but have never kissed. Sometimes you have ice cream with her at the shopping centre after you finish work. You have never had sex and get very uncomfortable if the doctor asks about this.

HOW TO PLAY THE ROLE

Although you have a very mild dysarthria, most people wouldn't be able to tell that you have a disability at first. You behave in a socially appropriate manner and have good self-care skills. Your intellectual function is roughly that of someone in about Grade 6, but you have had some life experience. However, you have difficulties expressing yourself verbally. This includes expressing your emotions. You are worried about what is happening to you – every time you have an episode you think you are going to die. If the doctor asks if you think the episodes you have been having could be related to worries about your parents' health, pause to think and agree that this could be possible, but you hadn't noticed a connection yourself.

You often don't realise that the doctor doesn't know things that you do. For example, you begin talking about Cathy or Cherie, without realising that the doctor has no idea who these people are. You are also vague about time frames, and can't provide a lot of details about things. You find open-ended or broad questions confusing. You get a bit lost when people use long sentences or big words. You want to please the doctor because they are a professional and will help you, so you sometimes say yes to things that you aren't sure about because this seems like the right thing to do. A few times in the interview, give inconsistent answers (e.g. say both 'yes' and 'no' when a question is asked more than once). You are agreeable, and say yes to anything the doctor suggests.

Model Answer

Psychiatric conditions are common in people with intellectual disability (see Box 21.3, page 349). They are often not picked up for many reasons, including diagnostic overshadowing and psychosocial masking. Communication difficulties may make it difficult to recognise a psychiatric illness, and the presentation of an illness may not conform to common diagnostic archetypes.

In this scenario, Mr O'Donnell does display fairly typical symptoms of panic disorder without agoraphobia (see pages 149–151), but the interview approach will need to be modified in light of his intellectual disability (ID). Mr O'Donnell, like many people with ID, has some difficulties understanding abstract concepts and emotions. He has somewhat limited verbal skills which make it difficult for him to communicate internal experiences. He is suggestible and wants to please authority figures. The candidate should adjust their language and communication accordingly (see Box 21.4, page 351). They should avoid leading questions, and use multiple choices when Mr O'Donnell has trouble with open-ended questions. Extra time may be needed for assessment, and further assessment sessions should be considered in the management plan if necessary. Collateral history from Mr O'Donnell's family is imperative, and it would be helpful to speak with the staff at Fraser House. The candidate should also speak with Mr O'Donnell's usual GP, Dr Lee, and discuss the management plan with him.

Mr O'Donnell will need a physical examination and appropriate investigations to screen for different causes of anxiety (see Box 10.2, page 150).

Treatment options should be discussed with Mr O'Donnell and his parents or guardian. As a general rule, management is the same as for people without an ID. Psychological techniques can be used in people with ID, depending on their abilities. Slow breathing exercises and relaxation strategies may be helpful for Mr O'Donnell, but they would be best taught by someone skilled in psychological approaches for people with ID.

It would be worth considering addressing Mr O'Donnell's fears about his parents' health, though these may be based in reality. This would depend on his ability to engage in a more cognitive approach. A selective serotonin reuptake inhibitor (SSRI) should be discussed with him and his guardian. Dosing should begin low and increases should be slow, as people with ID are, on the whole, more susceptible to side effects than the general population. Psychotropics also tend to take longer to work in people with ID. Mr O'Donnell may feel a bit worse initially on an SSRI, due to activating effects, and this should be factored into the management plan. For example, he could be taught deep breathing techniques before an SSRI is started. Benzodiazepines can be helpful in people with panic disorder, but if they are used, it should be with caution and only in the short term, in order to avoid tolerance and dependence.

If psychological treatment is chosen, Mr O'Donnell could be referred to a psychiatrist or a psychologist with an appropriate skill set. If treatment is initially commenced by a GP and an appropriately skilled psychologist, it would be prudent to involve a psychiatrist early on. This may take the form of a single assessment with a plan to re-refer Mr O'Donnell to the psychiatrist if he does not respond to treatment.

Chapter 22

SUBSTANCE USE DISORDERS

MICHAEL BAIGENT & DAN LUBMAN

A range of problems arise from the use of alcohol, tobacco, illicit substances or prescribed medications that are taken for non-medical purposes.

Substances of abuse

Alcohol

Alcohol affects the release of dopamine, noradrenaline, and endogenous opioids, producing an activated state that is pleasurable. It specifically acts at the GABA-A receptor, thus accounting for its anxiolytic properties. At higher concentrations, alcohol also blocks glutamatergic NMDA receptors, resulting in amnesia and further contributing to cerebral depressant effects. Ten grams of alcohol per hour will cause an increase in blood alcohol concentration levels to between 0.01 and 0.02%, with lower concentrations possible where there is marked tolerance, and higher concentrations found in females of small stature (see Table 22.1). Hazardous intake tends to lead to harm as a result of behaviours associated with acute intoxication (e.g. motor vehicle accidents, assaults, drownings and suicides), and is more common among young people. Long-term hazardous use can result in a broad range of physical complications, including hypertension, liver disease, pancreatitis and cancer. Dependent use can also lead to the development of a depressive syndrome, anxiety and psychosis (e.g. alcoholic hallucinosis and morbid jealousy).

Table 22.1

Alcohol effects

Blood alcohol concentration*	Effects
0.02–0.05	Cheerful, relaxed, reduced inhibitions, coordination and judgement beginning to be affected
0.06–0.10	Speech louder, very talkative, feels self-confident, less cautious, slowed reaction time, impaired coordination
0.20	Sedated rather than active. Clumsy, slurred speech, impaired cognitive functioning, amnesia
0.30–0.40	Semi-conscious or unconscious, bodily functions beginning to deteriorate, fatalities can occur
0.50	Fatalities common

*Blood alcohol concentration is grams of alcohol per 100 mL of blood.

Amphetamines

Amphetamines are a group of synthetic drugs that include 'speed' (amphetamine sulphate, dexamphetamine), 'meth' (methamphetamine or methylamphetamine) and 'crystal meth' (methamphetamine hydrochloride). They come in many forms (crystalline, paste, powder, pills) and in varying strengths. They are generally ingested or injected, although can be snorted or smoked depending on how they are prepared. They produce their stimulating effects through the release of dopamine and noradrenaline from pre-synaptic nerve terminals. Intoxication is associated with euphoria, increased physical activity, confidence, stamina and reduced need for sleep. Use that is above twice a week is more likely in dependent individuals. Dependence is also more likely among those who inject (50% likelihood). Long-term risks include those resulting from injecting if this is the mode of use. These include transmissible diseases such as hepatitis C and HIV. Teeth grinding, appetite suppression and weight loss, headache, chronic psychosis, mood instability, unpredictable behaviour and violence may also occur.

Benzodiazepines

Benzodiazepines act on GABA-A receptors, resulting in anxiolytic, hypnotic, sedative and anticonvulsant effects. The duration of effects varies according to the half-life of the benzodiazepine consumed. Abuse as a component of polysubstance abuse, dependence in conjunction with alcohol or other drug dependence, and long-term dependence in the context of long-standing repeat prescriptions, are the most common problematic patterns of use. Physiological dependence can follow 3 months of regular use, and in some instances has been noted to occur much earlier, particularly if there is already dependence on a sedating substance. Sleep impairment, sedation, cognitive impairment and falls in the elderly are some of the problems associated with dependence.

Cannabis

Cannabis is usually smoked, although it can be ingested. Delta-tetrahydrocannabinol (THC), the psychoactive component of the cannabis plant, binds to cannabinoid receptors (CB1) throughout the CNS. Intoxication is experienced within minutes of ingestion and lasts 3–4 hours. It produces transient euphoria and grandiosity, followed by sedation, lethargy, impaired short-term memory and concentration, slowed thinking, impaired judgement and motor coordination, perceptual distortions and a sense that time is passing slowly. Anxiety is a common unwanted effect. Dependence can develop. Cannabis use (especially if early onset) increases the risk of developing a psychotic disorder, as well as depression. It also impacts negatively on treatment outcomes in psychosis.

Cocaine

Cocaine inhibits the reuptake of noradrenaline, dopamine and serotonin. It tends to be either snorted in an intermittent binge pattern by mostly employed individuals or injected (less frequent) by those who inject other substances. The acute effects of cocaine are largely indistinguishable from amphetamine, although its duration of action is significantly shorter. Acute and chronic use may result in a number of serious cardiac complications. Chronic cocaine use can result in psychosis, mania, depression or anxiety.

Ecstasy

Ecstasy (N-methyl-3,4-methylenedioxy-amphetamine) is a synthetic compound that has both stimulant and hallucinogenic properties (due to its effects on noradrenaline, serotonin and possibly dopamine). Young people use ecstasy because it keeps them awake for long periods, increases sensory perception, confidence and energy levels, induces euphoria and makes them feel love, friendship and intimacy. It is usually sold as a tablet or capsule and taken orally, although some may also inject it. Young people predominantly take it in social settings in non-dependent patterns. It causes an increase in body temperature, which may, in combination with intense physical activity, a hot environment and minimal fluid intake, lead to severe heatstroke. With regular use, recurrent anxiety and panic disorders, as well as severe depression and psychotic symptoms (especially paranoid ideation) may also occur. There is evidence suggestive of neuronal damage to serotonin-producing neurons after prolonged heavy use.

Hallucinogens

Hallucinogens include a variety of substances, such as lysergic acid diethylamide (LSD), phenylalkylamines (mescaline), and psilocybin (from mushrooms). The effects are highly variable depending on the user, the expectations of the user and the situation in which it is taken. The central experiences of intoxication are perceptual distortions and hallucinations, as well as depersonalisation and derealisation. Synaesthesias may occur. Mood effects vary and anxiety can be prominent reaching panic. Delusions and agitation can occur. Tolerance rises, but withdrawal syndromes have not been described. Most use is intermittent. Flashbacks are distressing perceptual disturbances reminiscent of intoxication, which recur in the absence of continued use.

Heroin

Heroin is a short-acting opioid that in Australia is most commonly injected. Some smoke it. First-pass metabolism is extensive, so it is seldom taken orally. Unwanted effects include respiratory depression (can be fatal), pupillary constriction, nausea, vomiting and constipation. Associated hazards from use are secondary to the behaviours surrounding injecting (e.g. hepatitis C occurs in up to 15%), as well as the lifestyle associated with obtaining the substance. Approximately 30% of those who use heroin develop dependence. Heroin dependent individuals must use two to four times per day to avoid withdrawals due to the short half-life of the drug. Morphine and slow-release opioid preparations are also abused through supplies diverted after prescription. Methadone and buprenorphine are longer acting opioids prescribed for opioid dependence and those in chronic pain. They are also abused.

Inhalants

Inhalants are cheap and easily available. They comprise a wide range of household and commercial products (e.g. petrol, paint thinners, glues, solvents, spray paints). They are physically toxic, and long-term use is associated with significant neuro-cognitive disturbances. Deaths from acute inhalant use are largely associated with 'sudden sniffing death' (fatal ventricular arrhythmias) or accidental injury (related to impulsive risk-taking behaviours and impaired motor skills) while intoxicated. Dependence can occur.

Nicotine

Nicotine, the primary addictive component of tobacco, binds to nicotinic acetylcholine receptors, effecting the release of a number of neurotransmitters, including dopamine, noradrenaline and serotonin. A number of chemicals found in cigarette smoke are thought to be carcinogenic, while other chemical gases, such as carbon monoxide, impair oxygen transport in the body, or are irritants to the respiratory tract. The majority of smokers are dependent on nicotine. Those who smoke within half an hour of waking are likely to be dependent. There are much higher than expected rates of nicotine dependence in people with alcohol dependence and those with mental illnesses.

Caffeine

Caffeine is the most widely used substance in our community. A typical 150 mL cup of brewed coffee contains 100–150 mg of caffeine, instant coffee contains 30–100 mg of caffeine, and tea contains 30–100 mg of caffeine. A standard 250 mL energy drink contains 85 mg of caffeine, although some energy drinks contain up to 500 mg of caffeine per serve. Symptoms of caffeine toxicity include anxiety, insomnia, nausea and abdominal discomfort, diuresis, elevated blood pressure and heart rate. These symptoms occur at doses above 500 mg, or more if tolerant. Combining alcohol with energy drinks can mask the signs of alcohol intoxication, resulting in greater levels of alcohol intake, dehydration, more severe and prolonged hangovers, and alcohol poisoning. It may also increase engagement in risky behaviours (such as drink-driving), as well as alcohol-related violence. Caffeine dependence is common and withdrawal symptoms are most commonly headache and cognitive slowing.

Prevalence and costs

Epidemiological surveys consistently show that most people who report using substances do not do so on a regular basis (see Table 22.2). Experimental use is more common among adolescents and young people, while more frequent use is more prevalent in the 20–29-year-old age group. However, individuals with substance use disorders who present for treatment are typically older. While single episodes of use can cause problems (e.g. driving while intoxicated), individuals who use more frequently are more likely to experience deleterious mental and physical health consequences. Indeed, substance use and mental disorders frequently co-occur, and such comorbidity substantially impacts upon treatment outcomes for both conditions.

Substance use and misuse are important contributors to workplace injury, loss of productivity, relationship breakdowns, violence and crime, as well as illness and disease. The cost to our society is enormous, estimated in the tens of billions of dollars, with legal drugs accounting for the bulk of the costs (56% tobacco, 27% alcohol, 15% illicit drugs). Such figures are startling, and highlight the importance of early detection and treatment.

Patterns of use

An individual's pattern of substance use can range from experimental, through social to problematic use (i.e. a substance use disorder). It is important to consider the pattern of use in addition to the quantity of substance consumed. The terms abuse and dependence are used to describe patterns of problem use (see Table 22.3); dependence is generally regarded as the more reliable, robust and useful construct.

Table 22.2

Lifetime and recent (last 12 months) use of substances in Australia in those 14 years and over

Substance	% Population ever using substance	% Population using substance in the last 12 months
Alcohol	87.9	80.5
Cannabis	35.4	10.3
Pain killers/ analgesics/other opioids*	5.8	3.4
Ecstasy	10.3	3.0
Methamphetamine	7.0	2.1
Cocaine	7.3	2.1
Sleeping pills	3.2	2.1
Hallucinogens	8.8	1.4
Heroin	1.4	0.2

*for non-medical purposes
Source: National Drug Strategy, Household Survey 2010

Table 22.3

DSM–IV–TR criteria for abuse and dependence (adapted)

Substance abuse	Substance dependence
Maladaptive pattern of use in a 12-month period Impairment or distress >1 of: 1 Recurrent failure to fulfil role obligations 2 Recurrent use in situations in which it is hazardous 3 Recurrent substance related problems 4 Keeps on using despite problems 5 Not dependent	Maladaptive pattern of use in a 12-month period Impairment or distress >3 of: 1 Tolerance 2 Withdrawal 3 Takes substance in larger amounts or longer than intended 4 Limited control over use 5 Increased time spent obtaining or recovering from substance use 6 Gives up social, occupational or recreational activities 7 Keeps on using despite problems

Table 22.4

The CAGE questionnaire

CAGE questions	
C	Have you ever felt that you should cut down on your drinking?
A	Have people annoyed you by criticising your drinking?
G	Have you ever felt guilty about your drinking?
E	Have you ever had a drink first thing in the morning to steady your nerves or get rid of a hangover (an eye-opener)?

Screening and assessment

Given the high rate of morbidity associated with regular substance use, screening should be routinely conducted across all clinical settings. Presentations in which there are mental health issues, relationship or work problems, repeated requests for psychotropic medication (especially benztropine, anxiolytics or analgesics), and frequent attendances to different doctors, are all examples of when the clinician needs to be particularly mindful of the need to screen for substance use disorders.

Simple screening methods include:

- *CAGE questionnaire:* This screener consists of four questions, and scoring positive for two items is highly indicative of dependence on alcohol (see Table 22.4). It is useful as a very quick screen, but is not good at determining the severity of alcohol use, nor hazardous use that is non-dependent
- *Alcohol Use Disorders Identification Test (AUDIT):* This quick, 10-item questionnaire is good at identifying risky levels of alcohol use, as well as the severity of alcohol dependence

- *Alcohol, Smoking and Substance Involvement Screening Test (ASSIST):* This question-naire measures the frequency of substance use (lifetime and 3-month) across nine drug categories. There is also a brief intervention package associated with the screener which is freely available from the WHO website.

History

When assessing for substance use, it is imperative to take a non-judgemental approach during history-taking so as to avoid defensive answers. Alcohol should be quantified as the number of standard drinks (1 standard drink contains 10 g of alcohol), and all alco-holic beverages in Australia must now have this displayed on the label (see Figure 22.1). It is useful to understand the local street terms for available substances (e.g. 'ice', 'whiz' or 'goey' refer to methamphetamines), and to know the quantities by which they are con-sumed or purchased (e.g. methamphetamine is often sold as 'points', very loosely equating to 0.1 g). There is enormous variation in the purity of illicit substances, so the cost may be the best way to define the amount of substance being consumed.

The patient should be asked about use of all drugs of abuse (including non-medical use of prescribed medications) in a systematic manner (see Box 22.1). Use of more than one substance to problematic levels should be expected, as multiple drug use is common. It is particularly important to ask when the substance was last used, as this will often help identify current issues that the patient is presenting with (e.g. problems related to intoxi-cation or withdrawal). Features of intoxication vary depending on the substance con-sumed, and clinicians need to familiarise themselves with these effects (see below). Such

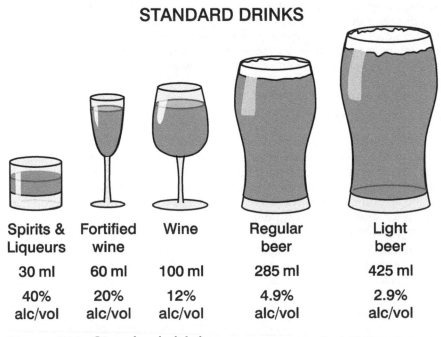

STANDARD DRINKS

Spirits & Liqueurs	Fortified wine	Wine	Regular beer	Light beer
30 ml	60 ml	100 ml	285 ml	425 ml
40% alc/vol	20% alc/vol	12% alc/vol	4.9% alc/vol	2.9% alc/vol

Figure 22.1 Standard drinks

Box 22.1
Substance use history

Areas of enquiry in a substance use history
Substance/s used (amount typically used or cost if undefinable otherwise)
When use began
What the pattern (frequency, mode of use) is now and recently
Route of administration, and history of safe injecting, if relevant
Features of DSM–IV–TR abuse or dependence
Consequences of use (physical, psychological, social, vocational, forensic)
Past treatment
Periods of abstinence
When last used
Reasons for use (typically related to enjoyment, socialising, peer pressure or to cope)
What the person wants to do now (readiness and confidence for change)
Psychiatric symptoms indicative of a co-occurring mental disorder

information also assists in the assessment of abnormal mental states, particularly if there is a history of a co-occurring mental disorder.

As with many areas of psychiatry, obtaining history from other sources can lead to a greater understanding of the extent of substance use, the effects of intoxication, as well as associated problems. Many people have difficulty recalling their intake spontaneously. It is often helpful to ask them to recount what they have consumed over the past week, working backwards on a daily basis, from yesterday to 1 week ago. You should establish whether the amount consumed was typical for them, and, if not, how it varies from their usual intake.

Mental state examination

Features to look for depend on the substance used, but can include: evidence of poor self-care, appearance and behaviour suggestive of intoxication (e.g. slurred or rapid speech, disinhibition, sedation, irritability or lability of affect, hallucinations (visual, auditory, tactile), persecutory beliefs, and cognitive impairment (acute or chronic)).

Physical examination

- Signs of intoxication (e.g. ataxia, pupillary constriction (opioids), dilatation (stimulants) or conjunctival injection (cannabis)) or withdrawal (e.g. sweating, tremor, piloerection or pupillary dilatation (opioids)).
- Signs of alcoholic liver disease.
- Evidence of injecting drug use (e.g. needle-tracks).
- Sequelae of injecting drug use (e.g. infected injecting sites, endocarditis and hepatitis).

Investigations

Clinical judgement should determine which investigations are relevant; however, the following should be considered depending upon the substance being used:

- Full blood count and liver function tests (about 75% of people with raised MCV and γGT are likely to have an alcohol disorder).
- Screening for viral hepatitis antigens and antibodies, and for HIV (consent should be obtained for these investigations).
- ECG (particularly relevant for patients taking methadone which can cause QT prolongation).
- Urine drug screen.

Substance-induced disorders

This important concept is defined in DSM–IV–TR as:
- a disorder directly caused by the effects of a substance
- the episode is above and beyond what would be expected during intoxication/withdrawal
- it develops within 1 month of intoxication or withdrawal
- it subsides once the substance is eliminated
- it is not due to delirium or other mental disorder.

It is important to note that heavy use of psychoactive substances can mimic the symptoms of almost any mental disorder (hence the importance of a substance use history during any psychiatric assessment), and should be considered a differential diagnosis for most presentations. Table 22.5 shows the range of disorders that can be induced by psychoactive substance use. In addition to induced disorders, many substances can cause symptoms suggestive of a syndrome, but not enough to justify a full diagnosis.

Management

Clinician attitude

Clinicians may experience a negative attitude when working with patients with substance use disorders, particularly those who are dependent. It is helpful to remember that these disorders may take a chronic relapsing course. Many respond well, with the majority improving over time. Rapid change may be more likely in patients with less severe conditions rather than if heavily dependent, but change is possible and frequently occurs even in those who appear to be the least capable of it. An approach that is non-judgemental, empathic and encouraging is necessary. It needs to occur within a harm reduction framework, appreciating that for some, complete cessation of harmful substance use is not possible.

Treatment options will depend upon parameters such as:
- the pattern of use – dependent or not
- negotiation with the patient of the treatment goals. Many would like to be able to continue to take the substance, but in safe controlled amounts. With most people who are dependent, the usual aim of treatment is abstinence rather than controlled intake due to the high rates of relapse when controlled use is attempted. Alternatively for some substances (e.g. opioid dependency), controlled substitution therapy may be the best option for reducing immediate risks (e.g. chaotic lifestyle and IV use), with the aim of drug cessation in the longer term

Table 22.5

Substance-induced mental disorders (adapted from DSM–IV–TR)

Substance	Anxiety disorder	Mood disorder	Psychotic disorder	Amnestic disorder	Sexual dysfunction	Sleep disorder
Alcohol*						
Cannabis						
Hallucinogen**						
Amphetamine***						
Cocaine						
Sedative, hypnotic, & anxiolytic*						
Opioid						
Caffeine						
Inhalant*						

*can also cause induced persisting dementia

**can also cause Induced Persisting Perception Disorder

***includes methamphetamine, ecstasy and other psychostimulants

Table 22.6

Stages of change and motivational enhancement techniques

Conceptual stage	Description	Consider approach
Pre-contemplation	The individual is not thinking about change	Provide factual information about the effects of substance use Avoid confrontation. Encourage considering change, offering an optimistic perspective
Contemplation	The individual is thinking about change within the next 6 months	Examine with the patient the pros and cons of change, as well as continuing intake Consider the compatibility of these with their broader life and health goals. Acknowledge ambivalence
Action	The individual has commenced attempts to change their use	Assist patient to enact strategies to change pattern of use
Maintenance	The individual has made a change	Assist patient to address ongoing ambivalence, rehearse relapse prevention strategies, and develop new skills
Relapse	The individual returns to aspects of previous behaviour (not always a full relapse)	Support the patient and assist them to re-engage with treatment as above

- the impact that the substance use is having on the person's life, and their awareness of the negative consequences
- their willingness and confidence to change, self-efficacy and identification of current goals
- the use of motivational enhancement, a useful therapeutic strategy for patients with a substance use problem, which can be used throughout treatment. It is helpful to use the stages of change approach to map where the patient is, and focus your therapeutic approaches accordingly (see Table 22.6). However, it is important to note that such stages are relatively fluid, and can rapidly change depending on psychosocial circumstances (e.g. break-up of relationship, resolution of crisis)
- co-occurring mental health disorders.

Substance use and mental disorders commonly co-occur, and integrated treatment should be offered for both conditions. This ensures that the patient understands the link between their substance use and mental disorder, and that common issues underpinning both disorders are addressed simultaneously.

Withdrawal management

The supervised management of withdrawal states is often referred to as 'detox' (detoxification), and should not be considered the main focus of treatment. In fact, only a very small percentage of patients subsequently remain substance-free in the long term or are able to continue to use in a controlled fashion. Nevertheless, detoxification may be a starting point for change, and other treatment strategies (see below) should also be offered. Stimulant-like substances (e.g. methamphetamines) produce withdrawal states characterised by lethargy and dysphoria. Sedative substances (e.g. alcohol and opioids) produce withdrawal effects of over-activation, such as anxiety and autonomic arousal (see Table 22.7).

Psychological strategies

Addressing the psychological processes involved in problem use is important, and should include concurrent treatment of co-occurring mental health issues.

- *Brief intervention:* an approach that is effective for non-dependent levels of use. It involves feedback to the patient about their consumption levels in relation to known safe levels of use, specific advice about how to change and achieve goals, encouragement, emphasising self-efficacy, and an optimistic perspective.
- *Motivational enhancement:* a therapeutic approach that avoids confrontation, acknowledges and examines ambivalence, and assists the patient to utilise inconsistencies in their present behaviours with identified goals, as a means of motivating change.
- *Relapse prevention:* a set of techniques learnt by the patient to prevent return to substance intake, particularly at times when there is high risk of use. It involves a behavioural analysis of substance-related behaviours, intervention that is tailored to the individual's needs and the acceptance that temporarily lapsing back to use is possible but not catastrophic.
- *Cognitive-behaviour therapy (CBT):* focuses on developing non-substance-related behavioural strategies, adaptive coping skills, and identifying and correcting any thinking errors.
- *Contingency management/behaviour modification:* provides positive reinforcement for abstinence in structured treatment programs.
- *Community reinforcement approaches:* a therapeutic approach that focuses on the individual's environmental and social factors that maintain drug intake and which discourage drug use.
- *Acceptance and commitment therapy:* learning to accept what is out of their personal control and to focus on whatever is within their control to improve their quality of life.
- *12-step facilitation:* supports working through the 12 steps to achieve abstinence in conjunction with attendance at Alcoholics Anonymous, Narcotics Anonymous, etc.
- *Therapeutic communities:* residential treatment programs that focus on abstinence-based outcomes, generally over weeks to months. They use both individual and group therapies to address entrenched patterns of thinking and behaving relevant to the person's substance use.

Table 22.7

Common withdrawal syndromes

Substance	Onset after last use	Main features and duration	Serious complications	Withdrawal management
Alcohol	8–72 hours	Uncomplicated: nausea, tremor, anxiety, insomnia, tachycardia, hypertension, sweating. Most withdrawals resolve within 3–5 days.	Complicated withdrawals: delirium, hallucinations, seizures, death.	General support measures are sufficient for most, which are mild in severity; benzodiazepines are the mainstay; antipsychotics may be necessary for psychotic symptoms. Always remember thiamine.
Benzodiazepines	Onset delayed if long half-life (e.g. diazepam), and can occur up to 3 weeks. More rapid for short half-life benzodiazepines (e.g. alprazolam) and withdrawals can occur after 12–24 hours.	Muscle spasms, insomnia, nightmares, anxiety, headache, tachycardia, hypertension, tremor, sweating, nausea. Acute symptoms can last up to 2 months. Clinically noticeable symptoms may persist for many more months depending on the dose and duration of use.	Protracted withdrawal, seizures, delirium.	Convert to an equivalent dose of diazepam (although usually 80 mg maximum) and taper. Long-term use may require a slow withdrawal over many months.
Heroin	6–24 hours (typically 8)	Sweating, nausea, vomiting, abdominal cramps, diarrhoea, muscle aches, fever, cold sweats, pupillary dilation, piloerection. Severe acute symptoms last less than 5–7 days. Milder complaints gradually subside over weeks.		Mild withdrawals may only require symptomatic treatment of withdrawal complaints (using temazepam, metoclopramide, diphenoxylate, ibuprofen, clonidine). More severe withdrawals may require buprenorphine regimen.

Methamphetamine	12–24 hours	Initial crash phase of oversleeping, eating excessively and exhaustion (1–2 days). Followed by more prolonged withdrawal with anxiety, dysphoria, sleeplessness, teariness, irritability, inability to concentrate, which can take weeks to resolve.	General supportive measures. Symptomatic relief of individual complaints.
Cannabis	Longer than 24 hours	Irritability, anxiety, anorexia, insomnia, sweating. No measurable physiological changes (4–7 days).	General supportive measures. Some may require symptomatic relief of individual complaints.
Nicotine	Begins after several hours	Irritability, restlessness, mood swings, sleep disturbance, anxiety, depression, poor concentration. Peak in first 24–72 hours, lasting 2–4 weeks.	Nicotine replacement therapies, bupropion and varenicline.
Caffeine	12–24 hours	Headache, drowsiness, fatigue, reduced concentration, 'flu-like' symptoms. Peaks at 1–2 days and may last up to 9 days.	Nil specific.

Table 22.8

Pharmacological treatments used in substance dependence disorders

Substance	Pharmacological options for management of dependence
Alcohol	Acamprosate, naltrexone, disulfiram
Benzodiazepines	Equivalent dose of diazepam and taper slowly
Heroin	Buprenorphine, buprenorphine/naloxone, methadone
Stimulants	Evidence lacking
Cannabis	Evidence lacking
Nicotine	Nicotine replacement therapies, bupropion and varenicline
Hallucinogens	Evidence lacking
Inhalants	Evidence lacking
Caffeine	Evidence lacking

Pharmacotherapy

There are evidence-based pharmacological approaches to some but not all substance dependence disorders (see Table 22.8).

Social aspects

Prohibition is a component of the policy adopted for substances such as heroin, cannabis and methamphetamines. Alcohol and tobacco are prohibited for people under certain ages in most states of Australia, and are subject to legislation and taxation to regulate their use.

Harm minimisation is another component of Australia's National Drug Strategy, and has three main elements:

- supply reduction (customs, police, courts, prisons)
- demand reduction (prevention)
- harm reduction (treatments and risk reduction). Prescribing methadone to patients with heroin dependence is an example of a treatment that has harm reduction as its principle aim.

Case studies: Substance abuse

Polydrug dependence

A 24-year-old unemployed man reported that he began using cannabis and alcohol after the death of his mother when he was 12. His mother had been the neutralising influence to his father's strict and unaffectionate parenting style. While still attending school he used cannabis almost daily and his alcohol intake steadily increased. He was expelled from school after repeatedly attending in an intoxicated state. He was an unreliable employee, and alienated himself from his father and siblings before eventually moving out of home. Injecting drug use began shortly

Continued

Case studies continued

afterwards, when he began experimenting with both heroin and amphetamines. He settled into a pattern of use that included benzodiazepines, intravenous amphetamines, alcohol and intermittent cannabis use. He had numerous encounters with the police for trivial offences related to intoxicated behaviour. He began to present to casualty departments from the age of 17 with suicide attempts, and brief psychotic episodes coupled with behavioural disturbance. He usually stayed for short periods only, before being discharged or leaving on his own accord. He was frequently urged to stop taking substances but didn't engage with treatment. When he tried reducing his use himself, he found that his anger and anxiety became overwhelming and he could not cope without feeling intoxicated. One day his sister tracked him down after some years of no contact. She pleaded with him to stop. He was shocked when she said he looked as though he would die soon and made him study his appearance in a mirror. With her persuasion he sought an admission for detoxification and withdrawal.

Treatment: Once detoxified, he was encouraged to aim for abstinence as an intermediate if not long-term goal. Psychological approaches included relapse prevention strategies and therapy aimed at improving his self-efficacy. Given the early age of onset, multiple drugs, social chaos and interrupted personality development, he required long-term rehabilitation, initially in a therapeutic community, followed by a residential program that involved learning basic life skills without drugs. Individual psychological work, addressing issues of anger, loss and mistrust (related to the death of his mother and perceived rejection from his family and community), was instituted.

Alcohol dependence with social anxiety

A 44-year-old man had received the disability pension for over 10 years. He had to stop work when his IT job required him to have more and more customer contact. He was very anxious that he may not know the answer to questions and would appear foolish. He had always drunk heavily on the weekends, but once he left work, his intake slowly increased until he was consuming at least 2 bottles of rosé per day (more than 15 standard drinks). He had the hallmarks of alcohol dependence, and had not had any significant periods of abstinence. His life had become constricted to staying at home and drinking alcohol. He could only leave his house if he was sure that he wouldn't encounter a situation in which he may need to ask a question. His GP reviewed him at home after being called by his family, and was appalled by the deteriorated state of his lodgings and the accumulated rubbish lying about. His GP prescribed an SSRI and acamprosate, but he had stopped taking the latter, feeling that it was not helpful.

He was aware that both alcohol and his anxiety were problems and he wanted to address them.

Treatment: As it was considered highly likely that he would experience withdrawal symptoms on cessation of his alcohol, he was admitted to hospital for detoxification and longer-term treatment planning. Part of this process was to engage a psychologist to assist with his anxiety symptoms, as relapse was felt to be highly likely if he was not able to learn to tolerate his anxiety symptoms. Treatment included motivational enhancement and relapse prevention for his alcohol dependence. Naltrexone was instituted to enhance his chances of remaining abstinent.

Heroin dependence

A 32-year-old woman had begun to smoke heroin when she was 26 years old after being introduced to the drug by her boyfriend. Initially she didn't like the nausea

Continued

Case studies continued

she experienced, but persisted using, even though she had to increase the amount she used each time to achieve the same effect. It wasn't long after that that she noticed she had a 'habit', and needed to use the drug two to three times each day. To maximise the experience, she began injecting the drug. The cost of using became prohibitive, so she began to work in the sex industry in order to sustain her heroin use. For various reasons she decided that she wanted to stop using, and had undergone detoxification a number of times in the previous year, although had relapsed within weeks.

Treatment: A maintenance/substitution program with either methadone or buprenorphine was instituted. The pros and cons of this approach were carefully explained, and additional psychosocial treatment provided.

REFERENCES AND FURTHER READING

Allsop, S. (Ed.), 2008. Responding to co-occurring mental health and drug disorders. Melbourne: IP Communications.

Baigent, M.F., 2003. Physical complications of substance abuse: What the psychiatrist needs to know. Current Opinion in Psychiatry 16, 291–296.

Hunter, B., Lubman, D.I., 2010. Substance misuse - management in the older population. Australian Family Physician 39, 738–741.

Kosten, T.R., O'Connor, P.G., 2003. Management of drug and alcohol withdrawal. New England Medical Journal 348, 1786–1795.

Lubman, D.I., Baker, A., 2010. Managing cannabis and mental health issues within primary care. Australian Family Physician 39, 554–557.

Lubman, D.I., King, J., Castle, D.J., 2010. Treating comorbid substance use disorders in schizophrenia. International Review of Psychiatry 22, 191–201.

Lubman, D.I., Sundram, S., 2003. Substance use in patients with schizophrenia: a primary care guide. Medical Journal of Australia 178, S71–S75.

Mathias, S., Lubman, D.I., Hides, L. 2008. Substance-induced psychosis: a diagnostic conundrum. Journal of Clinical Psychiatry 69, 358–367.

Miller, W.R., Rollnick, S. (Eds.), 2002. Motivational interviewing: preparing people for change. Guilford Press, New York.

Prochaska, J.O., DiClemente, C.C., Norcross, J.C., 1992. In search of how people change: applications to addictive behaviours. American Psychologist 47, 1102–1114.

Saunders, J.B., et al., 1993. Development of alcohol use disorders identification test (AUDIT): WHO collaborative project on early detection of persons with harmful alcohol consumption: II. Addiction 88, 791–804.

Schuckit, M.A., 2006. Drug and alcohol abuse: a clinical guide to diagnosis and treatment. Springer, New York.

A PATIENT NAMED PETER

CASE-BASED LEARNING

ANDREW GLEASON & JOEL KING

The following role-play requires two participants: one to play an intern (candidate) and another to play a patient named Peter Bergdorf and an examiner (actor).

OSCE Station Instructions

(Reading time: 2 minutes)

You are an intern working a night shift in an outer metropolitan hospital. At 2 am, you are paged by a nurse on the orthopaedics ward. The nurse asks you to prescribe a sleeping tablet for Peter Bergdorf, a 33-year-old who was admitted after a motor vehicle accident. He seems anxious and can't sleep.

You review his file. He was admitted about two days ago with left tibia and fibula fractures after his car went off the road into a ditch. His GCS was 15 when the ambulance arrived at the scene. He had an open reduction and internal fixation. He has no other injuries aside from some bruising and a forehead laceration which required suturing. He has no documented past medical or psychiatric history.

The most recent nursing entry reads:

18 May 20XX. 02:05

Patient admitted after MVA for ORIF of L tibia fracture. Non-weight bearing. On IV fluids. Patient seems anxious and requests a sleeping tablet. Intern informed. Patient looks sweaty. Obs: BP 140/85, HR 110, T 37.1, RR 12, O2 sats 99%.

L. Murphy, R.N.

His medications are:
- Oxycodone 5 mg qid
- Morphine 5 mg qid prn (he has had this four times in the last 24 hours).

Task (10 minutes)

- Interview Mr Bergdorf (8 minutes).
- After 8 minutes you have 2 minutes to present the most likely diagnosis, important differential diagnoses, and a management plan for the next 24 hours to the examiner.
- You do not need to perform a physical examination.

Actor role: Peter Bergdorf

You are 33 years old and live on your own in rental accommodation. You work as a plasterer.

HISTORY OF PRESENTING COMPLAINT

Three days ago you were driving home from work. You swerved to avoid a car that had come into your lane, ran into a ditch and hit a tree. You were driving about 70 kilometres per hour. You did not hit your head and can clearly remember what happened.

Explain to the doctor that you can't sleep. The ward is very noisy. The nurses keep walking by, and another patient is snoring really loudly. Your bed is uncomfortable. Last night you only got an hour or two of sleep. You also feel sick in the stomach and kind of nauseous. You attribute this to the morphine. However, you have not vomited. You feel anxious. You are alert and well oriented. If asked specifically about hallucinations, say that you saw some spiders on the ceiling a few hours ago, but you realised that there was nothing there. You have not had any illusions or hallucinations in other modalities.

You have not experienced any delusions. You have no symptoms of depression, aside from insomnia, which is relieved by 'a drink or two' before bed (only mention this if specifically asked about your sleep prior to coming to hospital).

You have no symptoms suggestive of infection or a pleural embolism, such as cough and shortness of breath.

PAST HISTORY

You have no past medical, surgical, or psychiatric history.

DRUG AND ALCOHOL HISTORY

If the doctor asks you if you drink, say 'socially'. Do not give any further information unless they enquire further.

You drink 10 to 15 bottles of beer (usually 375 mL) nearly every day after you get home from work. You also go out with your mates every weekend and have up to 10 bourbon and colas in addition to your usual 10 to 15 beers. You have maintained a similar pattern of weekend drinking since you were about 20. You first had a drink when your dad gave you a beer at the age of 13. Aside from getting drunk a few times at parties, you didn't drink regularly until you were 18. You began drinking during the week over the last five years, either at home or at the pub with mates from work. Initially this was a six-pack most days, but it increased over the last year or two. You drink from when you arrive home until you go to bed. You do get a bit shaky on days when you don't drink. Say, 'Actually, I'm feeling a bit shaky now, Doc.'

You find that it takes you more to get intoxicated than it used to. You do drink more than you intend at times, but you enjoy drinking and don't see it as a problem. Work is very important to you and you always show up, although you have been late a few times after a big night. Your boss thinks you do great work, so he tolerates the fact that you have been showing up late occasionally.

You would never drink and drive, and were not intoxicated when you had the car accident. You used to play footy on the weekends but stopped about a year ago because it was too difficult to get up for training if you'd had a big night. You never get angry when you are drunk, although if specifically asked about fights, admit that you did get into a fight in a bar once about six months ago and got a black eye. You have had no blackouts or seizures. You have never had any treatment for alcohol use. You drink because you enjoy it, and because it's what your mates do. If the doctor asks you if you feel you should cut down on your drinking, if you feel guilty about it, if people have criticised you for drinking, or if you need a drink first thing in the morning, say 'no', and get a little irritable.

You smoked marijuana occasionally at parties in the past, to the extent of once a month, but you haven't used any for years. You have taken ecstasy (MDMA) and cocaine a few times in your early twenties. You have never taken any other amphetamines, or used intravenous drugs, hallucinogens or inhalants. You have never taken benzodiazepines and don't smoke cigarettes.

FAMILY HISTORY

Your father was 'a bit of a drinker' and died at 71 of heart problems. Your mother is alive and well.

PERSONAL AND DEVELOPMENTAL HISTORY

You are an only child. You were an average academic student. You got in trouble because you couldn't stay seated in the classroom and found it difficult to concentrate, so you left after Year 10 and did an apprenticeship in plasterwork.

Your partner of eight years, to whom you were engaged, left you six months ago. If asked, say it happened out of the blue, but if pushed for more details, admit that you had been having arguments for about a year. If asked directly whether your drinking was contributing, reluctantly admit that this is a possibility, but only if the doctor seems very empathic. Do not mention this if you are not asked.

FORENSIC HISTORY

You have no forensic history.

HOW TO PLAY THE ROLE

Simulate a slight but noticeable tremor in your hands throughout the interview. You just want to get some sleep and wish the doctor would hurry up and give you a tablet. Your drinking isn't any problem from your point of view – it's what all of your mates do. If the doctor suggests that it might be a problem, you find this judgemental, and you get a bit irritable unless the doctor seems very understanding.

Statements you must make:

- Ask the intern at least three times to give you a sleeping tablet.
- 'Can you hurry up, Doc? I just want to get some sleep. Do you really have to ask so many questions?'

Model Answer

This patient gives a history of alcohol withdrawal. The candidate will consider a broad range of differential diagnoses, including a pleural embolism since this is an immobile post-operative patient who is tachycardic, but will recognise that alcohol withdrawal is the most likely cause of his symptoms (see Table 22.7, page 374).

The candidate should interview in a non-judgemental, empathic manner and take a systematic drug and alcohol history (see Box 22.1, page 369). In a patient with signs and symptoms suggestive of withdrawal, a screening test alone, such as the CAGE questionnaire (see Table 22.4, page 367), is inadequate. The lifetime pattern of drinking, current consumption, physical and psychiatric sequelae, problems related to drinking, past treatment attempts, and family history should be covered. Alcohol dependence is more likely than abuse, given the presentation of withdrawal. The candidate should be able to differentiate abuse from dependence (see Table 22.3, page 367). This patient describes tolerance, withdrawal symptoms, considerable time spent using, neglect of other activities in favour of alcohol use, and use despite problems, which is consistent with dependence.

It is important to screen for illusions and hallucinations, as well as delusions, in a patient in alcohol withdrawal. The candidate will also screen for depressive symptoms, but should recognise that a major depressive episode cannot be diagnosed with certainty in a patient with concurrent heavy alcohol use, as alcohol can also cause depressive symptoms. A cognitive examination should be performed to screen for delirium, which could suggest Wernicke's encephalopathy or another condition such as an undiagnosed neurological insult due to the motor vehicle accident.

A physical examination should be part of the management plan. This will include a neurological examination to look for signs of Wernicke's encephalopathy (ophthalmoplegia, nystagmus, ataxic gait), as well as signs of withdrawal (see Table 22.7, page 374) and disease related to chronic alcohol use.

Investigations should include a full blood count, looking for a raised MCV, and liver function tests, looking for a raised GGT. A raised INR may further indicate liver dysfunction.

The patient should be placed on an alcohol withdrawal scale (AWS). Regular diazepam and *pro re nata* diazepam, according to the AWS score, should be charted. *It is imperative that Mr Bergdorf is given thiamine.* He should not receive intravenous glucose before thiamine, as this could precipitate Wernicke's encephalopathy.

The candidate should include a discussion of their management plan with an appropriate senior doctor, such as a medical registrar or drug and alcohol registrar, and should inform the orthopaedics team of their findings and management plan.

FOR THE MORE ADVANCED LEARNER

Longer-term management is not addressed in this case. Nonetheless, the candidate should be aware of the broad range of psychological and pharmacological strategies for substance abuse, and should recognise that these need to be tailored to the patient's stage of change and personal preferences (see pages 370–376). For example, a brief intervention for Mr Bergdorf's alcohol use would be appropriate, but a rehabilitation program, or pharmacotherapy, such as disulfiram, naltrexone, or acamprosate, is unlikely to be of immediate use, given that he is at a pre-contemplative stage.

Index

Page numbers followed by 'f' indicate figures, 't' indicate tables, and 'b' indicate boxes.

A

ABC membrane transport proteins 215–16
abnormal illness behaviour 188
absorption 216
acceptance/commitment therapy 207
acetylcholine 122
acquired brain injury 76–8
   cognitive impairment 77–8
   frontal lobe syndrome 77, 77b
   mild TBI 76
   post-concussional syndrome 76, 76b
   post-traumatic amnesia 76
actuarial prediction 336
acute settings 287b
adaptive functioning domains 345
ADD *see* attention deficit disorders
ADHD *see* attention deficit hyperactivity disorder
adjunctive medications 249
adolescents *see* child and adolescent psychology
adrenal cortical disease 80–1
adrenal medullary disease 81
age *see specific age groups*
aggression
   instrumental 283
   management 284–7
   neurobiology of 284
   as psychiatric emergency 283
   psychosocial elements of 284
   reactive 283
   see also violence
agomelatine 215t, 228t
agoraphobia 152
   case example 154
alcohol 362
   effects of 363t
   standard drinks 368f
alprazolam 218, 218t
American Psychiatric Association
   DSM relating to 22
   foundation of 14
amines 120–2
amisulpride 235t
amitriptyline 222t
amnesia 76
amphetamines
   abuse of 363
   development of 16
AN *see* anorexia nervosa
The Anatomy of Melancholy (Burton) 7
anorexia nervosa (AN) 173–6
   case history 176b
   criteria for 174t
   description of 173
   DSM on 174t

ICD on 174t
   medical complications of 174b
   prevalence of 173
   thiamine deficiency from 176
   treatment of 173
      hospitalisation 175
      nutritional rehabilitation 175
anticholinergic medication 238
anti-convulsants 242
   doses and side effects 243t
   indications 242
   mode of action 242
   see also specific anti-convulsants
antidepressant medications 125
   for anxiety disorders 152b
   for bipolar disorders 114
   for bulimia nervosa 178
   clinical notes on 233b
   CYP enzymes relating to 216
   CYP isoenzyme inhibition by 215t
   for dementia 321
   doses, half-lives, and common side effects of 228t
   general comments on 220–1
   during pregnancy 248
   serotonergic 164
   suicide risk and 221b
   TCAs 226–7
   see also specific antidepressants
antipsychotic medication 232
   adverse effect frequency 235t–6t
   for bipolar disorders 114
   clinical notes on 240b
   for dementia 320–1
   EPS 238b–9b
   first generation 234, 237b
   general comments 232
   indications 234
   for OCD 164
   during pregnancy 248
   for schizophrenia 105
   second and third generation 234–40
   see also specific antipsychotics
anxiety/anxiety disorders
   anxiolytics for 218
   arousal, performance efficiency, and 148f
   case example 153b–4b
   case-based learning 157b–61b
   causes of 150b
      physical 150
      psychiatric 150
   of children 305, 306t
   classification of 67–9, 68b, 150t
   common elements of 149
   DSM on 150t

anxiety/anxiety disorders (Continued)
 in elderly 325
 GAD 68, 153–4
 ICD on 150t
 intellectual disability relating to 353
 neuroanatomy of 149b
 neurochemistry of 149
 panic attacks 148–9, 151b
 panic disorder 68, 149–51, 153–4
 phobic disorders 151–3
 SAD 152–3
 schizophrenia relating to 98
 symptoms of 148
 treatment of 151
  antidepressants 152b
  benzodiazepines 151
  clonazepam 219
anxiolytics 218t
 clinical notes on 218b
 indications of 218
 during pregnancy 248
arbitrary interference 269
Aretaeus of Cappadocia 5
arousal 148f
asenapine 235t, 240
Asperger's disorder 303
Asylum era 8
atomoxetine 246
attachment theory 270
attention deficit disorders (ADD) 246
 clinical notes 245b
 medications for 246t
attention deficit hyperactivity disorder (ADHD) 306–7,
  307t
atypical depression 116, 116b
auditory hallucinatory experiences 95
autism and autism spectrum disorders 303, 346–8
 aetiology 348
 criteria for 347b
 management 348
autoimmune diseases 79
 see also specific autoimmune diseases
autonomy
 concept of 27
 decisional capacity 28b
 ethics relating to 27
Axis II disorders 97

B
Bailey, Harry 23
Bandura, Albert 205–6
Battie, William 9
BDD see body dysmorphic disorder
Beck, Aaron 22, 205–6, 268
behaviour disorders 353
 see also specific disorders
behavioural therapy 267–8
 case example 267b–8b
benzhexol 238
benzodiazepines 74, 218–19, 238
 abuse of 363

adverse effects 153
 for anxiety disorders 151
 for bipolar disorders 114
 general comments 219, 242
 mode of action 219
 for PTSD 155
benztropine 238
bereavement 265–6, 266b
 see also grief
Berne, Eric 272
Bertillon, Jacques 17
binge eating disorders 178
 case history 179b
biological treatments
 absorption 216
 age relating to 217
 case-based learning 258b–63b
 drug interactions 215–16
 hepatic and renal dysfunction 216
 of OCD 164
 practical notes on 217b
 psychopharmacology 214
 for schizophrenia 105
 specific medications 217–40
biopsychosocial model 25
bipolar depression 140
bipolar disorders
 aetiology of 137–8
 brain in 139f
 case examples 136b–7b
 case-based learning 143b–6b
 in China 7
 clinical features of 132–7
 core elements of 132b
 course of 134–5
 depressed phase of 134
 differential diagnosis 137
 DSM on 132t
 in elderly 324
  case example 324b
 endocrine in 138
 features of 132t
 genetic factors of 137–8
 ICD on 132t
 management of 139–41
  antidepressant medications 114
  antipsychotic medications 114
  benzodiazepines 114
  biological interventions 141b
  clinical assessment 139
  lithium 324
  psychosocial interventions 141
  sodium valproate 324
  strategy summary 133b
 mania 132–4, 140
 medications for 140
 mixed bipolar states 136
 neurocognition 138
 neuroimaging 138
 neurotrophic factors of 138
 personality disorders relating to 137

prevalence of 131
psychosocial contributions 138
schizoaffective disorder relating to 136
signal transduction pathways 138
substance abuse and 137
sub-syndromal 136
types of 134f
bipolar spectrum disorders
classification of 66b
description of 66
management of 141
symptoms of 66
Bleuler, Eugen 18
blood tests
complete blood examination 53
physical examination 52–5
blood-injury phobia 153
BN *see* bulimia nervosa
body dysmorphic disorder (BDD) 164–5
Bowlby, John 270, 272
brain
in bipolar disorders 139f
in depressive disorders 120–2, 121b, 121f
disease 102–04
in schizophrenia 103b
breast feeding 247–8
see also pregnancy and lactation
brief cognitive screen 43b
brief psychodynamic psychotherapy 208
Bright, Timothy 7
bulimia nervosa (BN) 176–8
case history 178b
criteria for 177t
description of 176
DSM on 177t
ICD on 177t
medical complications of 177b
treatment of 177–8
antidepressants 178
psychological interventions 178
bupropion 215t, 228t, 248
Burckhardt, Johann 16
Burton, Robert 7
buspirone 218t, 219
clonazepam 219
general comments 219
mode of action 220

C
Cade, John 21
caffeine 365
cancer 98
cannabis 364
carbamazepine 242, 243t
during pregnancy 249
cardiovascular disorders 84
cardiovascular risk 98
Carlsson, Arvid 23
Castle Hill 12
CBT *see* cognitive behavioural therapy
cerebrovascular disease 78, 78t

character 199
definition of 199
child and adolescent psychology
adolescents and youth 309–11
case-example on 312b
depression in 117, 309–11, 310b, 310t
self-harm 311, 311t
aetiology 298–9
assessment 300–01, 300b
adolescents 301
children 300–01
case-based learning 313b–16b
classification of psychiatric disorders 302t
depression in 117
educational factors 299
family factors 299
forensic psychiatry 333
formulation and feedback 301
genetic factors relating to 299
infancy and early childhood 302–04
case example 303b
disorders of 303b
elimination disorders 304
intellectual disability 302–03
pervasive developmental disorders 303
management 301–02
medication 301–02
specific disorders 02
parental mental illness 299
parental separation and divorce 299
physical examination and investigations 301
primary school children 305–08
ADHD 306–07, 307t
anxiety disorders 305, 306t
case example 305b, 309b
conduct disorder 308, 309t
disorders of 305b
learning disorders 306, 307t
ODD 308, 308b
social and economic hardship 299
trauma 299
Chinese medicine 3
chlorpromazine 235t, 237b, 287
development of 21
cholinesterase inhibitors 320
chronic pain 85
chronic schizophrenia 99
circular questioning 276
citalopram 141, 215t, 223t, 248
civil arena forensic psychiatry 332–3
clinical judgement 336
clinician safety 289
clomipramine 164, 216, 222t
clonazepam 218t, 219, 287
intramuscular preparation 288
Cloninger, Robert
on personality 198
personality disorders relating to 201
clozapine 235t, 240b
cocaine 364
coercion 28

cognition 43
cognitive behavioural therapy (CBT) 269
  case example 270b
cognitive functioning 97
cognitive impairment 77–8
cognitive testing 320
cognitive therapy 268
  case example 269b
  mindfulness-based 207
  thinking traps 269b
commitment therapy 207
community care 25
comorbid intellectual disability 117
comorbidity
  developmental disorders and 348–50
  intellectual disability relating to 348–50, 349b
  personality disorders relating to 203, 203b
  PTSD relating to 98
  schizophrenia relating to 98
compensation neurosis 154
compulsory treatment 288–9
computerised tomography (CT) 55
  scanner 23
conditioned reflex 17
conduct disorder 308, 309t
confidentiality 30–1
  breaking, situations for 31b
  Duty to Protect 30
  Tarasoff I 30
  Tarasoff II 30
conflicts of interest 31
  other 32
  relationships with pharmaceutical companies 31–2
consent 28–9
  decisional capacity 28
  disclosure of information 28–9
  freedom from coercion or voluntariness 28
  Nuremberg Code 28
  requirements for 28
  to treatment 354
consequentialism 26
conversion disorder
  definition of 185
  specific treatment for 192t
countertransference 272
couple therapy 276
courts 334–5
criminal jurisdictions 333–4
CT see computerised tomography
current life situation 40
cyclopyrrolones 244
cyclothymia 67
Cytochrome p450 (CYP) enzymes/isoenzymes 215
  antidepressants relating to 216
  CYP1A2 252t–6t
  CYP2C9 252t–6t
  CYP2C19 252t–6t
  CYP2D6 252t–6t
  CYP2E1 252t–6t
  CYP3A3/4 252t–6t
  drugs metabolized by 252t–4t

inducers or inhibitors of 255t–6t
inhibition 215t

D
DBT see dialectical behaviour therapy
debriefing 155
decisional capacity 28, 28b
deep sleep therapy
  Bailey relating to 23
  Klaesi-Blumer relating to 19
defence mechanisms 274b–5b
delirium 71–3, 322
  case example 322b
  causes of 71–2, 73b
  description of 71
  intellectual disability relating to 352
  management of 72–3, 74b, 322
    haloperidol 322
  medications for 74b
  prevention 322
  symptoms of 72b
delusional disorders
  description of 96
  in elderly 325–6
  pathological jealousy 99
delusional perception 95
dementia 318–21
  assessment 318–20
  case example 321b
  causes of 75b, 318t
  clinical presentation 318
  cognitive testing 320
  description of 74
  family environment relating to 321
  history relating to 318–19
  intellectual disability relating to 352
  management 320–21
    antidepressants 321
    antipsychotic medication for 320–21
    risperidone 320–21
  medical conditions relating to 320–21
  mental state examination 319
  physical examination 320
  symptoms of 319b
demyelinating diseases 79
  multiple sclerosis 79
deontology 26
depression/depressive disorders
  in adolescents and children 117, 309–11, 310b, 310t
  aetiology of 120–3
  atypical 116, 116b
  bipolar 140
  brain in 120–2, 121b, 121f
  case examples 119b, 127b–30b
  in children 117
  classification of 67, 67b
  clinical features of 114–15
  comorbid intellectual disability 117
  core elements of 114b
  differential diagnosis 116–20
  DSM on 113t

ECT for 125
in elderly 117, 322–3
 assessment 323
 case example 324b
 clinical features 323
 management 323
endocrinology 122
episode features 113t
genetic factors of 120
grief relating to 116–17, 117b
hallucinations in 116
ICD on 113t
immunology 122
light therapy for 125
management of 123–5, 124b
 biological therapies 125
 in elderly 323
 medications for 125
 physical therapies for 125
 psychological therapies for 124
medical conditions associated with 118, 118b
mood changes in 114
natural history of 116–20
neurochemistry 120–2
neuroimaging 120
in pregnancy/post-partum 117
premenstrual dysphoric disorder 117
prognosis 126
psychological therapies for 124
psychosocial contributions to 122–3
psychotic 115–16
schizophrenia relating to 98, 118
self-care relating to 115
sleep relating to 122
social interaction in 115
subtypes of 115b
thinking in 114
vegetative functions in 114–15
see also antidepressant medications; suicidality
Descartes, René 8
desmethylvenlafaxine 215t, 225
desvenlafaxine 224, 228t
developmental disorders
 comorbidity and 348–50
 pervasive 97, 303, 346
dexamphetamine 246
DHA see docosahexaenoic acid
diabetes mellitus 81
diagnosis distortion 84
Diagnostic and Statistical Manual of Mental Disorders
 (DSM)
 on AN 174t
 American Psychiatric Association relating to 22
 on anxiety disorders 150t
 on bipolar disorders 132t
 on bulimia nervosa 177t
 on depressive disorders 113t
 on eating disorders 173t
 ICD classification compared to 62–3, 63t
 on intellectual disability 332–3, 333b
 multiaxial structure 45b

on personality disorders 200t
on schizophrenia 96t, 97b
on somatoform disorders 185t–6t
on substance abuse 367t
third edition of 25
dialectical behaviour therapy (DBT) 207, 270–1
 case example 209b
diazepam 218, 218t, 243t
dichotomous thinking 269
disclosure of information 28–9
 criteria for 29b
 Professional Practice Standard 29
 Reasonable Person Standard 29
 Rogers v Whitaker relating to 29, 29b
 Subjective Standard 29
 see also confidentiality
Discourse de la Methode (Descartes) 8
distortion of diagnosis 84
docosahexaenoic acid (DHA) 246
doctor avoidance 186
dopamine 121b
dopaminergic mechanisms 104
dothiepin 222t
downward arrow technique 268
drug interactions 215–16
DSM *see Diagnostic and Statistical Manual of Mental*
 Disorders
dual disability
 assessment issues 348
 clinical tips for 351b
 case examples 351b–2b, 354b
 case-based learning 357–61
 definition of 344
 diagnostic and classification issues 350
 intellectual disability 344–6
 management 354–6
 pharmacotherapy 354
 psychological treatments 355
 social interventions 355
 people involved in care of 355t
 process issues 348–50
 specific psychiatric disorders 352–3
duloxetine 215t, 224–5, 228t
 during pregnancy 248
Dutch Republic 8
Duty to Protect 30
dynamic risk factors 336
dysthymia 67

E
eating disorders
 anorexia nervosa 173–6
 binge 178
 bulimia nervosa 176–8
 case-based learning 181–3
 classification of 173t
 DSM on 173t
 ICD on 173t
 obesity 179–80
 other 178
economic hardship 299

ecstasy 364
ECT *see* electroconvulsive therapy
EEG *see* electroencephalography
ego boundaries 95
Egypt 3
eicosapentaenoic acid (EPA) 246
elderly 117
　suicide rates in 322
　see also old age psychiatry
electroconvulsive therapy (ECT) 249–51
　adverse effects 250–1
　contradictions 250
　for depression 125
　indications for use of 250
　mechanisms and action of 250
　nature of 249
electroencephalography (EEG) 55
electrolytes 53
elimination disorders 304
employment 106
endocrine and metabolic disorders 80–1
　see also specific endocrine and metabolic disorders
endocrine functions 85
　in bipolar disorders 138
　physical examination 53–4
endocrinology 122
Engle, George L. 25
EPA *see* eicosapentaenoic acid
epilepsy 80
　clinical features of 80
EPS *see* extrapyramidal side effects
Erikson, Erik 272
escitalopram 141, 215t, 248
ethical decision-making 26–9
　consequentialism 26
　deontology 26
　Kantianism 26
　utilitarianism 26
ethics
　autonomy relating to 27
　confidentiality 30–1
　conflicts of interest 31
　consent 28–9
　power imbalance and 26
　principle-based 27
　professional boundaries 32–3
　virtue 27
exercise 249
exogenous corticosteroids 81
extrapyramidal side effects (EPS) 238b–9b
　tardiv forms 239

F
family
　forensic psychiatry relating to 333
　history 39
　therapy 273–6
family environment
　child and adolescent psychology relating to 299
　dementia relating to 321
　schizophrenia relating to 102, 106

first generation antipsychotics 234, 237b
first onset schizophrenia 98
fitness to plead 334–5
　case example 334b–5b
flunitrazepam 218t, 242
fluoxetine 215t, 223t, 248
flupenthixol decanoate 236t
fluphenazine 235t, 237b
fluphenazine decanoate 236t
fluvoxamine 215t, 223t, 248
folic acid 249
forensic history 40
forensic psychiatry
　areas of work in 332–4
　　children and family 333
　　civil arena 332–3
　　courts and fitness to plead 334–5
　　criminal jurisdictions 333–4
　　secure psychiatric units 334
　case-based learning 339b–43b
　risk assessment 335–8
　　HCR-20 337, 337b
　　instruments 337–8
Frank, Jerome 264–5
freedom from coercion or voluntariness 28
Freud, Sigmund 272, 272b
　background on 18
frontal lobe syndrome 77, 77b
functional analysis of behaviours 336b
future developments 251
　light therapy 251
　magnetic stimulation therapy 251
　transcranial magnetic stimulation 251

G
GAD *see* generalised anxiety disorder
Galen of Pergamum 5
gastrointestinal disorders 84
gender 163
gene polymorphisms 120
generalised anxiety disorder (GAD) 153
　case examples 154
　description of 68
　treatment of 153
genetic factors
　of bipolar disorders 137–8
　child and adolescent psychology relating to 299
　of depression/depressive disorders 120
　of personality disorders 138
　of schizophrenia 102
George III (King) 9
Gladesville Macquarie Hospital 12
glutamatergic mechanisms 104
grief
　depression relating to 116–17, 117b
　management 265–6, 266b
Griesinger, Wilhelm 15
group therapy 208, 273
　advantages of 275b

H

habits 166
hallucinations 116
hallucinogens 364
haloperidol 74, 235t, 237b, 287
  for delirium 322
  intramuscular preparation 288
  intravenous administration 288
HCR-20 337, 337b
Hecker, Ewald 15
height 52
Heinroth, Johann 13
hepatic and renal dysfunction 216
heroin 365
history
  dementia relating to 318-19
  of depressive disorders, natural 116-20
  family 39
  forensic 40
  medical 39
  mental state examination 37-40
  past 38
  personal 39
  of presenting complaint 37-8
  psychiatric 38b
  of psychological medicine 2, 3t-25t
  of SSRIs 23
  substance abuse 39-40, 368-9, 369b
hoarding 163
hobbies 40
hospital for insane 7
Hounsfield, Godfrey 23
Human Acquired Immunodeficiency Virus 78
humane treatment 10
Huntington's disease 74-6
  clinical features of 74-5
  description of 74
  management of 75-6
hypericum perforatum (St. John's Wort) 217
hypnotics 242-5
  doses and half-lives 243t
  imidazopyridines 244
  see also benzodiazepines
hypochondriasis 165-6
  definition of 185
  specific treatment for 192t
hypothyroidism 80

I

ICD see Injuries and Causes of Death
ID see intellectual disability
identification 37
illness behaviour 188
  abnormal 188
imidazopyridines 244
  adverse effects 244
  general comments 244
  mode of action 244
imipramine 222t
  development of 22
immune function 84-5

immunology 122
impulse control disorders 166
India 3
indoleamines 244-5
  adverse effects 245
  general comments 245
  mode of action 245
Industrial Revolution 8
infants see child and adolescent psychology
infectious diseases 78-9
  see also specific infectious diseases
inhalants 365
Injuries and Causes of Death (ICD)
  on anorexia nervosa 174t
  on anxiety disorders 150t
  on bipolar disorders 132t
  on bulimia nervosa 177t
  on depressive disorders 113t
  DSM classification compared to 62-3, 63t
  on eating disorders 173t
  on personality disorders 200t
  on schizophrenia 96t, 97b
insight 42
instrumental aggression 283
insulin shock therapy 19
intellectual disability (ID) 344-6
  aetiology 345-6
  anxiety disorders relating to 353
  autism and autism spectrum disorders 303,
    346-8
  behaviour disorders relating to 353
  in children 302-03
  comorbidity relating to 348-50, 349b
  delirium relating to 352
  dementia relating to 352
  diagnostic and classification issues 350
  DSM on 344, 345b
  management 346
  mental health in severely disabled 353
  mood disorders relating to 352-3
  personality disorders relating to 353
  schizophrenia relating to 352
interpersonal psychotherapy (IPT) 270
interpersonal therapy 208
interview 37
intracellular signal transduction 122
intramuscular preparations 288
intravenous administration 288
iproniazid 22
IPT see interpersonal psychotherapy
isoniazid 22

J

jealousy 99
judgement
  actuarial prediction 336
  clinical 336
  mental state examination 43
  structured professional 336
Jung, Carl 272
  background on 18

K

Kahlbaum, Karl 15
Kantianism 26
Klaesi-Blumer, Jakob 19
Klein, Melanie 272
Kohut, Heinz 272
Korsakoff's syndrome 79b
Kraepelin, Emil 15
Kuhn, Roland 22

L

lactation *see* pregnancy and lactation
lamotrigine 141, 242, 243t
   during pregnancy 249
late onset schizophrenia 99
Lazarus, Richard 205–06
learning disorders 306, 307t
lie detector 19
life events 102
light therapy
   for depression/depressive disorders 125
   development of 251
lipids 54
lithium 241–2
   adverse effects 241–2
   for bipolar disorders 324
   Cade relating to 21
   clinical notes on 241b
   general comments 241
   indications 241
   medication blood levels of 54
   mode of action 241
   during pregnancy 248–9
liver function 53
lorazepam 74, 218t, 287
   intramuscular preparation 288
   intravenous administration 288
Lunacy Commission 14
lupus 79
Luria, Alexander
   lie detector relating to 19
   neuropsychology relating to 19

M

magnesium 249
magnetic resonance imaging (MRI) 55
magnetic stimulation therapy 251
major depressive disorder (MDD) 67
mania
   bipolar disorder 132–4, 140
   management of 140
MAOIs *see* monoamine oxidase inhibitors
Maudsley, Henry 14
Maudsley approach 36–7
MDD *see* major depressive disorder
medical conditions
   dementia relating to 320–1
   depression associated with 118, 118b
   psychological disorders and interaction with 84–6
   psychological responses to 83–4
   somatisation relating to 186

medical disorders *see* psychiatric disorders secondary to
      medical disorders
medical history 39
*Medical Inquiries and Observations upon the Diseases of
      the Mind* (Rush) 10
medication blood levels
   of lithium 54
   physical examination 54
   serology 54–5
   urine drug screens 55
   vitamin assays 55
medications
   absorption 216
   in acute setting 287b
   for ADD 246t
   adjunctive 249
   in America 10
   for bipolar disorders 140
   classification of 217
   doses, equivalents to diazepam and half-lives of
         anxiolytics 218t
   history of, psychological 2, 3t–25t
   oral 287
   during pregnancy/breast feeding 247–8
   recreational drugs relating to 217
   side effect management 217
   transport of 215–16
   see also biological treatments; *specific
         medications*
melatonin receptor agonists *see* serotonin receptor
      antagonists/melatonin receptor agonists
memantine 320
mensuration 52
mental state 36
mental state examination
   affect 42
   appearance and behaviour 40–1
   brief cognitive screen 43b
   case-based learning for 46–9
   cognition 43
   for dementia 319
   family history relating to 39
   forensic history relating to 40
   formulation 36, 44
   history 37–40
   identification 37
   insight 42
   interview 37
   judgement 43
   Maudsley approach to 36–7
   medical history relating to 39
   mood in 42
   overview of 41b
   perceptions 42
   personal history relating to 39
   presenting complaint 37–8
   psychiatric history
      overview 38b
      past 38
   psychiatric symptoms in 38
   speech in 41–2

substance abuse relating to 39–40, 369–70
  thought content 42
metabolic disorders *see* endocrine and metabolic
    disorders; *specific metabolic disorders*
metabolic functions 85
methylphenidate 246
Meyer, Adolph 270
mianserin 228t, 248
midazolam 288
  intravenous administration 288
mild traumatic brain injury (TBI) 76
mindfulness-based cognitive therapy 207
mirtazapine 215t, 228t, 248
mixed bipolar states 136
modafanil 247t
Moniz, António 17
monoamine oxidase inhibitors (MAOIs) 22,
    229–31
  adverse effects 229–31
  dietary restrictions 231t
  indications 229
  mode of action 229
mood
  in depressive disorders 114
  disorders 352–3
  in mental state examination 42
mood stabilisers 241–2
  during pregnancy and lactation 248 9
  see also specific mood stabilisers
Moore, Lawrence 30b
Morel, Bénédict 14
MRI *see* magnetic resonance imaging
multiple sclerosis 79

N
N-acetyl cysteine 249
narrative approach 276
NASAs *see* noradrenaline and specific serotonergic
    agents
neurochemistry
  amines 120–2
  of anxiety 149
  of depressive disorders 120–2
  intracellular signal transduction 122
  peptides and acetylcholine 122
  of schizophrenia 104
neurocognition 138
neurodevelopmental model 104
neuroimaging
  bipolar disorders 138
  CT 55
  depressive disorders 120
  MRI 55
  PET 56
  physical examination 55–6
  SPECT 55–6
neuroleptic malignant syndrome (NMS)
    238–9
neuroleptics 234
neurological disorders 166
neurological features 52

neurology 9
neuropsychology 19
neurosyphilis 79
nicotine 365
nitrazepam 243t
NMS *see* neuroleptic malignant syndrome
noradrenaline 121b
noradrenaline and dopamine re-uptake inhibitors
    227–9
  adverse effects 229
  indications 227
  metabolism 229
  mode of action 229
noradrenaline and specific serotonergic agents
    (NASAs) 226
  adverse effects 226
  general comments 226
  indications 226
  mode of action 226
nortriptyline 222t
NRIs *see* selective noradrenergic re-uptake inhibitors
Nuremberg Code 28

O
obesity 179–80
  classification of 179b
  prevalence of 179
  treatment for 179–80
observation 51–2
obsessive-compulsive disorders (OCD)
  case-based learning 168b–71b
  description of 162
  gender relating to 163
  hoarding 163
  management of 163–4
    antipsychotics 164
    biological treatment 164
    clomipramine 164
    psychological treatment 163–4
    serotonergic antidepressants 164
  prevalence of 163
  psychological domain 163–4
  subtypes of 163b
  symptoms of 163
obsessive-compulsive spectrum disorders (OCS)
    164–6
  BDD 164–5
  case examples 166b–7b
  description of 164
  hypochondriasis 165–6
  impulse control disorders 166
  neurological disorders 166
  symptoms of 68–9
  see also eating disorders
OCD *see* obsessive-compulsive disorders
OCS *see* obsessive-compulsive spectrum disorders
ODD *see* oppositional defiant disorder
oestrogen supplements 245–6
olanzapine 74, 235t, 287
  intramuscular preparation 288
olanzapine pamoate 236t

old age psychiatry
anxiety disorders 325
bipolar disorders 324
case-based learning 327b–31b
delirium 322
delusional disorders in 325–6
dementia 74, 318–21
depression 117, 322–3
schizophrenia 325–6
omega-3 fatty acids 246, 249
operational criteria 62–3
oppositional defiant disorder (ODD) 308, 308b
oral medications 287
organic disorders
classification of 65b
symptoms of 65
organic psychiatry
case-based learning for 88b–92b
psychiatric disorders secondary to medical
disorders 71–82
psychological disorders and interaction with general
medical conditions 84–6
psychological responses to general medical
conditions 83–4
organic psychoses 94
overgeneralisation 269
oxazepam 218t

P
pain, chronic 85
paliperidone 235t
paliperidone palmitate 236t
palpation 52
panic attacks
description of 148
features of 151b
habitual 149
panic disorder
case examples 153–4
description of 68, 149–51
paraneoplastic syndromes 79
parathyroid disease 81
parental mental illness 299
parental separation and divorce 299
paroxetine 215t, 223t, 224, 248
passivity phenomena 95
past history 38
pathological jealousy 99
Pavlov, Ivan 17
peptides 122
perceptions
delusional 95
mental state examination 42
performance efficiency 148f
pericyazine 235t
permeability of ego boundaries 95
personal history 39
personalisation 269
personality 198–9
Cloninger on 198

definition of 198
premorbid 40
personality disorders 199
aetiology 137–8
bipolar disorder relating to 137
case examples 202b
case-based learning 209b–13b
classification of 69–70, 199, 200t
Cloninger relating to 201
by cluster 201b
cognitively-derived theories on 205–06
comorbidity relating to 203, 203b
definition of 198
developmental factors relating to 204–05
differential diagnosis 203, 204b
DSM on 200t
genetic factors of 138
ICD on 200t
intellectual disability relating to 353
management of 206–07
crisis intervention 207b
crisis planning 206–07
specialised treatment 207–08
therapeutic alliance 206
neurobiological theories on 138
psychosocial theories on 205
social and cultural factors relating to 205
see also frontal lobe syndrome
pervasive developmental disorders 97, 346
in children 303
criteria for 347b
PET pethidine see positron emission tomography
P-glycoprotein (Pgp) 215–16
pharmaceutical companies 31–2
pharmacological management 287–9
intramuscular preparations 288
intravenous administration 288
oral medications 287
pharmacotherapy
for dual disability 354
for substance-induced disorders 376, 376t
phobic disorders 151–3
agoraphobia 152, 154
blood-injury phobia 153
description of 151
SAD 152–3
specific phobia 152
physical examination
blood tests 52–5
case-based learning for 57b–60b
of children and adolescents 301
context of 51
for dementia 320
EEG 55
electrolytes 53
endocrine functions 53–4
height 52
lipids 54
liver function 53
medication blood levels 54

mensuration 52
neuroimaging 55–6
neurological features, other 52
observation 51–2
palpation 52
reasons for 50–1
renal function 53
substance abuse 369
urine tests 52–5
waist circumference 52
weight 52
who performs 51
physical illness 188
physical restraint 286
physical treatments 249–51
  ECT 249–51
Pinel, Philippe 11
Poddar, Prosenjit 30b
positron emission tomography (PET) 56
post-concussional syndrome 76
  symptoms of 76b
post-Freudians 272b
post-traumatic amnesia 76
post-traumatic stress disorder (PTSD)
  case example 103b
  comorbidity relating to 98
  debriefing relating to 155
  schizophrenia relating to 98
  stages of 155b
  symptoms of 68, 69b, 155
  treatment of 155
    benzodiazepines 155
post-traumatic stress syndromes 154–5
power imbalance
  ethics and 26
  factors heightening 27b
pragmatic classification system 63–5, 64f
pregnancy and lactation
  antidepressants during 248
  antipsychotics during 248
  anxiolytics during 248
  breast feeding 247–8
  carbamazepine during 249
  depression during 117
  duloxetine during 248
  lamotrigine during 249
  lithium during 248–9
  mood stabilisers during 248–9
  risk of pharmacological treatment during 247b
  SSRIs during 248
  valproate during 249
premenstrual dysphoric disorder 117
premorbid personality 40
presenting complaint 37–8
principle-based ethics 27
professional boundaries 32–3
  in Australia 32, 32b
  non-sexual 33
  sexual 33
  slippery slope of 33

Professional Practice Standard 29
propranolol 238
psychiatric disorders secondary to medical
    disorders 71–82
  acquired brain injury 76–8
  autoimmune diseases 79
  cerebrovascular disease 78, 78t
  delirium 71–3
  dementia 74
  demyelinating diseases 79
  endocrine and metabolic disorders 80–1
  epilepsy 80
  Huntington's disease 74–6
  infectious diseases 78–9
  sleep disorders 82, 83b, 85
  speech and language disorders 81–2
  toxic disorders 80
  vitamin deficiencies 81
psychiatric emergencies
  aggression and violence 283
  case-based learning 293b–6b
  clinician safety 289
  compulsory treatment 288–9
  pharmacological management 287–9
  physical restraint 286
  seclusion 286–7
  suicidality 289–91
psychiatric history
  overview 38b
  past 38
psychodynamic psychotherapy 272–3
  brief 208
  case example 273b
psychoeducation 266–7
psychological disorders
  common investigations for first presentation of 51b
  interaction with general medical conditions
    and 84–6
  see also specific psychological disorders
psychopathy 338
psychopharmacology 214
psychosomatics 13
psychosurgery 16
psychotherapies
  behavioural therapy 267–8
  case study on 276b–8b
  case-based learning 280b–2b
  CBT 269
  cognitive therapy 268
  common features of 264–5
  couple therapy 276
  DBT 207, 270–1
  family therapy 273–6
  grief management 265–6, 266b
  group therapy 208, 273
  IPT 270
  psychodynamic 272–3
  psychoeducation 266–7
  supportive 265
  types of 265b

psychotic depression 115–16
PTSD *see* post-traumatic stress disorder

Q
Quakers 11
quetiapine 235t, 248

R
race 99–100
reactive aggression 283
Reasonable Person Standard 29
reboxetine 215t, 228t
recreational drugs 217
    see also substance abuse; *specific recreational drugs*
Reil, Johann 10
renal disfunction *see* hepatic and renal dysfunction
renal function 53
resistance 272
respiratory disorders 85–6
risk assessment 335–8
    instruments 337–8
risperidone 74, 235t, 287
    for dementia 320–1
risperidone depot 236t
Rogers v Whitaker 29, 29b
Rosenhan, David 24
Royal College of Physicians 7
Royal College of Psychiatrists 13
Royal Society 9
Rush, Benjamin 10

S
SAD *see* social anxiety disorder
safe restraint method 286b
Sakel, Manfred 19
schizoaffective disorder
    bipolar disorder relating to 136
    symptoms of 66, 96
schizophrenia
    aetiology 102–04
    anxiety disorders relating to 98
    Axis II disorders 97
    Bleuler relating to 18
    brain abnormalities in 103b
    as brain disease 102–04
    cancer relating to 98
    cardiovascular risk relating to 98
    case examples 98b–9b
    case-based learning for 107b–11b
    chronic 99
    classification of 65–6, 66b
    clinical features of 93–4
    cognitive functioning in 97
    comorbidity 98
    depression relating to 98, 118
    differential diagnosis 94–7
    dopaminergic mechanisms of 104
    DSM on 96t, 97b
    in elderly 325–6
    employment relating to 106
    environment relating to 102, 103b

epidemiology 99–101
    family environment relating to 102, 106
    first onset 98
    genetic factors of 102
    glutamatergic mechanisms of 104
    ICD on 96t, 97b
    intellectual disability relating to 352
    key aspects of 94b
    late onset 99
    life events relating to 102
    management 104–06
    neurochemistry of 104
    neurodevelopmental model of 104
    organic psychoses 94
    outcomes of 101–02, 101b
    pervasive developmental disorders 97, 346
    prevalence of 99
    PTSD relating to 98
    race relating to 99–100
    rates of 99–100
    risk markers in 335, 335b
    serotonergic mechanisms of 104
    social deprivation relating to 99–100
    substance abuse relating to 98, 100b
    subtypes of 97
    symptoms of 93–4, 95b, 95t
    treatment
        antipsychotic medication for 105
        biological 105
        family relating to 106
        psychological 105–06
        summary of 105
        vocational aspects 106
    see also delusional disorders
seclusion 286–7
second and third generation antipsychotics 234–40
    adverse effects 237–9
    cardiovascular side effects 240
    metabolic side effects 239–40
    mode of action 237
secure psychiatric units 334
selective attention 269
selective noradrenergic re-uptake inhibitors
        (NRIs) 225–6
    adverse effects 225–6
    general comments 225
    indications 225
    mode of action 225
selective serotonin reuptake inhibitors (SSRIs)
        221–4
    adverse effects 224
    dose ranges, half-lives, and common side effects
        of 223t
    general comments 221–4
    history of 23
    indications 224
    mode of action 224
    during pregnancy 248
self-care 115
self-harm 311, 311t
serology 54–5

serotonergic and noradrenergic re-uptake inhibitors (SNRIs) 224–5
  indications 224
  mode of action 225
serotonergic antidepressants 164
serotonergic mechanisms 104
serotonin 121b
serotonin receptor antagonists/melatonin receptor agonists 231–2
  adverse effects 232
  indications 232
  mode of action 232
serotonin syndrome 216b
sertindole 235t
sertraline 215t, 223t, 248
sexual professional boundaries 33
sick role 188
side effect management 217
signal transduction pathways 138
single photon emission computerised tomography (SPECT) 55–6
Skinner, Burrhus 205–06
sleep
  deep sleep therapy 19, 23
  depressive disorders relating to 122
  stages of 82b
sleep disorders 82, 83b, 85
smoking 365
SNRIs see serotonergic and noradrenergic re-uptake inhibitors
social and economic hardship 299
social anxiety disorder (SAD) 152–3
  generalised 153
  non-generalised 152
social deprivation 99–100
social interaction 115
social rhythm therapy (SRT) 270
sodium valproate 243t, 324
somatisation
  abnormal illness behaviour 188
  case example 188b–90b
  cultural variations of 188
  description of 187
  illness behaviour 188
  management of 190–1
    specific treatment 191, 192t
  medical conditions relating to 186
  physical illness relating to 188
  psychiatric disorders relating to 187b
  sick role 188
somatoform disorders
  causation 187
  classification of 67–9, 68b
  doctor avoidance of 186
  DSM on 185t–6t
specific phobia 152
SPECT see single photon emission computerised tomography
speech and language disorders 81–2
spirodecanediones 219–20
  buspirone 218t, 219

SRT see social rhythm therapy
SSRIs see selective serotonin reuptake inhibitors
St. John's Wort see hypericum perforatum
standard drinks 368f
static risk factors 335–6
STATIC-99 338
structured professional judgement 336
Subjective Standard 29
substance abuse
  alcohol 362
  amphetamines 363
  assessment 367–9
  of benzodiazepines 363
  bipolar disorders and 137
  caffeine 365
  CAGE questionnaire 367t
  cannabis 364
  case studies 376b–8b
  case-based learning 379b–83b
  cocaine 364
  cost 366
  DSM on 367t
  ecstasy 364
  hallucinogens 364
  heroin 365
  history 39–40, 368–9, 369b
  inhalants 365
  investigations 369–70
  lifetime and recent use of 366t
  mental state examination relating to 39–40, 369–70
  nicotine 365
  patterns 366
  physical examination 369
  prevalence of 366
  recreational drugs and medication 217
  schizophrenia relating to 98, 100b
  screening methods for 367–9
  urine drug screens for 55
substance-induced disorders 370–2, 371t
  clinician attitudes on 370–2
  management 370–2
  motivational enhancement techniques for 372t
  pharmacotherapy 376, 376t
  psychological strategies for 373
  social aspects of 376
  stages of change 372t
  withdrawal
    management 373–6
    syndromes 374t–5t
sub-syndromal bipolar disorder 136
suicidality 289–91
  in elderly 322
  management of 291b
  questions to assess 290b
suicide
  antidepressant medications and risk of 221b
  risk factors for completed 290b–1b
Sullivan, Harry Stack 270
sumatriptan 216
supportive psychotherapy 265
systemic lupus erythematosus 79

T
Tarasoff I 30
Tarasoff II 30
Tarban Creek Lunatic Asylum 12
tardiv akathisia 239
tardiv dyskinesia 239
tardiv dystonia 239
tardiv Parkinsonism 239
TBI *see* mild traumatic brain injury
TCAs *see* tricyclic antidepressants
temazepam 242, 243t
temperament 199
tetrabenazine 75–6
thiamine deficiency 176
thinking
    in depressive disorders 114
    dichotomous 269
    traps 269b
third generation antipsychotics 234–40
thought content 42
thyroid disease 80
    hypothyroidism 80
toxic disorders 80
transcranial magnetic stimulation 251
transference 272
trauma 299
Treatise of Melancholie (Bright) 7
Treatise on Madness (Battie) 9
trepanation 3
trichotillomania (TTM) 166
tricyclic antidepressants (TCAs) 226–7
    adverse effects 227
    doses, half-lives, and common adverse effects of 222t
    general comments 227
    indications 227
    mode of action 227
trifluoperazine 235t
trimipramine 222t
TTM *see* trichotillomania
Tuke, William 11

U
urine drug screens 55
urine tests 52–5
utilitarianism 26

V
valproate 242
    during pregnancy 249
vegetative functions 114–15
venlafaxine 215t, 225, 228t
violence
    management 284–7
    physical restraint 286
    prediction of 284, 285b
    as psychiatric emergency 283
    safe restraint method 286b
virtue ethics 27
vitamin assays 55
vitamin D 245–6, 249
vitamin deficiencies 81

W
waist circumference 52
weight 52
Wernicke's encephalopathy 79b
Wilbur, Cornelia 23
Willis, Thomas 9
withdrawal
    management 373–6
    syndromes 374t–5t
women 163
    premenstrual dysphoric disorder 117
    see also pregnancy and lactation

Y
Young, Jeffrey 206

Z
zimelidine 23
zinc 249
ziprasidone 235t, 240
    intramuscular preparation 288
zolpidem 243t
zopiclone 243t
zuclopenthixol acetate 236t, 237b
    intramuscular preparation 288
zuclopenthixol decanoate 236t